Surgery, Assisted Reproductive Technology and Infertility

Diagnosis and Management of Problems in Gynecologic Reproductive Medicine

Second edition

Surgery, Assisted Reproductive Technology and Infertility

Diagnosis and Management of Problems in Gynecologic Reproductive Medicine

Second edition

Gerard S Letterie, MD, FACOG, FACP
Medical Director, In Vitro Fertilization Program
Northwest Center for Reproductive Sciences
Seattle and Kirkland, Washington

Consultant
Department of Obstetrics and Gynecology
Evergreen Hospital and Medical Center
Kirkland, Washington

and

Associate Clinical Professor
Department of Obstetrics and Gynecology
University of Washington
Seattle, Washington

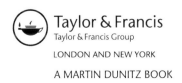

Taylor & Francis
Taylor & Francis Group
LONDON AND NEW YORK

A MARTIN DUNITZ BOOK

© 2005 Taylor & Francis, an imprint of the Taylor & Francis Group

The first edition of this text was originally published in 1998 by Blackwell Science,
Inc. as *Structural Abnormalities and Reproductive Failure.*

Second edition published in 2005
by Taylor & Francis, an imprint of the Taylor & Francis Group, 2 Park Square, Milton
Park, Abingdon, Oxon OX14 4RN

Tel.:   +44 (0) 20 7017 6000
Fax.:   +44 (0) 20 7017 6699
E-mail.:   info@dunitz.co.uk
Website: http://www.dunitz.co.uk

A CIP record for this book is available from the British Library.

ISBN 1-84184-341-5

Distributed in North and South America by
Taylor & Francis
2000 NW Corporate Blvd
Boca Raton, FL 33431, USA
Within Continental USA
Tel: 800 272 7737;   Fax: 800 374 3401
Outside Continental USA
Tel: 561 994 0555;   Fax: 561 361 6018
E-mail: orders @crcpress.com

Distributed in the rest of the world by
Thomson Publishing Services
Cheriton House
North Way
Andover, Hampshire SP10 5BE, UK
Tel: +44 (0)1264 332424
E-mail: salesorder.tandf@thomsonpublishingservices.co.uk

Composition by Wearset Ltd, Boldon, Tyne and Wear.

Printed and bound in Italy by Printer Trento.

Dedication

To the memory of Elizabeth and Joe

And once again:

To Theresa, Jan, Mia and Ava, whose signatures of kindness, so distinct in time and place, have shaped and enhanced my own sense of caring

Contents

Preface

Infertility evaluations and treatments have undergone remarkable and very positive evolutions over the past decade. Improvements have been made in virtually every way we diagnose and treat our patients. Innovations in imaging techniques and endoscopic procedures and markedly improved success rates with *in vitro* fertilization (IVF) have led to both subtle and dramatic improvements in care for our patients. Detailed information of structure and function of the reproductive tract has expanded what we do, and when we do it, to maximize the chances for pregnancy in an ever-expanding group of patients. Sensitive two- and three-dimensional ultrasound and magnetic resonance imaging techniques provide structural information. Microarray technology will refine our ability to evaluate function and genomic expression in an increasing number of settings. This technique is already providing insight into the pathophysiology of endometriosis and polycystic ovary syndrome.

Surgery, for so long the stand-alone treatment for infertility, has yielded in many circumstances to assisted reproductive technologies. The evolution of *in vitro* fertilization to a highly successful process has reduced the number of settings in which surgery is appropriate. Surgery has a continued, though redefined, role in infertility therapies. Though its role has been minimized in some settings, surgical intervention has expanded in two critical areas: in preparation for IVF in patients with factors possibly impacting outcomes negatively and as a conservative, organ-sparing procedure in patients for whom reproduction prior to ART was either not an option or a highly unsuccessful proposition at best. The challenge has been to match the most efficacious and cost-effective technique to that clinical setting where success is most likely. Careful patient selection is the order of the day.

The corollary to these improvements is the critical analysis of outcomes and better definition of populations most likely to benefit from these procedures. Success is improved not only by technical innovations but our ability to define who will and will not benefit. Decision trees guiding patient selection have evolved and matured. Our basis for making decisions has increasingly become data driven. Reliance on results of well-designed clinical trials has emerged as the contemporary paradigm of evidence-based medicine. The overall result of this reliance has been a remarkable improvement in clinical care, and improvements in the quality and cost-effectiveness of care.

This text presents contemporary techniques in diagnosis and management of the infertile patient. It describes the intersection of assisted reproductive technologies and surgery, increasingly two complementary techniques to achieve our patient's goals of family building. A balance between structure and function as cardinal to our understanding of normal and abnormal underpins the text. It is not intended as a surgical atlas, one to be used solely for guidance on the *how to* of a particular procedure. Instead, it provides guidance on not only *how to*, but also *when to* and *why* – the technical aspects of the diagnosis and explanations of appropriate treatment. The text stresses clinical and basic science data from both classic and contemporary research. Emphasis has been placed equally on etiology, diagnosis and management with surgery and assisted reproductive technologies. The rationale for choosing one technique over another is discussed. Most importantly, because the text is grounded in evidence-based medicine, it emphasizes outcomes analysis as a guideline for management.

The recommendations are literature-based. This approach de-emphasizes anecdotal data, intuition, or unsystematic clinical experience as sufficient grounds for clinical decision making. Instead, the text emphasizes practice and management guidelines based on reviews of the published data and on specific outcome measurements. Potential studies for analysis and review were identified by searching MEDLINE from 1971 to 2004. When possible, the recommendations in the text are based on randomized, controlled clinical studies. For several clinical problems, such data simply do not exist. In these circumstances, the recommendations are based on observational and descriptive studies with clearly defined outcome measures and an adequate follow-up interval. For certain clinically rare entities, limited trials, case series and case reports are used for guidance. In keeping with the trends and mandates of contemporary practice, reviews of costs for management are discussed. The bottom clinical line is recommendations for the most efficient and cost-effective diagnostic techniques and treatments.

A word about statistical analysis is appropriate. The literature describing outcomes in reproductive medicine is of extremely variable quality. Many of the early studies that provide insight regarding outcomes were observational, used the treatment groups as their own controls and provided very poor definitions of outcomes or successes. This profile makes calculating accurate statistics regarding success rates difficult. In only isolated circumstances could both odds ratios and confidence intervals be calculated to profile a particular therapy for a particular problem. In lieu of this more accurate and detailed analysis, the likelihood of success has expressed in the text as pregnancy rates and 95% confidence levels calculated where possible. In spite of these shortcomings these data do provide us with a gauge for the outcomes we can expect for a given procedure.

Hopefully the text will provide a keyhole view of the history of each disorder and give insight into what our predecessors did and how truly innovative they were. One tenet that underlies the text may be expressed as a rudimentary proverb (which I like to pass along to our residents and fellows);

> Read text before surgery,
> Avoid complications
> Read text after surgery,
> Understand them.

G.S.L.

Acknowledgments

The task of taking a textbook from initial concept to final publication is a complex and complicated enterprise. Several lines of effort by several individuals must converge at a common point at precisely the right moment if the project is to succeed. Such convergence prevailed in the case of this text. Several people were involved in this task and their efforts are herein acknowledged. A word of sincere gratitude is due to Bonnie Marston for her focused efforts in preparing the manuscript in a timely fashion (which she consistently does). Her ability to interpret various cut-and-paste formats and follow the road maps of early drafts carries my sincere compliments. My colleagues in the Medical Photography Department at Virginia Mason Medical Center, including Bob Riedlinger, Morris Ferensen, Terry King and Taylor Ubben, provided consistent support of a very high quality. Interpretation of the various images was aided by the staff of the Department of Radiology, who lent assistance in separating fact from fiction within the shades of gray of each study. Acknowledgments are also due to Dr. Joseph Mancini for his general counsel on the good and bad of it all and the general direction things should go to; Dr. Scott Rose for setting the bar so high – "you're where we all oughta be"; to Mr. Robert Hartfield for the humor; to Mr. Geoff Reiss for the referral to Mr. Tufte ("Edward who?" "Edward Tufte. Check out his depiction of Napoleon's army"); to Mr. John Holt for sharing insight, encouragement and definitions of friendship and partnership; to Drs Kennedy, Opsahl and Wiemer whose belief in an idea and willingness to step up, made it happen; thanks also to my friends and colleagues at Cook (Dan, Boz and Neal) for permission to use the artwork; and most importantly to my family, Jan, Mia and Ava, ever constant and present, who endured a preoccupation with the book and at times, its intrusion into our family life. These are very special people, unwavering and consistent. Their support cannot be overestimated. For the efforts of all these individuals, a sincere thanks is extended.

G.S.L.

1 Development of the Reproductive Tract

Ontogeny recapitulates phylogeny
— von Baer's law

Structure and function are tandem forces in reproductive medicine. Abnormalities in either within the reproductive tract may adversely influence reproductive potential. Clinical solutions to these problems and enhancements of fertility may require surgery and/or assisted reproductive technology (ART). These abnormalities vary in degree and etiology and provide a prism through which clinical care is viewed. Changes may be subtle and detected during an evaluation for infertility or poor obstetric outcome and require no immediate therapy or may be emergent presenting at puberty and require immediate surgical intervention. These abnormalities may be congenital such as the spectrum of uterine duplication, and vaginal agenesis, or acquired such as pelvic adhesive disease after acute pelvic inflammatory disease, intrauterine adhesions after a dilation and curettage or the progressive development of endometriosis or uterine myoma. Though of differing etiologies, congenital and acquired structural abnormalities impact function and share the common clinical expression of a relative or absolute compromise to reproductive potential. This textbook discusses the structural and functional aspects of congenital and acquired abnormalities of the reproductive tract, their diagnoses and management, and outcomes from surgery and/or ART.

Congenital abnormalities of the reproductive tract are surprisingly common with an incidence ranging from 1 in 200 to 1 in 600 women.[1] Approximately 25 to 35% of women with congenital uterine anomalies have impaired reproductive potential ranging from an inability to ever achieve a pregnancy to repeated pregnancy loss, malpresentation, and premature labor. Clinical problems associated with acquired changes such as ovarian endometriomas, pelvic adhesive disease, or tubal obstruction range from chronic pelvic pain and dyspareunia to infertility. Management may be surgical in select cases but increasingly relies on ART.

An understanding of normal embryology is essential to appreciate the significance of these abnormalities and the deviations in structure and function in clinical practice. The threshold issues in development of the female reproductive tract are the determination of genotype leading to a cascade of specific sequential anatomic and endocrine events that direct end-organ development.[2] Each embryonic landmark event must be met in a specific and precise fashion. Full functional differentiation and progression to sexual identity during puberty and adulthood are events that occur as a continuation of these early developmental events. The clinical consequences of perturbations of any one of these determinants may result in what is clinically observed as congenital, anatomic abnormalities and, in some cases, abnormal sexual development. This chapter outlines the key events at each stage of embryologic development and describes the congenital abnormalities that may result from any disturbance in this developmental sequence. The etiologies of acquired abnormalities are varied; they are discussed in the specific chapters dealing with them.

Development of the Mullerian Tract

Normal Sexual Differentiation

Wolff in 1760 and Muller in 1830 described paired structures present in early embryonic development that contributed to the formation of the male and female reproductive tracts, respectively.[3,4] The more generic terms, mesonephric and paramesonephric ducts, are used commonly in clinical parlance coincident with a trend from the tradition of using the names of investigators to designate anatomic structures. Both terms, however, are appropriate and continue in common usage. The terms "mesonephric" or "wolffian," and "paramesonephric" or "mullerian" designate laterally placed structures that develop between 5 to 16 weeks' gestation. These structures give rise to the male and female reproductive organs, respectively. The mesonephric ducts develop into the epididymis, vas deferens and seminal vesicles. The mullerian ducts are mesodermal derivatives of the paramesonephric duct and develop into the fallopian tubes, uterus, cervix, and probably the upper one-third of the vagina.

Early Development: The Genetics of Bipotential Gonad

The factors that contribute to the development of male and female anatomy and identity have intrigued investigators and clinicians for centuries. Theories progressed from the initial identification of the X and Y chromosomes to a focused search for ever smaller regions of the Y chromosome responsible for sexual determination (Table 1-1). Sexual dimorphism was one of the first characteristics to be shown to have a chromosomal basis.[5] Using *Drosophila* as a model, investigations in 1902 suggested that sex determination was based on the number of X chromosomes. This theory persisted through the 1950s, despite the discovery in 1923 of X and Y chromosomes in the human, and the suggestion that sex-role determination in the human, unlike that in *Drosophila*, may be based on the pairing of two different chromosomes. In 1959, however, the critical role of the Y chromosome in the development of males was determined. The entire Y chromosome was theorized in early studies as the determinant that triggered a cascade of events in the development of the genital ridges into testes rather than ovaries. This critical event, under the influence of testicular hormones,[6] resulted in the regression of

| Table 1-1.
Historical Aspects of Theories of Sexual Differentiation ||
Investigator	Comment
McClung, 1902	Sexual dimorphism on chromosomal basis
Painter, 1923	Existence of X and Y chromosomes
Jost, 1953	Hormonal influence of internal and external genitalia
Jacobs, 1959	Critical role of Y chromosome
Wachtel, 1975	H-Y antigen
Page, 1987	Testicular differentiating factor (TDF)
Palmer, 1989	Sex-determining region of the Y chromosome (SRY)

female internal anatomy and the development of male anatomy. Molecular technology, however, provided further insights into the exact factors determining sexual determination.[7]

Molecular Basis of Testicular Development

The possibility that sexual differentiation and the development of male and female reproductive organs depended on a specific part of the Y chromosome or a specific, male-related antigen associated with the Y chromosome and not the entire Y chromosome was initially suggested in the early 1970s. The H-Y histocompatibility antigen was described and the H-Y hypothesis was proposed in 1975.[8] This theory held sway for nearly a decade. Studies of intersex and abnormal sexual development yielded inconsistent results, suggesting that other factors may be responsible, and the H-Y theory was eventually abandoned.[9]

During the past 10 years, the search for the gene that switches development from the female to male pathway has focused on ever-smaller regions of the Y chromosome.[10] Evidence using deletion mapping suggests that genetic determinants of male and female differentiation and the subsequent development of the male and female reproductive organs may be related to limited, Y-related DNA located on the short arm of the Y chromosome. An early candidate was the so-called zinc finger protein of the Y chromosome (ZFY) that encodes for an immune-system protein found only in males (labeled testicular differentiating factor [TDF in humans, Tdy in mice]). Data for this theory came from two sources: XX men who had inherited a small fragment of the Y chromosome from their fathers, and XY females who had lost a crucial part of their Y chromosome. Additional study narrowed the focus further and suggested that ZFY had another small piece of the Y chromosome lying close to that previously described.[11] After intensive and provocative study by two

3

groups of investigators, it was subsequently established that this area located at the distal region of the short arm of the Y chromosome contained a single gene for the sex-determining region of the Y chromosome (SRY).[12]

The presence of SRY represents an essential, critical, and initial event in sexual development. Complete development of testicular or ovarian tissue is a complex series of events that involve migration of bipotential germ cells and stromal precursors to the genital ridge under the influence of genes and protein in addition to SRY. SRY is best thought of as a critical switch; its role is to direct development along one of two potential paths. With SRY as a moderator, a cascade of steps necessary to form a testis from an undifferentiated gonad are set in motion. SRY is a transcription factor that encodes a 204 amino acid protein that binds to double stranded DNA through its conserved domain, the high mobility group (HMG) box.[13] Other autosomal and X-linked genes, present in both male and female and capable of activation, are also required for testicular differentiation. Under these influences undifferentiated gonads develop into testes and the internal reproductive tract subsequently develops into the wolffian structures. In the absence of SRY, the gonads develop into ovaries and the reproductive tract subsequently develops along female lines or into the mullerian reproductive tract. With the establishment of the genetic sex and, specifically, the presence or absence of SRY, the bipotential or indifferent gonadal development develops into either testis or ovary (Figure 1-1).

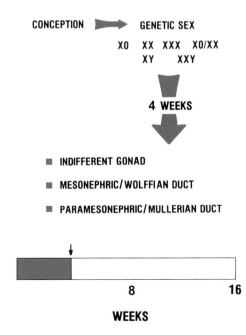

Figure 1-1   Establishment of the genetic sex at conception, and subsequent formation of an indifferent or bipotential gonad.

Despite 10 years of research, its biologic targets as well as its mechanism of action are complex and interdependent. Other important genes in addition to SRY may be involved in sex determination. Several other key regulators of male development have also been identified over the past decade.[14–16] Genetic factors such as SRY-related factor Sox9 appear to be key players in early testicular differentiation.[17,18] Sox9 belongs to a family of transcription factors, the Sox genes, that contain an HMG box similar to that of SRY. It has been shown that Sox9 binds to the same DNA targets in vitro as SRY.[19] Sox9 is highly conserved among mammals as well as other vertebrates.[20] High expression of Sox9 is always correlated with testicular differentiation and may act as a transcription factor in the Sertoli cells.[21,22] Though strongly implicated in testicular development, the precise and ultimate physiologic targets of Sox9 remain unclear. Numerous other factors have also been identified directing crucial steps in early gonadal development in both sexes, including Dmrt1, WT1, Sf1, Lm1, Lhx9, Emx2 and M33 (Table 1-2).[23–25]

Table 1-2. Transcription Factors in Gonadal Differentiation		
Gene	**Localization**	**Phenotypic Expression of Mutations**
Testicular Differentiating Pathway		
SRY	Xp11	XY gonadal dysgenesis
DAx1	Xp21.3	XY gonadal dysgenesis
Sox9	17q24	XY male-to-female reversal
SF1	9q33	Gonadal dysgenesis
WT-1	11p13	Deny-Dash and Frasier syndromes
Ovarian Differentiating Pathway		
FoxL2	3q23	Premature ovarian failure and eyelid defects

Molecular Basis of Ovarian Development

In contrast to the understanding of testicular development, ovarian development has remained relatively obscure. Female development is a default pathway in the absence of genetic male-promoting signals. Ovarian development proceeds in the absence of the genetic influences for testicular development. Genetic control of early ovarian development is largely unknown. Molecular regulation of fetal ovarian development depends on poorly understood signal pathways of cell differentiation. Though a few molecules have been implicated, their precise mechanisms and sites of action are undetermined. No genes have yet been demonstrated to play the equivalent role of

SRY or Sox9 genes. Development is dependent in part on the action of certain steroidal hormones and yet to be defined genes and target sites.

In female embryos, the germ cell lineage shows random X chromosome inactivation. On entry into the genital ridges, the silent X becomes reactivated so that both X chromosomes are expressed throughout oogenesis. Beyond these events, the molecular mechanisms involved in early ovarian differentiation and follicular development are poorly understood in spite of insights gained from several mouse models and the genetic study of patients with ovarian failure. The X-linked zinc finger gene (ZFX) is a candidate gene for ovarian maintenance that maps to the X chromosome.[26] X chromosomal abnormalities can result in gonadal dysgenesis and premature ovarian failure. Terminal deletions at Xp11 result in amenorrhea and premature ovarian failure in approximately 50% of affected patients. Deletions at Xq13 may result in primary amenorrhea.

Ultimately, in the ovarian anlage, in the absence of SRY, granulosa cells will develop. The granulosa cells become admixed with clusters of germ cells so that each surviving oocyte is surrounded by layers of flattened cuboidal cells forming the primordial follicle at approximately 16 weeks' gestation. The pool of primordial follicles is gradually depleted from this point forward. Seven million primordial follicles are initially present at completion of ovarian development. Two million are present in the newborn and 300,000 at puberty.

In summary, the sex-determining genes that direct the fate of the bipotential gonad into either testis or ovary can be placed into three categories: (1) transcription factors involved in early gonadal morphogenesis and throughout differentiation of sex-specific cell types; (2) initiators of testicular development; (3) antagonists of testicular development and potential promoters of ovarian development.[27–29] Study of human intersexes and sex-reversed patients may prove to be one promising model to gain insight into genes involved in the sex determination cascade.[30]

Gonadal Development

Under specific genetic guidance, gonadal development is a unique process with two possible organogenic outcomes: testis or ovary.[31,32] The gonads begin to develop when the embryo has a crown–rump length of 5 to 7 mm. The primitive gonad remains in an indifferent state until 4 weeks' gestation. Both paired mullerian and wolffian ducts are present at that time.[33] Complete differentiation of normal gonads depends on the migration of viable primordial germ cells from the yolk sac to the genital ridges on the dorsal mesentery. If the germ cells fail to arrive, the gonads do not develop; only fibrous streaks persist as remnants. After migration, the germ cells are then enveloped by coelomic epithelial cells. When the embryo has a crown–rump length of 7 to 9 mm, primitive sex cords from the coelomic epithelium and primitive germ cells from the yolk sac organize into a bipotential primitive gonad, with both cortical and medullary areas. These two anatomic regions of the primitive gonads, that is, the cortical and medullary areas, give rise to an ovary or testis, respectively.

The critical event for gonadal function is eventual enclosure of germ cells and somatic cells in specific germ-cell compartments. The primitive gonad at this point is composed of germ cells, somatic or epithelial cells destined to become either granulosa or Sertoli cells, and mesenchyme, destined to become either thecal or Leydig cells. At this point in development, essential, albeit rudimentary, architecture is present. As outlined above, male mammalian development is triggered by active signals from portions of the Y chromosome. Ultimate differentiation into an ovary or testicle depends on the presence or absence of the influence of the Y chromosome or Y-related segment of the Y chromosome (Figure 1-2). Chronologically, the formation of the testicle precedes any subsequent sexual development. Differentiation of the steroid-producing cells into Leydig cells influences subsequent development of the internal and external genital structures. Interstitial Leydig cells are formed from the mesenchyme or mesonephric-derived cells around the cords. These cells contain receptors for human chorionic gonadotropin (hCG) and produce testosterone at an early age, a critical next step in differentiation.[34]

Endocrine Events

At 4 to 5 weeks under any Y-related chromosomal influence, the indifferent gonads develop into testes and through a complex series of steps induce the development of the mesonephric or wolffian tracts. Simultaneously the

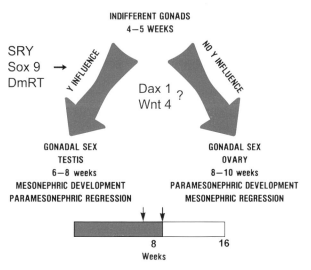

Figure 1-2   Under Y-related influence or the absence of such influence, leading to mesonephric or paramesonephric development, respectively, gonadal sex is determined to be either testicular or ovarian.

paramesonephric or mullerian ducts regress. The embryologic events of wolffian development and mullerian regression require two specific hormones produced by the testes at this critical point. The hormones are testosterone and mullerian inhibitory factor (MIF; also referred to as anti-mullerian hormone or mullerian inhibitory substance).

The discovery of endocrine influences on the development of the reproductive tract is a classic example of the intersection of basic science and clinical medicine. The mediation of the expression or regression of the mullerian or wolffian tracts by male-related hormones was described in 1930 by Alfred Jost.[35] In a series of classic and elaborate studies, Jost suggested that both local hormonal influence and the timing of this influence were essential and critical in the development of the internal reproductive tract. Jost initially demonstrated that testosterone was required for all steps of male genital differentiation, both internal and external. However, what induced mullerian regression remained a question. In studies in which a testosterone crystal was placed into a female embryo, masculinization of wolffian ducts occurred but no mullerian regression was noted, suggesting that not only was testosterone necessary for normal male development, but a second, then unknown, hormone was required to suppress mullerian development in the male. Further studies were needed to demonstrate that both hormones, testosterone and MIF, were essential for normal development of the male reproductive tract.

Studies by Jost also assessed the timing of the hormonal influences. He demonstrated that the removal of the testes prior to the twelfth day resulted in the development of female internal anatomy but removal of the testes after the twentieth day resulted in varying degrees of ambiguity. These results suggested that not only is the presence of two hormones required but that they must be secreted within a certain temporal window for normal development. These classical embryologic experiments suggested that phenotypic sex is correlated with the presence or absence of a testis in the embryo. These studies also implied that male mammalian development is triggered by active signals associated with specific chromosomes.

Although the testes are essential to the stimulation of male sexual development, female sexual development in the fetus does not depend on the presence of the ovaries. For example, the development of the mesonephric ducts in males may be disrupted if the testes are removed before differentiation of the genital ducts. In this circumstance, paramesonephric ducts develop. Removal of the ovaries of female embryos, however, has no effect on sexual development. These data further suggest that the testes impose the development of the wolffian ducts and repress the development of the mullerian ducts.

Normal male sexual differentiation is initiated by SRY, which directs testicular development in the gonadal ridge. SRY expression is characterized by the testicular secretion of MIF and testosterone. These two hormones are secreted (testosterone from the Leydig cells and MIF from the Sertoli cells) prior to the twelfth week of gestation. Both MIF, and testosterone, as well as the capacity to bind and metabolize them, are essential to normal development. MIF causes regression of the mullerian ducts during male embryogenesis. It is a member of the large transforming growth factor-β, (TGF-β,) multigene family of glyco-proteins involved in the regulation of growth and differentiation of tissue. It is precisely regulated at the transcriptional level by SRY and interacts post-trans-lationally with testosterone.[36,37] The receptor for MIF has been also described.[38] The secretion of MIF by the Sertoli cells stimulates the unilateral regression of the mullerian ducts by the eighth week. Defects in secretion of MIF result in persistence of the mullerian system and differentiation into uterus, tubes, and upper vagina. The secretion of testosterone by the Leydig cells stimulates the differentiation of the wolffian ducts into epididymis, vas deferens, and seminal vesicles and is a complex series of events involving five enzymes. Defects in each reaction have been described and may result in abnormalities of varying degrees in sexual differentiation. These defects may be either abnormal testos-terone biosynthesis or abnormal androgen action secondary to 5α-reductase, either a cytoplasmic receptor deficiency or a deficiency in nuclear chromatin receptors.

In the absence of any Y-related chromosomal influence, an ovary develops with the persistence of the paramesonephric or mullerian development and mesonephric regression. The development of the ovary in this setting occurs slightly later than the testicular development, at 8 to 10 weeks' gestation (Figure 1-2).

Development of Internal Genitalia and Genitourinary Systems

As noted above, two sets of potential duct systems develop simultaneously in both male and female embryos: the mesonephric and paramesonephric ducts. The dominance of one and regression of the other await specific hor-monal cues. The mesonephric urinary ducts are formed and connect at the caudal end of the urogenital sinus and the cloaca. Paramesonephric or mul-lerian ducts develop lateral and parallel to the mesonephric ducts. During their development, the paramesonephric ducts migrate until they lie side by side in the midline. The paramesonephric ducts develop initially at the cranial ends and communicate with the future peritoneal cavity. As the ducts develop caudally, they cross the ventral aspect of the mesonephric ducts to partially fuse in the midline, resulting in a Y-shaped structure.[39,40] The caudal portions of the paramesonephric ducts coalesce and form a discrete structure known as the *mullerian tubercle* (Figure 1-3). With downward growth, this tubercle protrudes into the upgrowing urogenital sinus. The caudal ends of the mesonephric ducts enter the urogenital sinus at either side of the muller-ian tubercle. Under the influence of the ovarian hormones (and the lack of any androgen influence) the paramesonephric ducts continue their develop-ment to form the genital tract while the mesonephric system regresses. Ves-tiges of the mesonephric ducts may persist in the adult, as Gartner's duct cysts, in the lateral vaginal wall.

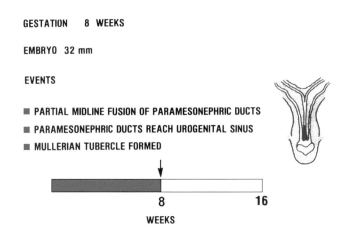

GESTATION   8 WEEKS

EMBRYO   32 mm

EVENTS

■ PARTIAL MIDLINE FUSION OF PARAMESONEPHRIC DUCTS
■ PARAMESONEPHRIC DUCTS REACH UROGENITAL SINUS
■ MULLERIAN TUBERCLE FORMED

8   16

WEEKS

Figure 1-3   Partial midline fusion of the paramesonephric ducts by 8 to 9 weeks'
gestation concomitant with the formation of the mullerian tubercle.

By 8 to 9 weeks' gestation, there is partial midline fusion of the paramesonephric ducts. At 10 weeks' gestation, there is full regression of the
wolffian duct (48-mm embryo) (Figure 1-4). At 12 weeks' gestation, the
ureterovaginal canal is formed and there is complete midline fusion of
the paramesonephric ducts (Figure 1-5). Continued downward growth of the
paramesonephric duct and upward growth of the vaginal epithelium occur
(69-mm embryo) (Figure 1-6). At 16 weeks' gestation, the final events in the
evolution of internal reproductive anatomy occur, full canalization of the
vagina and a fully unified single uterus (Figure 1-7).

The gradual unification of the uterine cavity may be followed through a
series of gradual steps from complete duplication of laterally placed paired
structures to midline fusion and eventual complete unification. Each clinical
abnormality such as septate and bicornuate uteri represents an arrest of
development at some point in the developmental pathway (Figures 1-8 and
1-9). As an interesting note in comparative anatomy, each stage of development of the uterus represents the normal reproductive anatomy of a lower
species. von Baer's law states that ontogeny recapitulates phylogeny. In this
theory, the embryonic development of a specific organ system progresses
through a step-by-step representation of the normal adult anatomy of lower
species within a group. A parallelism exists between the normal paired
reproductive anatomy in lower species and the various stages of embryologic development and uterine abnormalities in humans. Failure of fusion,
the commonality of each of the various congenital uterine abnormalities, has
a direct correlate in the normal reproductive anatomy of lower mammals
and in the various stages of development in the human. In mammals, starting with the lower species, all intermediate evolutionary stages have their
counterpart as congenital or developmental uterine abnormalities in humans
ranging from complete duplication to single unified uterus. Normal reproductive anatomy in lower species may be viewed as points of the continuum

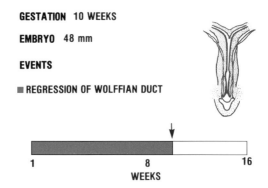

GESTATION 10 WEEKS

EMBRYO 48 mm

EVENTS

■ REGRESSION OF WOLFFIAN DUCT

1   8   16
WEEKS

Figure 1-4   Complete regression of the wolffian duct by 10 weeks' gestation.

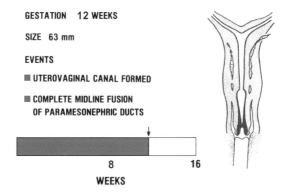

GESTATION   12 WEEKS

SIZE 63 mm

EVENTS

■ UTEROVAGINAL CANAL FORMED

■ COMPLETE MIDLINE FUSION
  OF PARAMESONEPHRIC DUCTS

8   16
WEEKS

Figure 1-5   Formation of the uterovaginal canal and midline fusion of the para-
                    mesonephric ducts by 11 weeks.

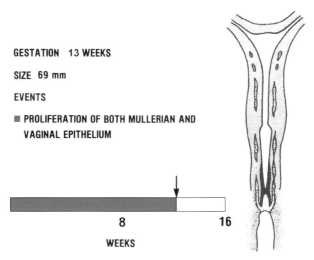

GESTATION   13 WEEKS

SIZE 69 mm

EVENTS

■ PROLIFERATION OF BOTH MULLERIAN AND
  VAGINAL EPITHELIUM

8   16
WEEKS

Figure 1-6   Proliferation of mullerian and vaginal epithelium and continued down-
                    ward growth of the paramesonephric and upward growth of the
                    vaginal epithelium by 12 weeks' gestation.

11

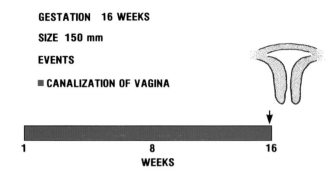

GESTATION   16 WEEKS

SIZE 150 mm

EVENTS

■ CANALIZATION OF VAGINA

1   8   16
WEEKS

Figure 1-7   Full canalization of the vagina and formation of a single uterine cavity at 16 weeks.

from complete duplication to a single uterine cavity. Beginning with the marsupials, in which paired vagina, cervix, and uterus constitute normal reproductive anatomy and progressing through lower mammals with paired uteri or arcuate uteri with single vagina to the primates with a single uterine cavity, each mullerian abnormality is represented.[41]

Development of the Urinary Tract

The development of the urinary tract is both anatomically and temporally closely related to the development of the mullerian tract. The ureteral buds grow laterally, both anteriorly and cranially, and approach the downward-growing metanephros to form the definitive kidney and ureters. The metanephrogenic mass is formed as a ureteral bud (or metanephric diverticulum) initially located in the pelvis. As the renal masses develop, they migrate cephalad to assume their position in the flank region. The bladder and urethra are derived from the urogenital sinus and adjacent splanchnic mesoderm. These embryologic events of renal development and maturation have important clinical significance and correlates. As much as one-third of patients with congenital mullerian abnormalities (depending on the specific abnormality) have concomitant renal abnormalities ranging from subtle renal malpositions and ureteral defects to complete absence.[43]

Development of the Vagina

Controversy exists concerning the embryology of the vagina. These issues have been debated since the 1930s when Koff and Minh attributed the origin of the vagina solely to the mullerian tubercle. The conflicting theories in this area suggest that the vagina is derived from mesonephric ducts, the urogenital sinus, or the paramesonephric duct. The most commonly accepted theory is that the upper one-third of the vagina forms from the fusion of the downgrowing paramesonephric ducts and the inferior two-thirds form from the urogenital sinus.[3]

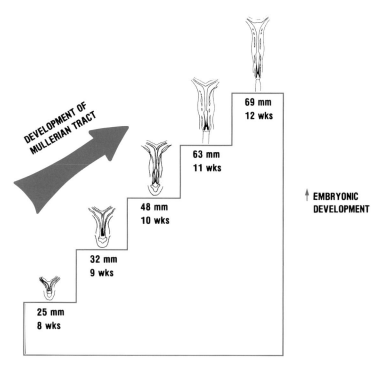

Figure 1-8   Summary of development of the mullerian tract.

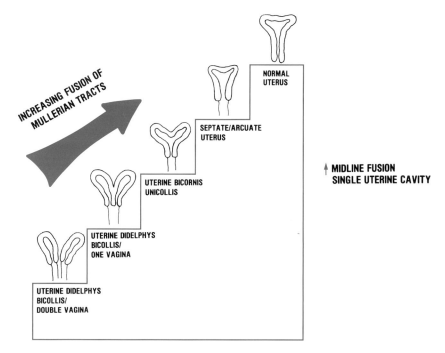

Figure 1-9   Progression of midline fusion from completely paired systems to a single unified midline structure. Note parallelism to embryonic events in Figure 1-8.

Development of the External Genitalia

External genital development proceeds along female lines except in the presence of androgens, an expression of the innate tendency of the embryo. The development of the external genitalia is intimately related with gonadal function, the secretion of testosterone and the presence of a system for the conversion of testosterone into a locally active form. The testosterone exerts its effects locally and directly on the mesonephric ducts as Jost demonstrated. Its effects on the external genitalia, however, are indirect and exerted by dihydrotestosterone (DHT) formed by the conversion of testosterone via a 5α-reductase enzyme.

Dihydrotestosterone is the primary androgen responsible for masculinization of the external genitalia in the male fetus. At the fourth week of gestation, the male and female external genitalia are similar and undifferentiated. Under the influence of androgenic stimulation, the genital tubercle, urethral folds, and labioscrotal swellings form the corpora cavernosa and glans of the penis, the cavernous urethra, and the scrotum, respectively (Tables 1-3 and 1-4). In the absence of Y chromosomal influence and androgen (testosterone and DHT) secretion, these structures form the clitoris, labia minora, and labia majora, respectively. Disorders of sexual development may arise by abnormal gonadal differentiation as in true hermaphroditism, X-Y gonadal dysgenesis, or mixed gonadal dysgenesis or by abnormal testosterone biosynthesis in which the production of testosterone is impeded by several enzyme deficiencies (five have been described: cholesterol desmolase; 3β-hydroxysteroid dehydrogenase; 17α-hydroxylase; 17,20-desmolase; and 17β-ketosteroid reductase). Abnormal androgen action, due to either an absence of receptors,

Table 1-3. External Genitalia		
Common Anlagen	**Male**	**Female**
Genital tubercle	Corpora cavernosa, glans penis	Clitoris
Urethral folds	Cavernous urethra	Labia minora
Labioscrotal swellings	Scrotum	Labia majora

Table 1-4. Internal Genitalia	
Structure	**Requirements**
Mullerian — uterus, fallopian tubes, upper vagina	Absence of Y influence
Wolffian — epididymis, vas deferens, seminal vesicles, ejaculatory ducts	Presence of Y-DNA, gonadal function

as in testicular feminization, or an absence of the enzymes necessary for conversion to DHT, as in 5α-reductase deficiencies, may also cause genital ambiguity. The former may be manifested by a completely normal-appearing habitus, blind vaginal pouch, and XY karyotype.[43] The latter may be manifested by varying degrees of abnormal-appearing external genitalia and, in some cases, abrupt change in sexual roles at adolescence.[44] The most common cause of genital ambiguity, however, is congenital adrenal hyperplasia, a disorder of adrenal steroid synthesis that leads to excessive secretion of androgens during critical phases of genital development.[45,46]

Etiology of Congenital Abnormalities

The exact causes of congenital abnormalities of the mullerian tract are not known. Several theories and hypotheses exist. All abnormalities have as their common defect a total or unilateral failure to develop or a failure of midline fusion. The association of other mesodermal defects in systems that develop concomitantly with the mullerian system, such as the urinary, alimentary, and cardiovascular systems, suggests a time-specific insult. There has, however, not been a specific teratogen associated with these abnormalities.

A genetic influence has been hypothesized. Most cases are sporadic and no specific genetic cause has been found.[48,49] Women with congenital abnormalities of the reproductive tract usually have a 46,XX karyotype. An abnormal karyotype is present in approximately 8% of women with these abnormalities. A polygenic or multifactorial inheritance pattern has been described showing a sex-linked autosomal dominant gene responsible for mullerian agenesis. Specific syndromes involving coincident congenital abnormalities of the reproductive tract and other system defects have been described. An autosomal dominant syndrome characterized by vaginal septum, hand anomalies, and urinary tract abnormalities is well described. Familial clustering, and autosomal, recessive, and dominant cases have also been described in case series and case reports. The most commonly accepted theory for any genetic basis is that congenital mullerian abnormalities are multifactorial, polygenic, and familial.

Specific Structural Abnormalities of the Female Reproductive Tract

Uterine Abnormalities

Structural abnormalities of the uterus occur in 0.1 to 2% of all women, in 4% of women with infertility, and in as many as 15% of women with recurrent pregnancy loss. More frequent use of hysterosalpingography, hysteroscopy, and sophisticated imaging techniques has led to an increase in the reported incidence of both congenital and acquired abnormalities. Because of the possibility of normal reproductive outcome, many cases will be asymptomatic

15

and escape clinical detection, making the above incidence figures somewhat lower than the number of abnormalities actually present.

The major congenital abnormalities of the mullerian tract related to reproduction are failure of fusion abnormalities of the uterus and vagina. The development of the uterus is best viewed on a continuum. Beginning initially as paired and laterally placed organs, the uterus undergoes a downward and medial migration eventually meeting in the midline as a single fused organ with a single cavity. Abnormalities at any point of the downward and medial migration can result in failure of midline fusion of the uterus. Uterine abnormalities vary from the complete absence, as in Mayer–Rokitansky–Küster–Hauser syndrome, through complete failure to fuse, as with bicornuate uteri, to subtle midline defects such as an arcuate uterus. Regardless of the exact abnormality, mullerian tract defects have as their common abnormality a failure of fusion. These failures may be manifested by a failure of lateral fusion, which consists of entities such as bicornuate bicollis uterus, to failure of vertical fusion such as a transverse vaginal septum.

Various classification schemes for uterine abnormalities have been suggested since Kauffmann's original description in the 1930s. The importance of a system of classification is twofold: to describe the specific influence of an abnormality on reproduction and the subsequent improvement (if any) that may result from intervention and to describe clinical anomalies in other systems associated with each abnormality. A mutually agreed-on system enables reliable and accurate discussion of these entities among practitioners and permits a uniform comparison of outcomes among clinical studies. The earliest classifications were primarily descriptive and made no attempt to correlate outcome with particular anomalies. The systems underwent successive modifications, none meeting with universal agreement. One currently used classification system was revised in 1983 and again in 1988.[50–52] The revised classification is based on a division of mullerian abnormalities into seven specific groups: type I: hypoplasia and agenesis (vagina, cervix, uterus, tubes); type II: unicornuate uterus (both patent and obstructed); type III: uterine didelphys; type IV: bicornuate uterus (partial and complete); type V: septate uterus (partial and complete); type VI: arcuate; and type VII: exposure to diethylstilbestrol (DES) (T-shaped uteri). This classification scheme represents one means of counseling patients regarding management and provides a common language for discussion. No system of classification of uterine abnormalities is perfect. Subtle variations in anatomy defy any specific categorization. Such cases must be managed individually and counseling extrapolated from data applicable to the most closely related abnormalities.

The most common acquired abnormalities of the uterine cavity include intrauterine adhesions secondary to intrauterine manipulation, usually dilatation and curettage (D&C). It is extremely unusual to encounter patients with an infectious etiology of intrauterine adhesions, though cases, particularly of tuberculosis, continue to be described in endemic areas.

Ovarian Abnormalities

Congenital anomalies of the ovaries are extremely rare. The most common disorders of gonadal development are gonadal dysgenesis (Turner's syndrome and Turner's mosaicism), pure gonadal dysgenesis, true hermaphroditism, and male pseudohermaphroditism. Nondevelopment or partial development of the ovary, supernumerary and accessory ovaries, frequently accompanied by anomalies of the mullerian and urinary tract, have also been described.[53] Abnormal locations of the ovary may occur at any point along the line of migration from the upper abdomen to the pelvis and are most commonly in conjunction with uterine abnormalities such as unicornuate uterus. The most frequent clinical ovarian abnormalities confronting the reproductive surgeon are acquired and include endometriomas, ovarian cysts, and morphologic changes, as part of the spectrum of changes of polycystic ovary syndrome.

Fallopian Tube Abnormalities

Congenital abnormalities of the fallopian tubes are complete absence of the tube and segmental absences in the isthmic portion of the fallopian tube. Salpingitis isthmic nodosa (SIN), a condition characterized by islands of tubal mucosa within the muscularis of the tube, is considered by some to be a congenital abnormality, though complete data to support this contention are lacking. The debate of SIN as a normal variant further complicate the discussion. The most common structural abnormalities of the fallopian tube confronting the reproductive surgeon are acquired and include obstruction, secondary to infection or tubal ligation. Of all structures in the reproductive tract, the fallopian tube is most susceptible to damage and alteration by infection. Tubal obstruction in this setting may be either in the proximal (i.e., cornual) or distal (i.e., fimbrial or ampullary) portions of the tube. The alterations in the structure and function of the tube after tubal ligation relate to the type of tubal ligation and ease of repair to the remaining tubal segments.

Vaginal Abnormalities

Congenital abnormalities of the vagina include complete absence as in vaginal agenesis or Mayer–Rokitansky–Küster–Hauser syndrome, and septate vagina, both transverse and longitudinal. Imperforate hymen, although not a true congenital mullerian abnormality, sometimes requires excision. Acquired abnormalities include stricture formation and contraction, usually after irradiation.

Cervical Abnormalities

Congenital absence of the cervix is rare but well described. These cases may be in association with congenital absence of the vagina. Intervention during adolescence is required for management of amenorrhea and pelvic pain secondary to hematometra and endometriosis. Acquired cervical conditions, such as hypoplastic cervix secondary to cone biopsy or exposure to DES and cervical incompetence and stenosis, are the most common abnormalities of the cervix. These circumstances pose challenges for transcervical embryo transfer in association with IVF.

Summary and Recommendations

Abnormalities of the reproductive tract may involve the uterus, tubes, and ovaries and may be secondary to congenital or acquired processes. Examples of the former process span a spectrum of changes from complete absence of all reproductive organs, as in mullerian aplasia, to complete duplication, as in uterine didelphys, to more subtle midline septal defects in the uterus. Examples of the latter process include tubal obstruction secondary to infection, cervical incompetence secondary to previous surgery, and more progressive and potentially debilitating processes such as endometriosis. The following chapters outline management plans according to evidence-based algorithms, a discussion of the various diagnostic modalities for each of the specific abnormalities, and descriptions of the therapeutic options of surgery and the assisted reproductive technologies to maximize reproductive potential for each clinical entity.

References

1.   Rock JA, Schlaff WD. The obstetric consequences of uterovaginal anomalies. Fertil Steril 1985;43:681–692.

2.   Crosby WM, Hill EC. Embryology of the Mullerian duct system. Obstet Gynecol 1962;20:507–515.

3.   Acien P. Embryological observations on the female genital tract. Hum Reprod 1992;7:437–445.

4.   Simpson JL. Genetics of the female reproductive ducts. Am J Med Genet 1999;89:224–239.

5.   Charlesworth B. The evolution of sex chromosomes. Science 1991;251:1030–1033.

6.   Bianchi NO. Sex determination in mammals. How many genes are involved? Biol Reprod 1991;44:393–397.

7.   Bowles J, Koopman P. New clues to the puzzle of mammalian sex determination. Genome Biol 2001;2:1025.

8.   Wachtel SS. Human sexual development. J Endocrin Invest 1984;7:663–673.

9.   Bogan JS, Page DC. Ovary? Testis? — A mammalian dilemma. Cell 1994;76:603–607.

10.   Page DC, Mosher R, Simpson EM, et al. The sex-determining region of the human Y chromosome encodes a finger protein. Cell 1987;51:1091–1094.

11. Palmer MS, Sinclair AH, Berta P, et al. Genetic evidence that ZFY is not the testis-determining factor. Nature 1989;342:937–939.

12. Sinclair AH, Berta P, Palmer MS, et al. A gene from the human sex-determining region encodes a protein with homology to a conserved DNA-binding motif. Nature 1990;346:240–244.

13. Haqq CM, King CY, Ukiyama E, et al. Molecular basis of mammalian sexual determination: activation of Mullerian inhibiting substance gene expression by SRY. Science 1994;266:1494–1500.

14. McElreavey K. Mechanism of sex determination in mammals. Adv Genome Biol 1996;4:304–354.

15. Jordan BK, Vilain E. Sry and the genetics of sex determination. Adv Exp Med Biol 2002;511:1–14.

16. Parker KL, Schimmer BP. Genes essential for early events in gonadal development. Ann Med 2002;34:171–178.

17. Kent J, Wheatley SC, Andrews JE, Sinclair AH, Koopman P. A male-specific role for SOX9 in vertebrate sex determination. Development 1996;122:2813–2822.

18. Raymond CS, Parker ED, Kettlewell JR, et al. A region of human chromosome 9p required for testis development contains two genes related to known sexual regulators. Hum Mol Genet 1999;6:989–996.

19. Marshall OJ, Harley VR. Molecular mechanisms of SOX9 action. Mol Genet Metab 2000;71:455–462.

20. Knower KC, Kelly S, Harley VR. Turning on the male–SRY, SOX9 and sex determination in mammals. Cytogenet Genome Res 2003;101:185–198.

21. Koopman P, Munsterberg A, Capel B, Vivian N, Lovell-Badge R. Expression of a candidate sex-determining gene during mouse testis differentiation. Nature 1990;348:450–452.

22. Taylor HS, Vanden Heuvel GB, Igarashi P. A conserved Hox axis in the mouse and human female reproductive system: late establishment and persistent adult expression of the Hoxa cluster genes. Biol Reprod 1997;57:1338–1345.

23. Parker KL, Schedl A, Schimmer BP. Gene interactions in gonadal development. Annu Rev Physiol 1999;61:417–433.

24. Kurita T, Cunha GR. Roles of p63 in differentiation of Mullerian duct epithelial cells. Ann N Y Acad Sci 2001;948:9–12.

25. van Lingen BL, Reindollar RH, Davis AJ, Gray MR. Further evidence that the WT1 gene does not have a role in the development of the derivatives of the mullerian duct. Am J Obstet Gynecol 1998;179:597–603.

26. Loffler KA, Koopman P. Charting the course of ovarian development in vertebrates. Int J Dev Biol 2002;46:503–510.

27. Lau YF, Zhang J. Sry interactive proteins: implication for the mechanisms of sex determination. Cytogenet Cell Genet 1998;80:128–132.

28. Huang B, Wang S, Ning Y, Lamb AN, Bartley J. Autosomal XX sex reversal caused by duplication of SOX9. Am J Med Genet 1999;87:349–353.

29.   Kwok C, Weller PA, Guioli S, et al. Mutations in SOX9, the gene responsible for Campomelic dysplasia and autosomal sex reversal. Am J Hum Genet 1995;57:1028–1036.

30.   Clarkson MJ, Harley VR. Sex with two SOX on: SRY and SOX9 in testis development. Trends Endocrinol Metab 2002 Apr;13(3):106–111.

31.   Pfeifer D, Kist R, Dewar K, et al. Campomelic dysplasia translocation breakpoints are scattered over 1 Mb proximal to SOX9: evidence for an extended control region. Am J Hum Genet 1999;65:111–124.

32.   Ostrer H. Sex determination: lessons from families and embryos. Clin Genet 2001;59:207–215.

33.   Wycoff GJ, Li J, Wu CI. Molecular evolution of functional genes on the mammalian Y chromosome. Molecular Biol Evol 2002;19:1633–1636

34.   Burgoyne PS, Lovell-Badge R, Rattigan A. Evidence that the testis determination pathway interacts with a non-dosage compensated, X-linked gene. Int J Dev Biol 2001;45:509–512.

35.   Jost A. Problems of fetal endocrinology: the gonadal and hypophyseal hormones. Recent Prog Horm Res 1953;8:379–418.

36.   Catlin EA, MacLaughlin DT, Donahoe PK. Mullerian inhibiting substance: new perspectives and future directions. Microsc Res Tech 1993;25:121–133.

37.   Taguchi O, Cunha GR, Lawrence WD, Robboy SJ. Timing and irreversibility of Mullerian duct inhibition in the embryonic reproductive tract of the human male. Dev Biol 1984;106:394–398.

38.   Grootegoed JA, Baarends WM, Themmen AP. Welcome to the family: the anti-mullerian hormone receptor. Mol Cell Endocrinol 1994;100:29–34.

39.   Gruenwald P. The relation of the growing Mullerian duct to the Wolffian duct and its importance for the genesis of malformations. Anat Rec 1941;81:1–19.

40.   Gruenwald P. Growth and development of the uterus: the relationship of epithelium to mesenchyme. Ann N Y Acad Sci 1943;15:436–440.

41.   Jarcho J. Malformations of the uterus. Review of the subject, including embryology, comparative anatomy, diagnosis and report of cases. Am J Surg 1946;71:106–166.

42.   Woolf RB, Allen WN. Concomitant malformations: the frequent simultaneous occurrence of congenital malformations of the reproductive and urinary tracts. Obstet Gynecol 1953;2:236–240.

43.   Griffin JE, Wilson JD. The syndromes of androgen resistance. N Engl J Med 1980;302:198–209.

44.   Imperato-McGilley J, Peterson RE. Male pseudohermaphroditism: the complexities of male phenotypic development. Am J Med 1976;61:251–272.

45.   New MI, Wilson RC. Steroid disorders in children: congenital adrenal hyperplasia and apparent mineralocorticoid excess. Proc Natl Acad Sci U S A 1999;96:12790–12797.

46.   Speiser PW, White PC. Congenital adrenal hyperplasia. N Engl J Med 2003;349:776–788.

47.   Olgemoller B, Roscher AA, Liebl B, Fingerhut R. Screening for congenital adrenal hyperplasia: adjustment of 17-hydroxyprogesterone cut-off values to both age and birth weight markedly improves the predictive value. J Clin Endocrinol Metab 2003;88:5790–5794.

48. Simpson JL. Genes and chromosomes that cause female infertility. Fertil Steril 1985;44:725–739.

49. Bercu BB, Schulman JD. Genetics of abnormalities of sexual differentiation and of female reproductive failure. Obstet Gynecol Surv 1980;35:1–11.

50. Buttram VC, Jr, Gibbons WE. Mullerian anomalies: a proposed classification (an analysis of 144 cases). Fertil Steril 1979;32:40–46.

51. Buttram VC, Jr. Mullerian anomalies and their management. Fertil Steril 1983;40:159–163.

52. The American Fertility Society. The American Fertility Society classifications of adnexal adhesions, distal tubal occlusion, tubal occlusion secondary to tubal ligation, tubal pregnancies, mullerian abnormalities, and intrauterine adhesions. Fertil Steril 1988;49:944–955.

53. Golan A, Langer R, Bukovsky I, Caspi E. Congenital anomalies of the Mullerian system. Fertil Steril 1989;51:747–755.

2 *Evidence-Based Medicine and Clinical Algorithms*

Therapeutic reports with controls tend to have no enthusiasm
and reports with enthusiasm tend to have no controls.
— *David Sackett, 1986*

For centuries, clinicians have evaluated and treated patients using information drawn from textbooks, formal training, consultation, and personal experience. Traditional decision making involved definition of a problem, reference to a database (usually personal experience), and formulation of a therapeutic plan after discussion with the patient. An inherent part of this process was accepting a certain degree of uncertainty regarding the plan, and so it remained until the widespread availability of medical journals. Guidance to reduce this uncertainty was then sought in the medical literature. However, reference to a bibliographic data base was complicated by difficulties identifying relevant published studies and discovery that the studies were poorly designed, with recommendations based on little or no valid data. In spite of publications of increasing number and focus sound clinical data existed for only 50% of clinical practice. Forty percent of this evidence demonstrated effectiveness for a particular modality, while 60% of the evidence suggested a *lack* of value of current clinical interventions.[1] Such was clinical decision making for most of the twentieth century.

Contemporary paradigms for practice and decision making have changed in both bold and subtle ways. Guidelines for assessing the quality of published clinical data, improved methods of information access, and recommendations for best practices are now well-established reference tools.[2] Rapid evolution in diagnostic and therapeutic choices has created the need for ongoing assessment and prioritization in clinical care using these new paradigms. These changes are particularly important and relevant in infertility and reproductive medicine. The diagnostic and therapeutic range of options in reproductive medicine has markedly increased with advances in surgical techniques and instrumentation and in assisted reproductive technologies, particularly in vitro fertilization.

Reproductive medicine continues to evolve in response to these changes and provide carefully crafted recommendations for surgery, ART or both that are tailored to a patient's unique clinical profile. This chapter addresses this unique perspective and reviews two shared aspects of reproductive surgery and assisted reproductive technologies: the assessment of clinical literature describing diagnostic and therapeutic options, and a standardization of definitions of treatments, successes, and patient selections for the most effective application of these options. As background information, this chapter discusses the past and current trends in clinical literature, their influences on contemporary practice and clinical paradigms for management.

Past Trends in Clinical Literature

Clinical algorithms in reproductive medicine have undergone rapid change and transition from past patterns. Recommendations for treatment were previously based on a sequential process of making laboratory observations, formulating clinical plans, and observing outcomes on a random case by case basis. If a therapy appeared to work after an appropriate interval of trial and error, regardless of study design, it was incorporated into clinical care and considered dogma. Seldom was the quality of the data or study design questioned. In many cases, it should have been. By several accounts, the quality of the reports in the early literature of obstetrics and gynecology has been disappointing. Randomized studies were the exception and a reliance on descriptive and anecdotal data, the rule.

The hazard of relying on descriptive observational data becomes clear with scrutiny of diethylstilbestrol (DES) in clinical care (see Chapter 7). In the mid-1940s, early observational and retrospective data suggested that DES during pregnancy would prevent first-trimester loss and preeclampsia.[3] These observations led to the recommendation for widespread use of DES early in gestation. Contrary to these recommendations, the publication in the early 1950s by Diekemann of a prospective, randomized, placebo-controlled study showed no positive benefit of the use of DES.[4] Nonetheless, because of a growing clinical need to treat these problems and an established trend in clinical care, DES became well-entrenched as a clinical modality for the prevention of first-trimester loss and other obstetric complications. The final outcome after 20 years of using DES is well-known medical history.

Scrutiny of publications on treatment for infertility reveals a similar pattern. Early literature describing outcomes for infertility therapy through the 1980s was primarily in the form of case reports and limited case series. The data were typically descriptive and observational without proper study design or controls. Though important for clinical practice as the only available database, methodologic limitations in study design weakened the validity and conclusions of these reports and at times led to different solutions for seemingly identical problems. Clinical confusion resulted when reports on identical therapies yielded conflicting conclusions. The explanation lay in study design and limited understanding of the problems. Variable outcomes resulted from differing methodologies, data collection, and reporting. In addition, limited knowledge of a clinical problem led to inappropriate patient assignment in studies. An example is the management of infertility secondary to endometriosis and ovarian endometriomas. What is optimal management for either: laparoscopic surgery or IVF? The answer is: *it depends* (on multiple variables). In this case, early studies included any patient with endometriosis stratified by stage and assumed that all study groups were otherwise homogeneous. Better understanding of the patho-physiology of endometriosis associated infertility suggest that these groups are quite heterogeneous and comparisons limited. As ART has become increasingly effective, the balance between surgical intervention and ART has become more delicate. It has become essential to study effectiveness of each option in a more systematic fashion through clinical trials or epidemio-logic studies. The ultimate goals of such study are to define populations and describe the relative risks, benefits, cost-effectiveness, and appropriateness of each option for a given condition and patient profile.

A definitive trend away from descriptive reports to studies that incorporate randomization, control, and outcome analysis has become a standard in medicine in general and in reproductive medicine in particular. Recent evid-ence suggests this shift. An analysis of trials from one journal published over 30 years (between 1953 and 1983) revealed only 44 reports on therapeutic trials.[5] Only three of these trials were of a randomized, controlled design. A gradual increase in the number of reports on therapeutic trials with defined endpoints was noted between 1983 and 1987.[6] Seventy reports (excluding those on in vitro fertilization) of therapeutic trials were reported during this five-year interval. Six of these reports using pregnancy as an outcome were of a randomized, controlled design. The increase in the number of clinical publications during the more recent interval primarily included non-ran-domized or retrospective studies. However, even studies intended to be truly randomized and prospective may have design flaws. In one series, 82% of articles reviewed in the obstetric and gynecologic literature between 1990 and 1991 had errors in study design (such as poor randomization technique and blinding) and had no mention of a methodology text or reference.[7,8] Most clinical practice when viewed from the quality of clinical data on which the practice is based merits only a class "C" or "III" recommendation. Gradual improvement in study design, prioritization for publication of controlled trials and emerging concepts of evidence-based medicine have reversed this trend over the past decade.[9]

In addition to the varying quality in study design in the literature, further uncertainty was caused by variable definitions and endpoints to assess the effectiveness of a given intervention. The problem of assessing the effective-ness or calculating a success rate in reproductive medicine is a complex process.[10,11] Any definition of success in treating the infertile patient must include a precise definition of a pregnancy, define the age of the population of interest and the specific clinical problem, and equally important, indicate the complications and duration of follow-up for any intervention. Previous literature lacked this precision and used a variety of definitions for preg-nancy rates, such as biochemical and crude pregnancy rates, for outcome after surgery and in vitro fertilization. These differing endpoints made it dif-ficult to extrapolate and compare results for specific clinical conditions.

Similar limitations apply in the interpretation of outcomes for other problems in reproductive surgery. For example, various definitions for success have been used in the management of vaginal agenesis in past literature. These outcomes range from an anatomically correct neovagina to broader and fuller definitions of success including favorable psychological profiles and sexual satisfaction. Variable endpoints characteristic of previous literature brought into focus the need to establish standard definitions of success and effectiveness in assessing any intervention in reproductive medicine and surgery and the assisted reproductive technologies. Efforts of professional organizations such as the Society for Assisted Reproductive Technology and the European Society for Human Reproduction and Embryology have set standards for these definitions in contemporary practice.

Contemporary Trends in Clinical Literature

Assessing the Quality of Evidence

Much has changed since Cochrane initiated his discussions on the necessity to base clinical care on data from randomized, controlled trials in 1979.[12] An increasing awareness of the role for data from prospective, randomized trials has guided clinical decision making in contemporary practice. This evolution represents a much needed improvement away from reliance on descriptive, retrospective studies characteristic of the earlier literature. Interpretation of data from clinical trials in contemporary practice may be made with reference to what Chalmers calls a "hierarchy of evidence".[13] Simply put, this hierarchy maintains that not all data from clinical trials are created equal. The reliability of data from a simple, extended, case series, though interesting, is hardly sufficient for formulating clinical recommendations. Case reports or limited series remain an important part of clinical literature and provide important insights into potential trends. They should not, however, dictate management. Clinical trials meeting minimal standards have become the hallmark of reliable clinical reporting (Table 2-1). Among trials meeting such criteria, prospective, randomized, and blind studies stand out as most reliable.[14]

Results from randomized, controlled clinical trials are the standard for comparison among the various types of study design. These studies frame the relative efficacy of different treatment regimens for specific problems and specific populations to guide clinical care. Guidance for management decisions on the basis of data from randomized, controlled studies is fast becoming the standard of care.[15,16] When data from such trials are not available, an assessment of the quality of the existing data may be made and the literature categorized to provide insight into the reliability of the conclusions and recommendations. Study design for assessing effectiveness for any treatment in reproductive medicine has evolved to the point that confounding

Table 2-1.
Minimum Standards for Reports of Randomized Trials

Trial hypothesis

- o   Formulation of a primary trial hypothesis
- o   Power calculation based on that hypothesis

Randomization

- o   Type of randomization (e.g., simple, blocking, stratified)
- o   Method of generation of randomization sequence (e.g., table of random numbers, computer)
- o   Method of allocation concealment (e.g., telephone, pharmacy, opaque sealed envelope)

Table of baseline characteristics

- o   Inclusion of important prognostic variables
- o   Measures of central location and dispersion of prognostic variables (e.g., mean and SD; median and interquartile range)
- o   Description of exclusions after randomization

Ascertainment of outcomes

- o   Description of efforts to blind those assessing outcomes

factors should be controlled. In addition outcome analysis and cost considerations should be incorporated as part of the study design.

Quality of data is ranked according to the type of study generating the data.[17] When possible, these studies should guide care and a discussion of the quality of data and strength of recommendations should be incorporated into all patient consultations. Randomized clinical trials yield the highest quality data and most reliable results and recommendations. Following randomized controlled trials, prospective cohort studies, retrospective studies, case control studies, and case reports or case series are ranked in order of decreasing reliability. The sequence of an assessment of the quality of evidence and strength of ranked recommendations based on the evidence is at the cornerstone of evidence-based medicine (Table 2-2).[18,19] Patient counselling for any procedure should reference the quality of the literature on which a recommendation is made.

Evidence-Based Medicine

Analysis of Clinical Data

Evidence-based medicine is a clinical paradigm initially described in the 1600s in French literature. Evidence-based medicine has become a contemporary standard to guide clinical decision making and practice. This paradigm is a marked departure from practice patterns of even the recent

Table 2-2. Assessment of Quality of Evidence for Health Intervention and Grades of Recommendations	
Quality of Evidence	
I	Evidence obtained from at least one properly designed randomized, controlled trial
II_1	Evidence obtained from well-designed controlled trials without randomization
II_2	Evidence obtained from well-designed cohort or case control analytic studies, preferably more than one center or research group
II_3	Evidence obtained from multiple time series with or without the intervention. Dramatic results in uncontrolled experiments could also be regarded as this type of evidence
III	Opinions of respected authorities based on clinical experience or descriptive studies, or reports of expert committees
Strength or Confidence of Recommendations	
I	Directly based on category I evidence
II	Directly based on category II evidence or extrapolated from category I
III	Directly based on category III evidence or extrapolated from category I or II
Grades of Recommendation for a Specified Level of Baseline Risk	
A_1	Randomized, controlled trials (RCTs) with homogeneous results, with all confidence intervals (CI) on one side of the number needed to treat (NNT)
A_2	RCTs with homogeneous results, with CIs overlapping threshold NNT
B_1	RCTs with heterogeneous results, with all CIs on one side of threshold NNT
B_2	RCTs with heterogeneous results, with CIs overlapping threshold NNT
C_1	Non-RCTs in observational studies, with all CIs on one side of threshold NNT
C_2	Non-RCTs in observational studies, with CIs overlapping threshold NNT

past. Previous, classic paradigms held that an individual practitioner provided comprehensive and continuous care to a patient. Treatment was frequently based on consensus and personal opinion as to what constituted optimal care. Contemporary practice patterns represent a shift from so-called *consensus-based medicine* to decision making based on integrated information from clinical trials, to guide clinical decisions, so-called *evidence-based medicine*.

Evidence-based medicine is defined as the conscientious and judicious use of current best evidence in making decisions about the care of individual patients.[20–22] Its cornerstone is the interpretation of data, preferably data collected through randomized, controlled trials or systematic review and meta-analysis, and application of these data to the formation of management guidelines for each specific clinical problem.[23] A tremendous effort in all specialties is being placed on establishing guidelines for evidence-based medicine; nowhere is this more evident than in reproductive medicine and surgery and the assisted reproductive technologies.[24–26]

Interest in evidence-based medicine has resulted in several new texts and a dedicated journal, *Evidence-Based Medicine*, published as a joint effort between the American College of Physicians and the British Medical Journal Publishing Group. These resources describe trends and address the issue of effectiveness in clinical literature. A broader collaborative effort, the *Cochrane Collaboration*, is a systematic review of published and unpublished literature during the past 50 years including over 1 million randomized, controlled trials of various medical treatments.[26] The *Cochrane Collaboration* is an offspring of a British-based effort initiated in 1976 and directed in part towards reviewing randomized clinical trials in reproductive medicine. Between 1978 and 1984, a systematic poll of practitioners in women's health care was undertaken, as part of this collaboration, in a deliberate search of any trials or data that had not been published. The goal was to discover both positive and negative trials and gain a more balanced view of the true effectiveness of different therapies and interventions. The effort revealed approximately 3500 trials, of which 600 were properly conducted with valid data for interpretation.[27]

Surgery, Assisted Reproductive Technology and Evidence-Based Medicine

The gold standard for the evaluation of any surgical therapy is the randomized, controlled trial of sufficient size to prevent false positives (alpha error) and false negatives (beta error) with proper randomization schemes. Ideally, such a trial should include some assessment of cost and cost comparison between the two modalities or agents being compared. Meeting this standard has been the exception. Only 10% of surgical technologies have been evaluated using this approach. There are unique aspects, however, to evaluating surgical therapies that are not evident in evaluating medical therapies and pose difficulties in reaching this standard. Trials of medical therapies are usually comparing two drugs in well defined populations. The first randomized clinical trial was reported in 1948 and evaluated streptomycin in the treatment of pulmonary tuberculosis. Those clinical circumstances that are most easily evaluated by such trials are comparisons of drug therapies in which drug A is compared to drug B and a decision made regarding which is better for the treatment of condition C. Implicit in these studies are reliable methods of randomization, blinding, and a standardization of the therapy under investigation. Surgical trials differ from this model in several critical aspects. Surgical trials have been based primarily on clinical impressions, case reports, and case series without controls and case studies with controls. In one review of published literature on surgical research only 7% of reported data derived from randomized trials. Forty-six percent were case series, followed by animal experiments accounting for 18%. This shortcoming in research design leaves several hypotheses and practice patterns untested. False inferences have been generated from these studies as frequently as 50–60%. Several inherent aspects of surgical practice explain these early findings.

Historically, the introduction of new surgical procedures resulted from the initiative of individual surgeons who designed a new piece of equipment or developed a novel technique. This approach posed several problems in evaluating these new therapies as randomized controlled trials. Among these difficulties the inability to have a true placebo group is the most significant. As the only true placebo is a sham operation, placebo controls for any surgical trial are not possible. In addition, a learning curve varies substantially for a single surgeon, depending on where he/she is on the curve (intra-surgeon variability), and different skill levels among surgeons at different institutions (inter-surgeon variability), making multi-center trials difficult. Randomization to a new procedure arm of a study may also introduce a selection bias. Hence, the application of randomized controlled trials to any surgical specialty, reproductive surgery included, is somewhat more problematic than the simple comparison of drug A or drug B for the treatment of condition C.

Without a randomized trial (a common scenario in reproductive medicine), the overall confidence on which a therapeutic decision is based may be limited depending on the clinical problem. When two possible therapies exist in the absence of comparative data, decisions may not be straightforward. A reasonable plan of treatment is still possible without data from randomized trials. But limitations exist. This database may be impossible for certain clinical problems. For example, in vaginal agenesis, guidance is available from a review of outcomes from non-comparative, descriptive trials. Clinical decisions involve tradeoffs and compromises when solid data are lacking. In reproductive medicine, these frequently focus on patient circumstances such as personal choices, financial circumstances, the clinical assessment of data, quality of the recommendations, and increasingly, society's input as types of therapies may impact more far reaching issues of overall health care costs related to outcomes such as the cost of ectopic pregnancies from tubal surgeries or multiple births from IVF.

Contemporary Paradigms in Reproductive Medicine

Outcome Analysis

Approximately 9% of women 15 to 44 years of age or 5 million women will have an impaired ability to have children. This condition accounts for $1 billion in expenditures for medical care. A unique aspect to reproductive surgery and ART is the variable coverage by medical insurers for any diagnostic or therapeutic interventions. The reality for many couples is that these costs must be paid through their personal finances. This aspect must be frequently factored into any clinical decision making. Clinicians are faced with achieving a balance between appropriate timely and clinically effective therapies and the cost of these decisions for a given couple. Medical coverages may be variable ranging from 100% to offering options at extra cost to complete out-of-pocket payment. Payment plans are also influenced by locale where coverage may be determined by state specific laws.

The most cost-effective means of planning infertility services remains a question with several answers. Financial modeling to assess outcomes, utilization of services, and cost of achieving the outcome is one approach. Economic analysis is not a new phenomenon in health care in general, or in reproductive medicine in specific. A role for cost assessment as part of a clinical study design is essential. According to one study, economic analyses should be incorporated into current clinical trials when a large amount of resources are at stake, when a new technique is likely to become widespread in the near future, and when a shortage of resources forces a choice between options for care. Economic analyses provide a prism through which clinical data may be viewed and may lead to recommendations somewhat different than if based solely on clinical outcomes. Very few studies in reproductive medicine incorporate a formal economic analysis. In a review of 100 studies in reproductive medicine, none included any economic evaluation. In approximately one-half, analyses would have been useful. An example of the potential role of such analysis in reproductive medicine is comparison between in vitro fertilization and surgery for tubal obstruction or endometriosis. The cost differences between these two strategies might focus not only on the cost of the procedure itself, but also on the possible costs of ectopic pregnancies and higher order multiples are factored into the final analysis.

Outcome analysis and research has evolved into a subspecialty within the health care environment. Multidisciplinary efforts involve health services, researchers, epidemiologists, economists, sociologists, statisticians, and ethicists. The focus on outcomes research is ultimately to provide the most effective treatment available to a patient under the most cost-effective terms. The first tenet requires a precise definition of success or what is sometimes referred to as outcome measures. Outcomes or the measure of success of a therapy may be clinical events, economic events such as the cost of individual medical care, or humanistic events such as the quality of life.

Frequently, all three are influential in formulating a therapeutic plan. In reproductive medicine, these variables ultimately translate to define a success as a singleton pregnancy at the lowest cost using the simplest and most efficient clinical plan. How best to determine this plan will be based on collaborative data collection and analysis, enabled in no small part by computer technology.

Concomitant with these changes in definitions and guidelines for clinical practice through evidence-based medicine and outcomes analysis, computer technology is an indispensable tool in clinical practice.[28] Computers and user-friendly software enable the establishment of large databases for the dual purpose of data analysis of large-population-based studies and near-immediate feedback for practitioners seeking access to such databases. On-line services and CD-ROM technology make large databases available to all, regardless of practice or location. Computer access to information provides an important resource for assistance in clinical decision making in the practice of evidence-based medicine. The two significant ways that computers can influence practice are rapid access of medical information through on-line technologies, providing practitioners with a near-immediate electronic consult, and the pooling of data, providing comparison and assessment of treatment effect or adverse reactions.[29,30] In addition to bibliographic databases, there are several on-line databases for full textbook information and practice guidelines.[31,32] Practice paradigms are readily available on-line to guide both physician and patient in selecting the best treatment. The emergence of computer technology has made assessment of outcomes a clinical reality. This technology will enhance the tracking of success rates for ART. Real-time reporting of clinical outcomes to a central agency (such as the Society for Reproductive Technology) will provide clinicians with a tool for evaluating outcomes and patients with an independent, contemporary view of overall and clinic specific success rates. The real-time format will reduce the lag in publishing clinical and multiple pregnancy rates. Live birth rates may be layered on at a later date.

Translating Clinical Data into Clinical Practice

Success in formulating any plan for diagnosis and therapy revolves around a precise definition of clinical problems, the patient population, and end point for therapy. These definitions and an assessment of the quality of the literature form the essentials of a clinical plan. Optimal therapies should then be tailored to the individual patient. However, given the media coverage of infertility therapies, a treatment plan based on available outcomes can be somewhat complicated. Though unproven therapies may seem appealing, practical problems in dealing with patient requests to try unproven therapies is a daily reality in reproductive medicine. Practice should be based on clinical data from well-designed studies, but the clinician frequently must confront reports labeled "breakthroughs" that appear on the television news or in tabloids. Many of the reports are based on isolated cases or small case series and have no role in dictating therapies or in deviating from recommendations grounded in solid clinical data. Patients may pressure clinicians to proceed with the "newest" technique, often prompted by a friend's success or tabloid tale. The task at hand, then, becomes deciding what is new, useful, and worth pursuing versus what is new but without merit.

The focus of therapy in reproductive medicine should be to restore structure and function to as near a normal state as possible and/or enhance fertility. A broad range of clinical problems may be encountered with widely variable goals. Intervention may be warranted to enhance structure, function and fertility or strictly to restore structure and function. For example, management of structural abnormalities of the reproductive tract may include the correction of congenital abnormalities such as vaginal agenesis to enable normal coital activity, or excision of ovarian endometriomas or endometriosis to relieve pain, restore function and structure. Similarly, therapies to enhance fertility in the case of tubal obstruction may focus strictly on restoring function and enhancing fertility. Clinicians have an extensive array of therapies, both medical and surgical, with which to manage these problems. The difficulty is frequently in assessing the patient profile accurately, establishing endpoints for success and outcomes, and accurately defining the problem. This section defines the demographics of patients seeking care for reproductive problems, specifically for infertility, and reviews the various definitions for success and failure in these circumstances. Based on these parameters, more accurate patient selection is possible.

Definition of the Demographics of Reproduction
A progressive trend has occurred in the patterns of childbearing during the past century: fewer births later in life per person and a decline in fertility. These changes have been even more pronounced over the past two decades. Women are delaying childbearing to their mid- to late thirties in increasing numbers. The trend to have children between the ages of 25 and 34 years peaked in the mid-1960s. Since then, maternal age for firstborn has continued to increase dramatically.[33] Two sets of data are reviewed to provide a broad overview of these trends over time: an early set from 1970 to 1980 and the most recent data yet compiled by the Center for Disease Control and Prevention's National Center for Health Statistics (NCHS) under a collaborative arrangement with the United States Census Bureau for 1990 to 2001. In the first set of data, two concomitant age-related events described: a gradual decrease since 1970, from 86 to 72% among those who realized fertility plans, and a gradual increase among women with their first birth at an age older than 34 years.[34] Between 1972 and 1982, the first-birth rate (i.e., age of first delivery) for women aged 30 to 34 years increased from 7 to 15% per 1000 women; for women aged 35 to 39 years, the rate was 1.8 to 3.3% per 1000 women, an 83% increase. Similar changes were also noted in second-birth rates for women in their thirties, increasing by more than 60% between 1972 and 1982. Changes in fertility rates are also reflected in a trend in women in the 38 to 42 years age range. The fertility rate rose slightly from 67 births per

1000 women aged 18 to 44 years in 1976 to 71 per 1000 in 1980. The most notable increases occurred among women who were 30 years and older. Almost one-half the births to college graduates over age 30 were first births, indicative of delayed childbearing among this group of women. These data demonstrate a persistent and progressive shift in childbearing into older reproductive-age groups.

The second set of data are from 1990 to 2001. The birth rate for age groups from 20 to 29 years decreased 9% and 6% respectively. In contrast, the birth rate for all ages from 30 to 49 years increased over the interval from 1990 to 2001 ranging from 14% to 47% (Table 2-3). Most notably, the birth rate for women aged 45 to 49 years more than doubled from 0.2 in 1990 to 0.5 in 2001. These changes reflect in part the increased use of oocyte donation to fulfill the reproductive needs of the age group. The additional demographic data for this group describes a stability in the number of women greater than 40 years over the observation interval suggesting that the increases in birth rate were real and not a reflection of population increases. Data describing live birth order reflect changes in the age of women pursuing pregnancy at advanced reproductive ages. These recent statistics corroborate the observations of two decades ago. First birth rates for women decreased by 11% and 8% during the interval 1990 to 2001 for ages 20–24 and 25–29 years respectively. In contrast, first birth rates increased by 25% and 36% for women aged 30–34 and 35–39 years respectively. Remarkably, increases of 70% were described for women aged 40–44 years.

This diminution in fertility rates is reflective in part of delayed childbearing. Since the interval of 1945 to 1965 (the so-called baby boom), the total number of births to women aged 30 to 44 years has decreased steadily (Figure 2-1).

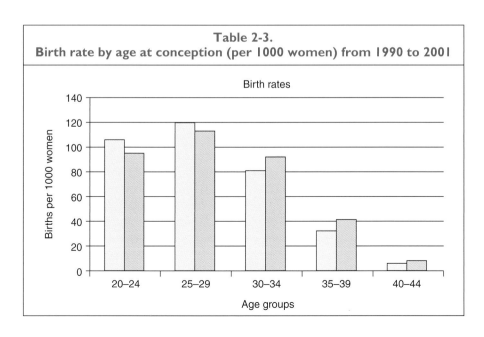

Table 2-3.
Birth rate by age at conception (per 1000 women) from 1990 to 2001

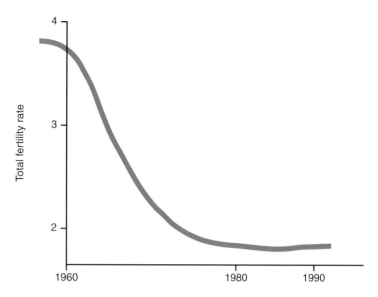

Figure 2-1   Fertility rate in the United States from the baby boom and through the early 1960s to current plateaued rates through.

The decrease in fertility reflects factors that are partly age-related phenomena.[35] U.S. Bureau of Census projections suggest that the female population in the age range of 35 to 49 years increased progressively through the 1990s, reaching an estimated 20 to 30 million through the early part of the 21st century. Further estimates suggest that the increasing number of women in this age bracket seeking to achieve a pregnancy will ultimately result in an increase of approximately 75% of the proportion of total births for populations between the ages of 35 to 49 years.[36] Because of the well-described influence of age on fertility, the number of women in this age range will increasingly seek consultations to discuss reproductive issues.

Several lines of clinical evidence support an age-specific adverse influence on reproductive potential including outcomes and observations from assisted reproductive technology.[36,37] Historical data suggest that in a population not using contraception, one-third to one-half of couples will remain involuntarily childless when the woman marries in her late thirties or early forties. Fertility diminishes when the median age of the female partner is approximately 40 years.[38,39] The data derive from two sources: an older set of studies from religious groups and a more recent, though dated, set of studies from therapeutic donor insemination. These two data sets are in remarkable agreement. Data from studies of religious groups, such as Hutterites, suggest a gradual decline in fertility through the mid-1930s and 1940s (Figure 2-2).[40] These data were insightful and unique but did not control for other factors potentially contributory to fertility–coital activity, a possible male factor, or additional female factors such as anovulation. The 1982 report on therapeutic donor insemination from CECOS further substantiated the decline in fertility for

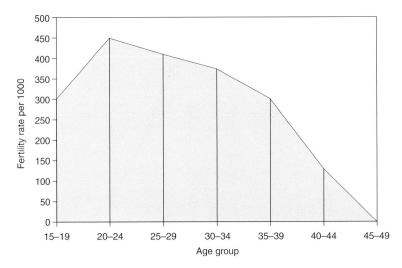

Figure 2-2   Fertility rates by 5-year age groups.

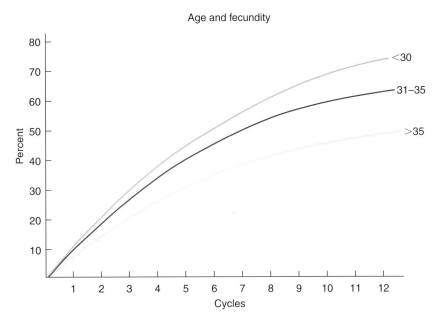

Figure 2-3   Percentage of pregnancies through 12 cycles as a function of age by 5-year age groups.

women older than age 30. Though dated, the study provides further, more controlled insight into reproductive potential. In this study the fecundity was reported as a function of age through an analysis of over 2000 women under-going artificial insemination.[41] The cumulative pregnancy rates by age after 12 cycles were 26 to 30 years, 74%; 31 to 35 years, 62%; and 35 years and older, 53.6% (Figure 2-3). Data also suggest a steady increase in impaired fecundity, which tripled from a level of 12% for women aged 20 to 24 years to 34% for women aged 35 to 39 years.[42]

These observations have significant implications in counseling infertile couples. Care is required in discussions with patients to balance therapeutic options and a patients age. Counseling must be tempered to a specific couple's circumstances, balancing age of the female partner, duration of infertility, the number of concomitant and possibly contributory factors to the infertility, and the couple's interest in the intensity of therapy. Of all possible factors, age has emerged as the most significant. For many couples, advanced age beyond 35 years leads to requests for evaluation and at times aggressive therapies after abbreviated attempts at natural conception. Extreme care in counseling is essential. Because more than one-third of infertile couples may conceive within 2 to 7 years of discontinuing fertility therapy and because couples with potential age-related factors feel a greater pressure to conceive within a short period of time, a definition of infertility as the inability to conceive with 1 year combined with a lower threshold for seeking treatment could overstate the incidence of infertility in this group of women. Despite this possibility, intervention is appropriate earlier in the evaluation than a standard 12 months trial, particularly for patients older than 38 years.

Definition of the Problem

A variety of definitions for infertility have been used (Table 2-4). These definitions can confuse both the interpretation of the literature in reproductive

Table 2-4. Definitions Associated with the Problem of Infertility	
Term	**Definition**
Fertility	The rate of live births expressed per 1000 women aged 15–44
Fertility rates	Live births/1000 women of the same age
Total fertility rate	The number of births that 1000 women would have in their lifetimes if at each year of age during the reproductive span they experienced the birth rates per 1000 women that occurred in that calendar year (the age-specific birth rate)
Infertility	Inability of couple to obtain clinically recognizable pregnancy, to achieve fertilization of gametes
Clinical definition	Couple does not achieve clinically or biochemically recognizable pregnancy after 12 months of intercourse
Fecundity	Ability of a couple to have a live-born child
Infecundity	Inability of couple to achieve live birth
Clinical definition	No pregnancy resulting in live birth after 12 months of unprotected intercourse
Resolved infertility	Infecundity (subfertility or subfecundity)
Clinical definition	Episode that is eventually followed by conception or birth
Unresolved infertility or infecundity	Episode that is not followed by conception or birth

medicine and the discussion and counseling between clinician and patient. The problem is compounded by the tendency to apply one definition to all patient populations. For example, infertility is clinically defined as an inability to achieve a pregnancy after 12 months of unprotected intercourse. However, the duration of 12 months may be extended in some circumstances to 18 or 24 months for patients younger than 30 with favorable profiles and an interest in a conservative approach, or shortened to 6 months for patients older than 35 with several factors. Regardless of the definition used, infertility is a common and increasing problem. Approximately 10 to 15% of couples from ages 15 to 44 years have impaired fertility. The upward trend in infertility has been similar since 1965 to the present, and the number of patients seeking care continues to increase as the trend in delayed childbearing continues.

There are multiple factors for infertility. A World Health Organization task force, in a broad view of the problem, revealed the following causes of infertility in women: tubal factor, 36%; ovulatory disorders, 33%; endometriosis, 6%; and no demonstrable cause, 40%.[43] The incidence of unexplained infertility will continue to diminish as improvements in diagnostic techniques provide better insight into etiology. In other circumstances, clinical assessment and investigations are designed to confirm ovulation, establish normal uterine tubes, ensure adequate coital pattern, and exclude processes affecting fertility such as tubal disease, pelvic adhesive disease, and endometriosis.[44] Any definition of the problems contributing to infertility must exclude these contributory factors but must also take into account two additional critically important factors: age of the female partner (or *ovarian reserve*) and duration of infertility. Fecundity in women decreases after the age of 30 years; infertility accelerates after age 35 years. The age of the woman and the role assisted reproductive technologies may play must be assessed at the initial evaluation.

Oocyte quality and duration of infertility are among the more significant factors. The reason for age-related decline in reproductive potential in women is primarily ovarian. The term *diminished ovarian reserve* is related to age, and the quality and quantity of oocytes.[45] Insight into the latter may be gained through markers of ovarian reserve such as serum concentrations of FSH on menstrual cycle day 3 and antral follicle counts. Both are important predictors of outcome. Age relates to oocyte quality. FSH concentration relates to oocyte quantity. The effect of nonovarian components, such as uterine aging or the condition of the endometrium, probably has little influence on the likelihood of conception.[46] Diminished ovarian reserve may not be identifiable by traditional clinical parameters such as menstrual cycle regularity, ovulatory pattern, or progesterone secretion. Ancillary factors responsible for age-related changes may be an increasing incidence of intercurrent problems such as endometriosis and ovulatory disorders as well as the overall aging of the hypothalamic-pituitary axis.[47] However, the most compelling reason for the decrease in age-related fecundity is clearly the age and quality of the oocytes.

Duration of infertility is the second important variable in determining the chance of pregnancy. This influence is expressed by a high rate (44 to 96%) of treatment-independent pregnancies for a group of patients with problems that include ovulatory dysfunction, endometriosis, tubal and cervical factors, and idiopathic infertility.[48,49] A spontaneous conception without treatment is possible for patients who have been attempting pregnancy for less than three years when only mild factors potentially contributory to a failure to conceive are present. These data are based on a definition of infertility as a failure to achieve pregnancy after 12 months. Patients in these categories may have conditions that contribute to a delay in, but not absolute prevention of, fecundability and represent a group at the low extreme of normal distribution of fecundability. More serious conditions, such as severe hydrosalpinges or severe male factor, or age-related infertility are excluded from this consideration and should be considered for immediate therapy. For patients with a duration of fertility greater than three years, the likelihood of a spontaneous conception is low regardless of age of the female partner.

Definition of Success

Reporting success rates has been one of the most controversial issues in any reproductive therapy, whether medical or surgical. The definition of pregnancy live birth, the ultimate goal, is at times unclear and vaguely defined or absent in reports.[50] The controversy about pregnancy rates, what a pregnancy is or is not, has been so widespread that it gained the attention of the political process in the 1990s. Hearings were held in Washington, DC on reproductive outcomes for IVF before the Subcommittee on Regulations and Business Opportunities. These hearings and government intervention led to the Fertility Clinic Success Rate and Certification Act of 1992.[51] The goal of this process is to provide information to satisfy the public demand for accurate, clinic-specific information, standardized for all the known variables.

Outcome measures of various therapies for infertility are difficult to compare unless uniform conventions, such as strictly defined patient populations, are used and the numerators and denominators in calculating the rates clearly defined (Table 2-5).[52–54] The most common and simplest calculation for fertility trials (the calculation used in earlier studies) is the simple or crude pregnancy rate. This value is defined as the number of pregnancies divided by the number of patients treated. Of all methods of analysis, it is the easiest to perform but the most difficult to interpret reliably. Two shortcomings are inherent in this definition: the calculation does not adjust for confounding variables or other factors that may affect a couple's fertility (so-called sample bias), and calculation depends on the length of follow-up. The critical interval may range from as short as 3 months in some studies to as long as 36 months in others. The longer the follow-up, the higher the pregnancy rates. Given the increasing number of women older than age 35, this variable is essential to consider. It is unreasonable to offer a couple a therapy that requires

Table 2-5. Definitions of Success Rates		
Term	**Definition**	**Shortcomings**
Simple or crude pregnancy rate	Number of pregnancies divided by the number of patients treated	No adjustment for confounding variables that may affect a couple's fertility or length of follow-up
Corrected pregnancy rates	Number of pregnancies divided by the number of patients treated, excluding patients with additional infertility factors	No control for follow-up intervals
Life-table analysis	Estimation of the percentage of study subjects that will conceive at any given period of follow-up	No correction for non-pregnant drop-outs
Pregnancy rate by ART cycle	Percent of cycle starts, oocyte retrievals or embryo transfers resulting in a pregnancy	No insight into complexity of population treated; number of cycles may influence percent success

Table 2-6. Success Rates with ART, 2001*				
Type of Cycle	**Age of Women (in years)**			
	<35	**35–37**	**38–40**	**41–42**
Fresh embryos from nondonor eggs				
Pregnancy rate in per cent	40.6	34.4	26.2	17.3
Live birth rate per retrieval	38.9	33.1	23.8	13.2
Percentage of pregnancies with twins	33.1	28.6	22.7	14.5
Percentage of pregnancies with triplets or more	8.1	7.8	6.2	2.9
Frozen embryos from nondonor eggs				
Percentage of transfers resulting in live births	26.0	23.3	19.4	15.8
Donor eggs	**Fresh embryos**		**Frozen embryos**	
Percentage of transfers resulting in live births	47.0		27.3	

*Data available at http://www.cdc.gov/reproductivehealth

an interval of 18 months' follow-up to realize maximal pregnancy rates and then, if unsuccessful, consider other assisted reproductive technologies such as IVF for which age is such a critical factor to success. Corrected pregnancy rates are calculated similarly, stratified by specific variables such as age or etiology; restriction of study populations to those with similar profiles enables comparisons of more homogeneous populations. This method, like crude pregnancy rates, does not control for the follow-up intervals. These calculations are meaningful for comparison in calculation for example of pregnancy rates with IVF stratified by age and/or etiology (Table 2-6).

Cumulative pregnancy rate

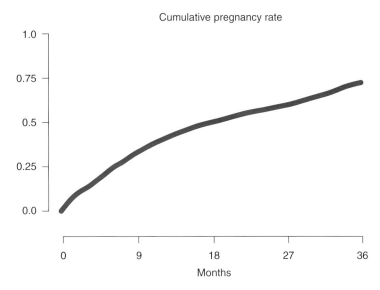

Figure 2-4   Life-table analysis of cumulative pregnancy rates during 36 months of follow-up.

Crude and corrected pregnancy rates are easy to calculate but do not address length of follow-up. A method of graphic display, called the life-table, provides more precise description of the likelihood of success as treatment duration increases. The life-table also compensates for the problem of variable follow-up (Figure 2-4). The purpose of the life-table in fertility trials is to estimate the percentage of study subjects who will conceive at any given period of follow-up. The data can be rearranged by months of follow-up. For each month of follow-up, a certain number of women are expected to achieve a pregnancy. The life-table has the advantage of identifying the rate of conception at any particular time after the initiation of treatment. It does not suffer from any assumptions of uniformity of success from month to month. Life-tables are best applied to treatments in which single intervention produces long-term result. A classic example is pregnancy rates after tubal surgery in which follow-up intervals may be as long as 3 years.

Although the life-table represents an improvement over the calculation of simple pregnancy rates, there is one potentially misleading facet of the technique: when using life-table analysis, there must be reasonable assurance that *censored patients* do not differ substantially from *noncensored patients*. If patients drop out of the study without conceiving, the *censored patients* can be mathematically corrected for and an estimate calculated to describe what would have happened if all patients had continued in the trial. For large patient numbers, the life-table often takes on the appearance of a relatively smooth curve. As the number of patients decreases with increasing length of follow-up, the variance for each data point increases. The life-table is best considered as a visual device for estimating cumulative pregnancy rates. To use the life-table for comparative purposes, it is necessary to create a mathematic model that describes the curve and provides parameters for comparison.[55] Despite its complexities, life-table analysis provides a more realistic and reliable assessment of the likelihood that a particular therapy will benefit a couple than do crude or corrected pregnancy rates.

Accurate and precise definitions of success in reproductive medicine are essential for calculating accurate condition-specific measures for outcomes and in formulating patient-specific measures for outcomes. These outcome measures should be discussed in sufficient length and detail with the patient at the outset so that clear expectations are established. Because of possible changes in expectations on the part of couples, discussions must be a recurrent exercise to continually reestablish goals and priorities. The need for ongoing discussions is essential particularly in patients over 38 years for whom time investment in any therapy must be carefully weighed.

Patient Selection

Clinicians are increasingly confronted with complex decisions regarding optimal therapy for a particular patient or couple. Whom does one treat, when does one treat, and how does one treat are the three key questions. Delay in childbearing and low age-related fertility rates in this group force the clinician to make decisions regarding what therapy may be most efficacious, based on the amount of time of follow-up required, especially for any surgical therapies for fertility, in which pregnancy rates do not fall to 0 until after 2 to 3 years of follow-up. What may be appropriate therapy for a 25–year-old may be inappropriate for a 35–year-old. Therapies should carefully assess the influence of the age of the female partner and the detrimental effect age has on reproduction on outcome. Fortunately, some parameters can be used to further guide the decision making.[56,57]

The likelihood of success, and optimal management plan are critical points for counseling any patient prior to settling on any intervention. Adequate discussion of options is essential. Four aspects are essential to consider in any discussion. These are the approximate 12 to 15% fecundability per month of an untreated normal population in age less than 35 years, the possibility of treatment-independent pregnancies for those couples with mild factors and a duration of infertility less than three years, the success rate and duration of follow-up required after any intervention for a specific problem, and the role of the more complex and expensive assisted reproductive technologies. The choice of whether therapy is necessary or if observation is an option should involve an assessment of the potential contributing factors to infertility, the age of the female partner, cost of treatment and the attitude of the patient (perhaps the most critical variable). In those circumstances where a clearly defined and treatable condition is present, calculation of the success rate for any intervention must carefully factor in the duration of follow-up required, for maximum success the duration of follow-up a patient can afford (based on age), and whether the success rate stratified for age will exceed that offered by IVF. The issue of age in this circumstance is critical, as success for in vitro fertilization follows a clearly downward trend with advancing age.[58,59] The discussion for the surgical management of a specific condition must balance the likelihood of success through surgery against that for IVF. Interestingly, age may have implications on male outcome.[60]

Ovarian Reserve

Assessment of ovarian reserve (or functional ovarian age) at the time of the discussion should be made to further refine the influence of age and oocyte quality on the likelihood of success with in vitro fertilization. Basal follicle-stimulating hormone (FSH) levels are the most common means of assessing ovarian reserve.[61,62] There is an age-related increase in the early follicular phase (day 3) serum concentration of basal FSH. There is a decrease in the pregnancy rate for aggressive assisted reproductive technologies especially with increasing FSH levels on day 3 (Figure 2-5). The parameters are applicable regardless of whether one or two ovaries are present. The reason for the elevated FSH is probably related to the quality of the oocytes, the need for increasing stimulation to set in motion the process of folliculogenesis, and diminished feedback within the pituitary-ovarian axis. In addition, serum FSH concentration greater than 15 mIU/mL on day 3 has been shown to be associated with extremely low pregnancy and high first trimester loss rates. There is laboratory-to-laboratory variation regarding the sensitivity and

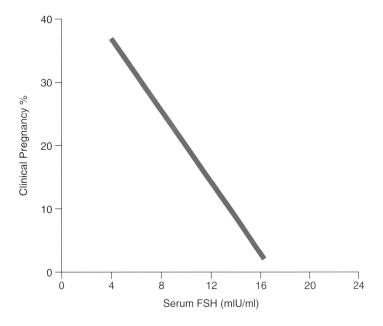

Figure 2-5   Day 3 FSH concentrations and clinical pregnancy rates.

specificity of FSH testing on day 3, but in general, serum concentrations greater than 15 mIU/ml and an age greater than 35 years, have been associated with extremely poor outcomes.

A second common method of assessing ovarian reserve is the clomiphene citrate challenge test (CCCT).[63,64] In this test clomiphene citrate 100 mg is used on cycle days 5 through 9. Levels of FSH are drawn on days 3 and 10. Any elevation of FSH on day 3 or day 10 is predictive of a poor outcome. This method may be used in patients in whom age-related infertility is suspected but basal FSH concentrations are normal. The CCCT identifies two times the number of patients than does standard FSH testing on day 3. The CCCT is an accurate back up for patients who have a normal FSH concentration on day 3.

Basal FSH and age are indicators of oocyte quantity and quality, sometimes referred to as *ovarian reserve*. FSH may be a better and possibly independent predictor of cycle cancellation for ART and pregnancy after in vitro fertilization than age. Patients with elevated FSH levels are often advised not to proceed with in vitro fertilization because of low success rates secondary to diminished ovarian reserve.[65–68] Patients should not uniformly be considered to have limited ovarian reserves who have an elevated FSH level. This finding may not always be synonymous with advanced ovarian aging, diminished egg quality, and diminished ovarian reserve. An increasing number of reports suggest that patients less than 35 with elevated FSH levels can achieve reasonable pregnancy rates both with and without assisted reproductive techniques.[69] This outcome of in vitro fertilization may differ between patients older than 40 years of age with normal FSH levels and relatively young patients with elevated FSH levels. In a study comparing patients older than 41 years with normal (less than 15 mIU/mL) FSH levels and patients younger than 40 years with elevated FSH levels, the high FSH group experienced more cycle cancellations due to absent follicular growth than did the high age group. However, the high FSH group had better implantation rates per embryo. Hence, the decision to proceed with in vitro fertilization should not be based solely on age or FSH level but a combination of the two. Elevated FSH levels on day 3 are associated with lower numbers of growing follicles. Advanced age appears to be more strongly associated with low implantation rates and low pregnancy rates per embryo transfer, reflecting diminished oocyte quality.

The low success rates predicted by an elevated FSH, particularly in younger women, may be overcome through in vitro fertilization. In true limited ovarian reserve, elevated FSH levels represent quantitative and qualitative limitations in follicular development. These may not always, however, occur simultaneously. One possible explanation for elevated FSH levels is a variant of the FSH receptor. In this variant, the enzyme asparagine of the receptor protein is replaced by serine at position 680.[70] This change leads to a slightly less active FSH receptor that required higher FSH levels for normal function and is probably not related to reproductive aging.[71,72] This etiology of elevated FSH may be over-represented among patients with subfertility who have elevated FSH levels.[73] Ironically, assisted reproductive technologies and, in particular, in vitro fertilization may be the only way to overcome infertility in this group of patients. Routine screening of patients for basal FSH levels is still an essential first step. However, this screening should be accompanied by attempts to differentiate among the various possible causes of elevated basal FSH concentrations. Future studies should be able to identify the genotype of FSH receptors to help us differentiate those patients for whom in vitro fertilization offers the best option for achieving a pregnancy. Antral follicle counts are useful for identifying diminished ovarian reserve. These counts may be used as a stand alone assessment and have the advantage that the interval for observation is broader than the rigidly defined criteria for day 3 or CCCT.[74,75] Antral counts are assessments of follicles with a diameter range of 2 to 10 mm (measured in two dimensions) imaged by transvaginal ultrasound examination. These follicles represent a cohort that may be recruited during stimulation with gonadotropins. As such, these numbers provide insight into ovarian reserve and the likelihood of a clinical pregnancy. This study may also be used as a complementary assessment with FSH testing. Antral counts are measured early in the menstrual cycle and may range from 5 to 18–20 follicles per ovary. The counts are related to age and ovarian reserve.[76] When several examiners are doing the ultrasounds, coordination among examiners is essential. Using additional testing other biochemical markers such as anti-mullerian hormone inhibin and FSH isoforms may provide further insight into the causes of elevated FSH levels in these patients. This screening ultimately will lead to better patient selection and more effective counseling.

Formulating a Plan

Reproductive plans should be discussed early in any patient's care plan. For women who are older than 35 years and present for routine gynecologic care, discussion of specific fertility plans should be included as part of the routine and annual health care. A 1-year trial at conception for these patients is inappropriate. A 6-month trial strikes a balance between overly aggressive and premature intervention and the loss of valuable time in patients older than age 35. Immediate evaluation should be considered, however, if these patients have clear-cut risk factors such as a history of pelvic inflammatory disease or extensive pelvic surgery or endometriomas identified on ultrasound examination. Patients who are at risk for a failure to conceive secondary to decreased ovarian reserve and age require extensive counseling and discussion of options including oocyte donation.

Summary and Recommendations

The formulation of a plan of therapy for any couple requesting evaluation in reproductive medicine should include a clear definition of the problem and success of therapy and an analysis of the options available, the attendant costs, and the risks associated with each therapy. Regardless of the clinical problem, considerable attention and skill must be devoted to defining the most cost-effective and efficacious solution. Counseling should be based on data from randomized, prospective studies whenever possible, with a trend away from formulating plans based on anecdotal or empiric evidence or descriptive data in the literature (Table 2-8). The advent of evidence-based medicine, outcome analysis, and computer-accessed databases should help make these recommendations a reality.

Planning for infertility therapy has progressed from recommendations based on anecdotal or empiric evidence to clinical studies that clearly support not only the benefits and likelihood of a positive outcome but also the potential long- and short-term complications. In clinical practice, patients frequently confront clinicians with a demand for some sort of therapy, even in the absence of a clearly defined problem or clear-cut therapies. In these circumstances, a wide spectrum of options are available; some are best considered empiric, and, at worst, some a detriment, especially if the patient's age is a major consideration. For example, certain types of tubal surgery or prolonged evaluation and therapy for a cervical factor or luteal phase defect in a 38-year-old woman are inappropriate.

An effective evaluation for a couple includes not only appropriate diagnostic studies but also a formation of a plan that takes into account the efficacy, safety, and cost of a particular treatment plan. Any couple presenting for evaluation and therapy in reproductive medicine should have three specific criteria fulfilled: an adequate definition of the problem, an adequate definition of outcomes analysis, and a discussion of the costs of the therapeutic options and the likelihood of success for each option (Table 2-7). In patients with an age greater than 35 years, any discussion of potential therapies should also take into account the future role that other assisted reproductive technologies may play. In this group of patients, the discussion of options should be extended to include not only conservative options but also the role that IVF may play in their overall, long-term plan. As part of any discussion with patients with mild factors, the possibility of treatment-

Table 2-7. Factors Influencing Reproductive Potential		
	Prognosis	
Factor	**Good**	**Poor**
Diagnosis	Unexplained	Multiple factors
Duration of infertility	1–3 yr	> 3 yr
Pregnancy history	Successful with previous partner	Unsuccessful with previous partner
Age of female partner	< 30 yr	> 30 yr

Table 2-8.
Counseling and Minimal Basic Evaluation for Women Older Than 35 Years

Counseling

Discussion of fertility plans during routine care

1-yr trial at conception: inappropriate

6-mo trial if unremarkable history after assessment of ovarian reserve

Immediate evaluation if history is significant (e.g. PID, IUD, unsuccessful prior attempts)

Aggressive therapies including assisted reproductive technologies

Evaluation

o   Imaging

   Hysterosalpingogram
   Transvaginal ultrasound

o   Laboratory

   Clomiphene challenge test or Day 3 FSH and estradiol

   TSH

   Prolactin

   Semen analysis

o   Questionable (if any) role for endometrial biopsy and for histologic dating and postcoital testing

o   Endometrial biopsy for luteal function (e.g., integrin concentrations)

o   Early laparoscopy to rule out moderate-to-severe endometriosis or hydrosalpinx if history or ultrasound is suspicious

o   Recent cervical cytology and mammogram

FSH = follicle-stimulating hormone; IUD = intrauterine device; PID = pelvic inflammatory disease; TSH = thyroid-stimulating hormone

---

independent pregnancy should also be discussed. For any patient older than 40 years, the possibility of oocyte donation should be discussed by comparing success rates for any therapy with clinic-specific rates for oocyte donation.[42,43] It may be appropriate to proceed directly to oocyte donation and forego other options with unacceptably low rates of success; in select circumstances, patients may need to be counseled about the futility of further therapeutic trials. For patients less than 35 years, an extended interval of observation without therapy is an option for any couple with mild reproductive problems. Though supported by several studies describing treatment independent pregnancies, non-intervention is a difficult option for any group of patients. It should however be discussed for completeness. Otherwise, in younger patients, it is possible to invest more time in conservative options without compromising success with ART should that option be needed.

References

1.   Haynes RB. Some problems in applying evidence in clinical practice. Ann N Y Acad Sci 1993;703:210–224.

2.   Wasson JH, Sox HC. Clinical prediction rules: have they come of age? JAMA 1996;275:641–642.

3.   Noller KL, Fish CR. Diethylstilbestrol usage: its interesting past, important present, and questionable future. Med Clin North Am 1974;58:793–810.

4.   Dieckmann WJ, Davis ME, Rynkiewicz LM, Pottinger RE. Does the administration of diethylstilbestrol during pregnancy have therapeutic value? Am J Obstet Gynecol 1953;66:1062–1081.

5.   Olive DL. Analysis of clinical fertility trials: a methodologic review. Fertil Steril 1986;45:157–171.

6.   Tulandi T, Cherry N. Clinical trials in reproductive surgery: randomization and life-table analysis. Fertil Steril 1989;52:12–14.

7.   Grimes DA, Schulz KF. Methodology citations and the quality of randomized controlled trials in obstetrics and gynecology. Am J Obstet Gynecol 1996;174:1312–1315.

8.   Johnson NP, Proctor M, Farquhar CM. Gaps in the evidence for fertility treatment–an analysis of the Cochrane Menstrual Disorders and Subfertility Group database. Hum Reprod. 2003;18:947–954.

9.   Schulz KF, Grimes DA, Altman DG, Hayes RJ. Blinding and exclusions after allocation in randomised controlled trials: survey of published parallel group trials in obstetrics and gynaecology. BMJ 1996;312:742–744.

10.   Jansen RP. Elusive fertility: fecundability and assisted conception in perspective. Fertil Steril 1995;64:252–254.

11.   Schieve LA, Reynolds MA. What is the most relevant standard of success in assisted reproduction? Human Reprod 2004;19:778–782.

12.   Cochrane AL. 1931–1991: A critical review with particular reference to the medical profession. In: Teeling Smith G, ed. Medicines for the year 2000. London: Office of Health Economics, 1999:1–11.

13.   Chalmers I, Dickersin K, Chalmers TC. Getting to grips with Archie Cochrane's agenda. BMJ 1992;305:786–788.

14.   Grant JM. Randomised trials and the British Journal of Obstetrics and Gynaecology: minimum requirements for publication. Br J Obstet Gynaecol 1995;102:849–850.

15.   Richardson WS, Detsky AS. Users' guides to the medical literature. VII. How to use a clinical decision analysis. B. What are the results and will they help me in caring for my patients? Evidence Based Medicine Working Group. JAMA 1995;273:1610–1613.

16.   Grimes DA. Introducing evidence-based medicine into a department of obstetrics and gynecology. Obstet Gynecol 1995;86:451–457.

17.   Daya S. Pitfalls in the design and analysis of efficacy trials in subfertility. Hum Reprod 2003;18:1005–1009.

18.   US Preventive Services Task Force. Guide to Clinical Preventive Services. An Assessment of the Effectiveness of 169 Interventions. Baltimore: Williams & Wilkins, 1989.

19.   Guyatt GH, Sackett DL, Sinclair JC, et al. Users' guides to the medical literature. IX. A method for grading health care recommendations. Evidence-Based Medicine Working Group. JAMA 1995;274:1880–1884.

20.   Epstein RS, Sherwood LM. From outcomes research to disease management: a guide for the perplexed. Ann Intern Med 1996;124:832–837.

21.   Taubes G. Looking for the evidence in medicine. Science 1996;272:22–24.

22.   Sackett DL, Rosenberg WM, Gray JA, et al. Evidence based medicine: what it is and what it isn't. BMJ 1996;312:71–72.

23.   Dickersin K, Scherer R, Lefebvre C. Identifying relevant studies for systematic reviews. BMJ 1994;309:1286–1291.

24.   Sackett DL, Rosenberg WM. The need for evidence-based medicine. J R Soc Med 1995;88:620–624.

25.   Collins JA. New treatments, preliminary results, and clinical practice. Fertil Steril 1993;60:403–405.

26.   Evidence-based medicine. A new approach to teaching the practice of medicine. Evidence-Based Medicine Working Group. JAMA 1992;268:2420–2425.

27.   Schulz KF, Chalmers I, Grimes DA, Altman DG. Assessing the quality of randomization from reports of controlled trials published in obstetrics and gynecology journals. JAMA 1994;272:125–128.

28.   Detmer WM, Shortliffe EH. A model of clinical query management that supports integration of biomedical information over the World Wide Web. Proc Ann Symp Comput Appl Med Care 1995;9:898–902.

29.   Zelingher J. Medicine on the Internet, summer 1996. MD Comput 1996;13:295–297.

30.   Glowniak JV. Medical resources on the Internet. Ann Intern Med 1995;123:122–131.

31.   Pallen M. Introducing the Internet. BMJ 1995;311:1422–1424.

32.   Taubes G. Science journals go wired. Science 1996;271:764–766.

33.   Westoff CF. Fertility in the United States. Science 1986;234:554–559.

34.   Hansen JP. Older maternal age in pregnancy outcome: a review of the literature. Obstet Gynecol Surv 1986;41:726–742.

35.   van Noord-Zaadstra BN, Looman CW, Alsbach H, et al. Delaying childbearing: effect of age on fecundity and outcome of pregnancy. BMJ 1991;302:1361–1365.

36.   Wright VC, Schieve LA, Reynolds MA, Jeng G, Kissin D. Assisted reproductive technology surveillance. MMWR Surveill Summ 2004 Apr 30;80:1–20.

37.   Menken J, Trussell J, Larsen U. Age and infertility. Science 1986;233:1389–1394.

38. Collins JA, van Steirtegham A. Overall prognosis with current treatment of infertility. Human Reprod Update 2004;10:309–316.

39. Berkowitz GS, Skovron ML, Lapinski RH, Berkowitz RL. Delayed childbearing and the outcome of pregnancy. New Engl J Med 1990;322:659–664.

40. Stein ZA. A woman's age: childbearing and child rearing. Am J Epidemiol 1985;121:327–342.

41. Schwartz D, Mayaux MJ. Female fecundity as a function of age: results of artificial insemination in 2193 nulliparous women with azoospermic husbands. Federation CECOS. New Engl J Med 1982;306:404–406.

42. Mosher WD, Pratt WF. Fecundity and Infertility in the United States, 1965–1988. Advance Data From Vital and Health Statistics, No. 192. Hyattsville, MD: National Center for Health Statistics, 1990.

43. Healy DL, Trounson AO, Andersen AN. Female infertility: causes and treatment. Lancet 1994;343:1539–1544.

44. Evers JL. Female subfertility. Lancet. 2002;360:151–159.

45. Navot D, Bergh PA, Williams MA, et al. Poor oocyte quality rather than implantation failure as a cause of age-related decline in female fertility. Lancet 1991;337:1375–1377.

46. Meldrum DR. Female reproductive aging — ovarian and uterine factors. Fertil Steril 1993;59:1–5.

47. Fitzgerald CT, Seif MW, Killick SR, Elstein M. Age related changes in the female reproductive cycle. Br J Obstet Gynaecol 1994;101:229–233.

48. Habbema JD, Collins J, Leridon H, Evers JL, Lunnenfeld B, le Velde ER. Towards a less confusing terminology in reproductive medicine: a proposal. Human Reprod 2004;19:1497–501.

49. Collins JA, Wrixon W, Janes LB, Wilson EH. Treatment-independent pregnancy among infertile couples. N Engl J Med 1983;309:1201–1206.

50. Buckett W, Tan SL. What is the most relevant standard of success in assisted reproduction? The importance of informed choice. Human Reprod 2004;19:1043–1045.

51. Fertility Clinic Success Rate and Certification Act of 1992, Report 102–624, 102nd Congress, US Congress, 1992.

52. McDonnell J, Goverde AJ, Vemeiden JP. The place of crossover design in infertility trials: a maximum likelihood approach. Human Reprod 2004;30:14–20.

53. Wheeler JM. The emperor (or rather his statistician) has new clothes. Fertil Steril 1990;53:220–222.

54. Wilcox LS, Peterson HB, Haseltine FP, Martin MC. Defining and interpreting pregnancy success rates for in vitro fertilization. Fertil Steril 1993;60:18–25.

55. Isaksson R, Tutinen A. Present concept of unexplained infertility. Gynecol Endocrinol 2004;18:278–290.

56. Bancsi LF, Broekmans FJ, Eijkemans MJ, et al. Predictors of poor ovarian response in in vitro fertilization: a prospective study comparing basal markers of ovarian reserve. Fertil Steril 2002;77:328–336.

57. Scheffer GJ, Broekmans FJ, Dorland M, et al. Antral follicle counts by transvaginal ultrasonography are related to age in women with proven natural fertility. Fertil Steril 1999;72:845–851.

58. Akande VA, Fleming CF, Hunt LP, et al. Biological versus ageing of oocytes, distinguishable by raised FSH levels in relation to the success of IVF treatment. Hum Reprod 2002;17:2003–2008.

59. Chuang CC, Chen CD, Chao KH, et al. Age is a better predictor of pregnancy potential than basal follicle-stimulating hormone levels in women undergoing in vitro fertilization. Fertil Steril 2003;79:63–68.

60. De La Rochebrochard E, McElreavey K, Thonneau P. Paternal age over 40 years: the "amber light" in the reproductive life of men? J Androl 2003;24:459–465.

61. Van Rooiz IAJ, Bansi L, Broekmans FJM, et al. Women older than 40 years of age and those with elevated follicle-stimulating hormone levels differ in poor response rate and embryo quality in in vitro fertilization. Fertil Steril 2003;79:482–488.

62. Lambalk CB. Value of elevated FSH levels and the differential diagnosis during subfertility work-up. Fertil Steril 2003;79:489–490.

63. Martin J, Nisker J, Jeffrey A, et al. Future in vitro fertilization potential in women with variably elevated day 3 FSH levels. Fertil Steril 1996;65:1238–1240.

64. Scott RT Jr, Illions EH, Kost ER, et al. Evaluation of the significance of the estradiol response during the clomiphene citrate challenge test. Fertil Steril 1993;60:242–246.

65. Lambalk CB. Value of elevated basal follicle-stimulating hormone levels and the differential diagnosis during the diagnostic subfertility work-up. Fertil Steril 2003;79:489–490.

66. Erdem M, Erdem A, Biberoglu K, Arslan M. Age-related changes in ovarian volume, antral follicle counts and basal follicle stimulating hormone levels: comparison between fertile and infertile women. Gynecol Endocrinol 2003;17:199–205.

67. Klein J, Sauer MV. Assessing fertility in women of advanced reproductive age. Am J Obstet Gynecol 2001 Sep;185:758–770.

68. Barnhart K, Osheroff J. We are overinterpreting the predictive value of serum follicle-stimulating hormone levels. Fertil Steril 1999;72:8–9.

69. Esposito MA, Coutifaris C, Barnhart KT. A moderately elevated day 3 FSH concentration has limited predictive value, especially in younger women. Hum Reprod 2002;17:118–123.

70. Perez Mayorga M, Gromoll J, Behre HM, et al. Ovarian response to follicle-stimulating hormone (FSH) stimulation depends on the FSH receptor genotype. J Clin Endocrinol Metab 2000;85:3365–3369.

71. Jurema MW, Bracero NJ, Garcia JE. Fine tuning cycle day 3 hormonal assessment of ovarian reserve improves in vitro fertilization outcome in gonadotropin-releasing hormone antagonist cycles. Fertil Steril 2003;80:1156–1161.

72. Randolph JF, Ginsburg KA, Leach RE, et al. Elevated early follicular gonadotropin levels in women with unexplained infertility do not provide evidence for disordered gonadotropin-releasing hormone secretion as assessed by luteinizing hormone pulse characteristics. Fertil Steril 2003;80:320–327.

73. Sudo S, Kudo M, Wada S, et al. Genetic and functional analyses of polymorphisms in the human FSH receptor gene. Mol Hum Reprod 2002;8:893–899.

74. Chow GE, Criniti AR, Soules MR. Antral follicle count and serum follicle-stimulating hormone levels to assess functional ovarian age. Obstet Gynecol 2004;104:801–804.

75. de Vet A, Laven JS, de Jong FH, et al. Antimullerian hormone serum levels: a putative marker for ovarian aging. Fertil Steril 2002;77:357–362.

76. Frattereli JL, Lauria-Costa DF, Miller BT, et al. Basal antral follicle number and mean ovarian diameter predict cycle cancellation and ovarian responsiveness in assisted reproductive technology cycles. Fertil Steril 2000;74:512–517.

3 Diagnostic Procedures Prior to Surgery and Assisted Reproductive Technology

A method whereby patency of the tubes could be accurately documented without surgical means is eminently desirable.
— I. C. Rubin, 1920

Any infertility evaluation of reproductive potential includes both direct and indirect evaluations of structure and function with radiologic and endoscopic techniques and emerging molecular technologies. Interest in using images to evaluate the female reproductive tract dates to the start of the clinical use of x-rays. These attempts progressed from intrauterine insufflation with oxygen, as described by Rubin in the 1920s, through hysterosalpingography (HSG) in the 1930s to contemporary sensitive and specific cross-sectional imaging techniques such as two- (2-D) or three-dimensional (3-D) transvaginal ultrasound, sonohysterography, and magnetic resonance imaging (MRI).

In 1920, Rubin described the injection of O_2 into the uterine cavity as a means of assessing tubal patency without contrast media, known at that time for their unpleasant side effects.[1] Rubin's method was notable in that it provided the first reliable method of nonoperative assessment of tubal patency. Its limitations and the availability of safe and better-tolerated contrast media led to the widespread use of HSG. Early HSG techniques used a contrast medium of 40% iodine in poppy-seed oil (Lipiodol).[2] This contrast medium was a variation on iodized oil introduced in France at the turn of the century and initially had rapid applications to neurosurgery for myelography and subsequently to gynecology as a means of assessing tubal patency. This agent yielded better-quality images with improved diagnosis of tubal patency, tubal architecture, and uterine anatomy.[3] So widespread was the use of Lipiodol and HSG in early gynecologic practice that they were used as a means of early pregnancy diagnosis. Lipiodol subsequently gave way to water-based media (such as Salpix) and improved oil-based media (such as Ethiodol, a 37% iodine solution).

The armamentarium for diagnostic imaging of the reproductive tract has expanded markedly during the past 10 years. Current imaging techniques include 2- and 3-D transvaginal and transabdominal ultrasonography, MRI of the pelvis, and transvaginal sonohysterography.[4,5] Molecular technology has expanded dramatically and rapidly. Progress has been made with fluorescence in situ hybridization, polymerase chain reactions and rapidly emerging microarray technology. These molecular techniques provide valuable insights into function and should emerge as integral aspects in the evaluation of infertility.

In spite of improved accuracy of imaging, a need for direct visualization of reproductive anatomy continues into the 21st century. Operative investigation of reproductive anatomy using hot light sources for culdoscopy remained the mainstay until contemporary endoscopic equipment and cold light fiberoptic cables became available. With the advent of sophisticated endoscopic units and data suggesting the importance of endoscopy in the infertility evaluation, both laparoscopy and hysteroscopy became essential tools in the evaluation of reproductive abnormalities.[6] Laparoscopy remains an operative standard.[7] However, the marked improvement in success with ART calls into question its role as a standard for all cases.[8,9] This chapter describes the diagnostic techniques for evaluating the structure and function of the reproductive tract with imaging in two or three dimensions and with emerging molecular technologies. The techniques include radiographic studies of HSG, sectional imaging by ultrasound and MRI, the endoscopic techniques of laparoscopy and hysteroscopy and the molecular tools of microarray technology.

Hysterosalpingography   *18~ a screening test*

HSG

Hysterosalpingography remains a standard in any evaluation for infertility. Though other studies such as hysteroscopy and laparoscopy are available to evaluate the uterine cavity and tubal patency, HSG remains one of the most useful and cost-effective tools.[10,11] Contemporary techniques for HSG use one of several water- or oil-based contrast media.

The advantages and disadvantages of water- or oil-based media for improved images and enhanced pregnancy rates have been debated since the 1960s.[12,13] Several limited, retrospective studies compared water-based and oil-based contrast media; enhanced fertility with oil-based agents was noted.[14–16] A meta-analysis of data on the subject also showed a beneficial effect.[17] The issue of improved fertility with an oil-based contrast medium remained a compelling though much debated reason to use these media for two decades.

The controversy focuses on study design and definitions of success. Claims that diagnostic tests for tubal patency with *any* media could in themselves enhance fertility were made up to 50 years ago. Multiple reports of variable quality on the therapeutic aspects of oil-soluble contrast media have been published since the 1960s. The shortcomings of earlier studies include their retrospective nature, the failure to include life-table analyses in the assessment of pregnancy rates, the failure to include other potential causes of infertility, and poorly matched populations. Contemporary studies have attempted to control for these factors, and both improved pregnancy rates and term deliveries have been noted (Figure 3-1). This effect appears to persist in a variety of clinical settings. Increased pregnancy rates have also been demonstrated after tubal lavage with oil-based contrast media performed at laparoscopy.[18] In this setting, laparoscopic evaluation of pelvic anatomy controlled for any additional anatomic factors such as adhesions or endometriosis.

Randomized controlled trials are of more recent origin. In prospective, randomized studies comparing the two media, a definitive therapeutic effect of oil-based contrast media was demonstrated.[19] Interestingly, a companion article to this study demonstrated slightly better image quality with water-based media and better patient tolerance with oil-based contrast media.[20] A doubling of conception rate in 4 months after hysterosalpingography with oil-based contrast media has been reported. There is also evidence of effectiveness that tubal flushing with oil-based contrast media increases the odds of pregnancy versus no intervention or flushing with water-based contrast media.[21] Tubal flushing with oil-based contrast media may represent a simple, less invasive, and more economic alternative prior to more aggressive options for couples with unexplained infertility. Apart from pregnancy rates, oil-based contrast media may offer other advantages, as follows: (1) the slow filling of the fallopian tubes owing to the higher viscosity; (2) sharper radiographic images; (3) and possibly less pain at time of injection. Robust randomized trials comparing oil- and water-based contrast media are required to provide convincing evidence as to whether the technique should be accepted into widespread clinical practice where a live birth is considered the primary outcome.

The exact cause of the enhanced fertility is unknown, The previously proposed mechanism of tubal lavage and flushing of debris is doubtful because in comparative studies lavage is carried out with each agent. One hypothesis suggests inhibition of peritoneal fluid lymphocytes and immune cell function by HSG oil-based contrast media enhances fertility.[22] Ethiodol contrast medium has been shown to inhibit macrophage phagocytosis and adherence

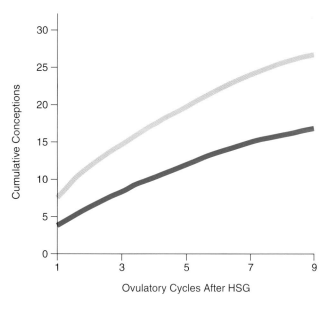

Figure 3-1   Cumulative conceptions versus ovulatory cycles after HSG with oil-based (red line) and water-soluble contrast media.

by altering membrane electronegativity and microviscosity. Alteration of membrane function may be caused by a reduction of membrane negative surface charge and microviscosity.[23] These mechanisms suggest a possible explanation for the therapeutic effect of oil-based contrast hysterosalpingograms in women with unexplained infertility. The pregnancy rates for oil-based and water-based contrast media range from 28 to 30% and 13 to 15%, respectively, with follow-up intervals of 3 to 6 months. The upper age limit for this enhancement has not been established.

✳ In the Cochrane database, tubal flushing with oil-based contrast media was associated with a significant increase in the odds of pregnancy (odds ratio 3.75, 95% confidence interval 1.76–7.23).[24] Subgroup analysis by cause for infertility show the odds of pregnancy for couples with unexplained infertility was significantly increased following hysterosalpingography with oil-based contrast media versus no treatment. The sensitivity analysis for whether the interventions in the trials were performed primarily for diagnostic or therapeutic purposes suggested that the odds ratio for diagnostic purposes was 3.02 with 95% confidence intervals of 1.41–6.8 and primarily as therapy the odds ratio was 9.74 with 95% confidence intervals of 1.50–63.18.

✳ Tubal flushing with oil-based contrast media in the Cochrane database showed a significant increase in the odds of a live birth versus flushing with water-based contrast media.

HSGs are used to assess the uterus, tubes, and, indirectly, the peritoneal cavity for abnormalities potentially contributory to infertility. The sensitivity and specificity of HSG is influenced in part by the anatomic area being evaluated and the specific abnormality noted. For example, an abnormal HSG may be highly predictive of severe distal tubal disease when the tubes are obstructed and markedly dilated, but relatively insensitive when used to assess pelvic adhesive disease. Abnormal HSGs are sufficiently reliable for diagnosing distal tubal obstruction, when characteristic hydrosalpinges are noted, that counseling for treatment options does not require diagnostic laparoscopy. Patients with suspicious or equivocal HSGs do, however, have a significant likelihood of tubal or associated pelvic disease.[25]

Patients with equivocal results may require confirmatory laparoscopy. This decision turns in part on the role IVF may ultimately play and the significance of the tubal segments. Normal HSG has a high negative predictive value for distal tubal disease and the assessment of the uterine cavity. However, the incidence of additional pelvic disease, particularly mild pelvic adhesive disease and endometriosis, in the normal HSG group is sufficiently high to warrant discussion of diagnostic laparoscopy versus ART if conservative options fail. A meta-analysis of 20 studies on the accuracy of HSG suggested that HSG was an adequate test for assessing tubal obstruction and an inadequate test for assessing peritubal adhesions.[26] As a method to assess tubal patency after any tubal surgery, HSG has a high false-negative and false-positive rate and is not recommended.[27]

HSG, however, is not as sensitive for proximal obstruction, with a false-positive rate as high as 30 to 35%.[28] Suspected proximal tubal obstruction may be either organic (true-positive) or functional (false-positive) obstruction of the fallopian tubes. Differentiation is important: true obstruction is caused by intrinsic disease. Functional obstruction or occlusion may be due to spasm at the uterotubal junction and amenable to simple medical management or selective salpingography.

To maximize the sensitivity and specificity of the test for proximal obstruction, a variety of pharmacologic agents and intervention have been used. Prostaglandin antagonists (aspirin), β_2 agonists (such as terbutaline), or both, as well as glucagon nonsteroidal anti-inflammatory drugs (NSAIDs) and selective salpingography have been used to reduce the incidence of false positives for proximal tubal obstruction.[29,30] HSG after premedication with aspirin, selective salpingography, or both, revealed false positives and functional tubal obstruction in 60% of patients after an initial conventional HSG suggested proximal obstruction.[31] Other agents, such as atropine, amyl nitrate, dihydroergotamine, diazepam, and nitroglycerin, have been used in the past with variable success. No agent is absolutely reliable in reversing proximal obstruction suspected to be secondary to spasm. The most effective method of reducing false positives for proximal tubal obstruction during HSG is by premedication with an NSAID such as 800 mg of ibuprophen one [1 hour] hour prior to HSG.

A single HSG demonstrating proximal obstruction is not an indication for immediate referral to IVF. Proximal tubal obstruction on HSG should prompt further evaluation with selective salpingography. In approximately 40% of patients with proximal tubal obstruction, selective salpingograms demonstrate patent fallopian tubes despite as many as two previous HSGs demonstrating proximal obstruction. In these circumstances, transvaginal catheter dilatation successfully recannulized the proximal portion of the tubes in 82% of the patients. In 80% of the patients at 6-month follow-up, the tubes remained patent. Coexisting distal disease was diagnosed in 20% of the patients. The diagnosis of proximal obstruction on the basis of one HSG should be approached cautiously. One abnormal study requires confirmation with a second study, preferably after premedication with a nonsteroidal agent and with appropriate plans for selective salpingography if necessary. Interventional radiography or immediate referral for IVF for proximal obstruction should not be planned solely on the basis of one study.

A key component to HSG interpretation is fluoroscopy. Close assessment of filling patterns and areas of obstruction is important. Considerable variation in inter-observer interpretation of the HSG has been described, emphasizing the need for careful review of fluoroscopy by the clinician directing care of the case and, when appropriate, for consultation with a radiologist.[32] Cooperation between radiologist and clinician is essential. Both members should be present for the study.

Technique

A nonsteroidal agent as preoperative analgesic to minimize the degree of cramping is recommended. Prophylactic antibiotics are indicated depending on history.[32] Doxycycline in patients with a negative history is debatable. HSG is best performed in the early follicular phase to avoid the possibility of pregnancy and to avoid any endometrial debris that may obscure a detailed evaluation of the endometrial cavity. The procedure is performed after a sterile preparation of the vaginal vault. A rigid cannula or a disposable catheter system (Ackrad Labs. Co., Cranford, NJ) may be attached to a 30-ml syringe to inject the dye. Care should be taken to flush all air from the cannula or tubing before injection to minimize the likelihood of an air bubble causing a suspicious finding. Caution, however, must be exercised when using a disposable system and oil-based media because the rubber may degenerate when exposed to the oil. Selective salpingography or β_2 agonists such as subcutaneous terbutaline should be available for immediate use if proximal tubal obstruction is noted, but are not absolute prerequisites.

The cornerstone to interpreting HSG is the information obtained at the time of fluoroscopy. Hence, the study is best done with the gynecologist in attendance.[33] For an initial injection, 5 to 20 mL of contrast medium may be required. The amount of contrast required may vary depending on the volume of the uterine cavity and amount of reflux encountered. The contrast medium is injected under *gentle* thumb pressure on the syringe. Careful attention to the degree of patient discomfort is essential. If extreme, pausing during injection may be necessary. If distressed, the procedure should be discontinued. The uterine cavity is observed during the filling phase for any potential defects, best noted during the *early* filling phase of the procedure because continued intrauterine filling may obscure subtle defects.[34] Tubal filling and patency are then assessed. Particular attention is paid to the distal aspects of the tubes and the rugal markings of the distal tubal segments. These aspects have predictive value regarding future fertility (Figure 3-2). Clear intraperitoneal spill must be demonstrated. If spill is equivocal, rotating the patient from side to side or gentle abdominal pressure by hand may increase the likelihood of demonstrating intraperitoneal dispersion of the dye. As the contrast medium disperses throughout the peritoneal cavity, loops of bowel may be outlined as crescent collections of contrast or form beaded collections if an oil-based medium is used (Figure 3-3).

Oblique films may be required to assess potential filling defects within the uterine cavity and to assess the distal tubal segments should there be any question of intrauterine defects or intraperitoneal spill, respectively (Figure 3-4). In cases of questionable fill or in cases in which there is the possibility of spill into an area of loculation, delayed films (15 to 30 minutes or as long as 24 hours) after the procedure are recommended to further assess the possibility of complete intraperitoneal spill. A comparison of 1-hour and 24-hour follow-up radiographs has shown them to be comparable in the detection of

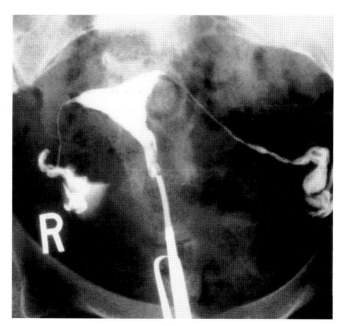

Figure 3-2   Normal hysterosalpingogram demonstrating a normal endometrial cavity and tubes with a thin isthmic segment, and slightly dilated distal ampullary segment. Note rugal markings in the distal tubal segments consistent with normal distal segments.

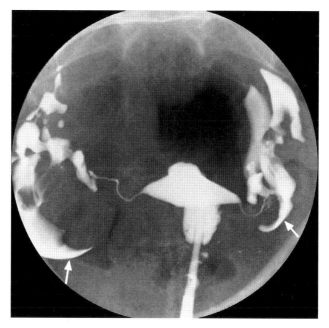

Figure 3-3   Hysterosalpingogram demonstrating bilateral intraperitoneal spill. Note layering of the contract medium around the loops of bowel, thus rendering a crescent appearance (arrows).

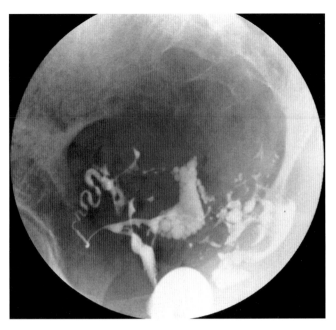

Figure 3-4   Oblique view of a hysterosalpingogram. Note intrauterine filling defects occupying the upper one-third of the uterine cavity and the bilateral intraperitoneal spill with a beaded appearance as the oil-based contrast medium mixes with the peritoneal fluid.

tubal patency and pelvic adhesive disease. The most useful role for delayed films is in the detection of adnexal adhesions and loculation of contrast media.

HSG is usually well tolerated, easy to perform, and well suited as an out-patient procedure. The most common complication is cramping at the time of injection of the contrast. Febrile morbidity following HSG is the second-most-common complication. Serious infections occur in 0.3% to 1.3% of patients undergoing this procedure.[35] A history of previous pelvic infection requiring hospitalization or outpatient antibiotics increases the risk. Chlamydia trachomatis antibody testing is a simple, inexpensive technique to evaluate for previous infection prior to HSG if the history is negative. If testing is positive, antibiotic therapy is warranted.[36] This testing may be included as part of the investigation prior to HSG, for patients suspected to be at high risk for tubal-factor infertility.[37] Intravasation into the myometrium and intravenous injection of the contrast medium are usually of no significance (Figure 3-5).[38] Its detection during fluoroscopy, however, warrants discontinuation of the procedure. Cerebral embolization and coma with recovery following injection of Lipiodol has been described.[39] During the procedure described in this report, intravasation of the contrast medium was noted. Allergic reactions may also occur. An allergic reaction to an iodine-based contrast injected intravenously does not preclude performing the HSG, but

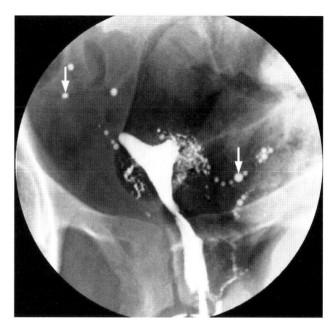

Figure 3-5   Hysterosalpingogram demonstrating bilateral tubal obstruction, myometrial blush greater on the left than on the right, and intravenous injection of the contract medium bilaterally (arrows).

pretreatment with a combination of prednisone and diphenhydramine is required. Retained contrast in the pelvis has been described 20 years after the HSG when an oil-based contrast was used (Figure 3-6).[39]

Any potential risk attendant to x-rays is proportional to the radiation dose to the pelvis. Radiation exposure during HSG depends on the fluoroscopic time and the number of radiographs. Both are influenced by whether the HSG is normal or abnormal, and by increased time and images required to evaluate abnormal findings. Total exposure time may range from 1 to 2 minutes, depending on findings. To minimize radiation risk, the distance between the roentgenogram tube and the pelvis should be kept at 30 to 45 cm, and a field of 4 x 4 should be used whenever possible. The Committee of the National Academy of Sciences on the Biologic Effects of Ionizing Radiation (BEIR Committee) concluded that the risk from radiologic exposure is extremely low when radiation time is limited and equipment properly calibrated.[40] The maximum radiation exposure, even for more extensive studies, has been established as 0.27 rad per minute, with maximum permissible time of 10 minutes.[41] Following these limits, complications from radiation are extremely low or even nonexistent.

If the patient reports a pregnancy at some point immediately after the HSG, with a suspicion that the HSG was performed while she was pregnant, immediate consultation with the radiation safety committee is essential.[42] No

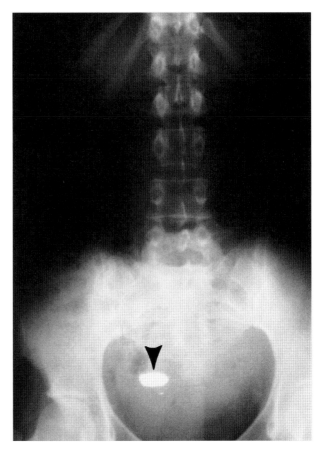

Figure 3-6   Scout radiograph of the abdomen and pelvis demonstrating retained contrast medium (arrowhead) in the right adnexal 12 years after a hysterosalpingogram performed with oil-based contrast medium.

immediate decisions regarding the viability of any pregnancy after exposure to radiation in this setting should be made. Careful and precise dating of the pregnancy and calculation of the amount of radiation is essential in counseling in this circumstance.

Ultrasound Imaging in Reproductive Medicine

Transabdominal and Transvaginal Ultrasonography

Ultrasound imaging of the cervix, uterus, tubes, and ovaries has become an integral part of any evaluation for infertility. Ultrasound examinations may be either transabdominal or transvaginal in two or three dimensions. The frequencies of commonly used transabdominal scanners are 3.5 to 5 and 6.5 MHz; transvaginal scanners (TVS) have higher frequencies of 5.0 to 7.5 and

10.0 MHz. Probes for TVS have scanning angles ranging from 60° to 180° within a single probe. Transvaginal ultrasound images provide details of the pelvic anatomy not possible with transabdominal scanning because of higher frequency probes and the near constant probe-to-target distance not possible with transabdominal scanning. Advantages of vaginal ultrasonography are its ease of performance, immediate availability (no bladder-filling phase is needed), constant image quality regardless of body habitus, and the ability to incorporate the procedure into a routine gynecologic examination performed in the office or the emergency room. With a high-resolution transducer, detailed images of uterine anatomy, ovarian architecture, and adnexa can be obtained to rule out defects such as uterine fibroids and endometrial polyps and, at times, to exclude mullerian abnormalities such as a bicornuate or septate uterus and ovarian cysts or endometriomas.[43,44] Tubal anatomy is reliably demonstrated, but in select circumstances (severe hydrosalpinges, for example) images may suggest tubal obstructions.[45,46] A major application of transvaginal imaging is in the assessment of early pregnancy and to rule out or rule in intrauterine versus an ectopic pregnancy. Transvaginal real-time ultrasound scanning provides a means to detect cardiac motion that is particularly useful in early first-trimester transvaginal exams. Fetal heart motion can be detected as early as 5 weeks.

The disadvantage, however, is in a relatively restricted view of pelvic structures. Wider angle probes of 180° provide increased field of view, but in cases where a large area such as an ovarian mass or large uterine fibroids is of clinical concern, transabdominal scanning is required. Transabdominal scanning provides a fuller and broader image of the pelvic anatomy in evaluating large masses, but sacrifices some of the detail of the highly focused transvaginal approach. These approaches are considered complementary and, depending on the structure of interest, both may be required for complete evaluation and assessment of dimensions of character.

Three-dimensional ultrasound facilitates the evaluation of the antral follicles, ovarian volume, ovarian stroma, and analysis of the intensity of ovarian stromal blood flow as a prelude to in vitro fertilization.[47,48] Given the impact of antral follicle number influencing outcome, patient selection, and live birth rates, this provides another sensitive indicator of ovarian reserve in addition to basal FSH levels. Three-dimensional ultrasound can also be used as a screening method for the detection of uterine abnormalities. It is a sensitive screening tool in the detection of congenital uterine abnormalities, submucous leiomyomata, endometrial polyps particularly with sonohysterography, and intrauterine adhesions prior to in vitro fertilization. In gynecologic and infertility practice, it is a study that is complementary to 2-D ultrasound. It has an evolving role and maybe useful as an intraoperative adjunct.

Technique

Any scanning routine should involve three basic motions with the vaginal probe. The scanner may be angled to aim the tip in any direction, advanced into the apex of the vagina to focus the structure of interest, and rotated to change the scanning plane from longitudinal to transverse. Conventional TVS scanning is two dimensional. To assess pelvic structures in a third dimension the probe must be rotated using a 2-D probe. The procedure may be incorporated into any routine gynecologic examination whenever the suspicion of an anatomic abnormality exists. A transvaginal examination may be completed in 5 to 10 minutes. A detailed explanation of the examination with demonstration of the vaginal probe eases the patient and facilitates the examination. The patient's bladder should be empty, and the ultrasound scanning performed with the patient supine with her thighs abducted and knees flexed. A standard gynecologic examination table is ideal. The probe should be covered with a condom with a small amount of imaging gel placed in the condom for contact between the transducer and the condom face. Generous use of lubricating (K-Y) jelly on the outside of the condom facilitates insertion.

The technique of transvaginal ultrasound scanning involves a systematic assessment of the pelvic structures. The uterus should be evaluated looking at the endometrium, myometrium, and the serosa. The appearance of the endometrium varies depending on the day of the menstrual cycle and may range from a homogeneous, thin appearance to a characteristic trilaminar appearance (Figures 3-7 and 3-8). Peristalsis within the endometrium may be noted prior to or during menses. The myometrium is examined with particular attention to any rounded distortions suggestive of leiomyoma or adenomyosis. The adnexa are systematically examined for the presence or absence of cysts and follicles and measuring the ovaries in three dimensions. The cul-de-sac is checked for any fluid. After this survey, a directed examination may be performed to look for particular details in the structures of interest.

The ovaries are evaluated next. Characteristics of the ovarian stroma, cortex, and any ovarian cystic structure are noted. The ovaries may be located using the artery and vein as prominent landmarks (Figure 3-9). A lateral movement from the uterus toward the pelvic side wall usually brings the ovary into view. The ovary is scanned from medial to lateral poles. Any other cystic structures in the adnexa are closely examined. Antral follicle counts prior to ART are essential. Antral counts provide an additional assessment of ovarian reserve and prediction of outcome after ART. All follicles in a 5- to 12-mm range in two dimensions should be counted. Follicle counts in the range of 12 to 15 are considered normal. High follicle counts, particularly if the follicles are located in the periphery of the ovary surrounding a hyperechoic core, suggest a polycystic morphology and may be part of polycystic ovary syndrome. A hydrosalpinx should be considered if an enlarged curvilinear cystic

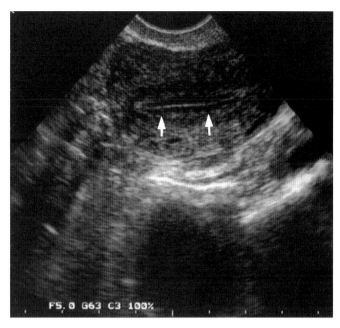

Figure 3-7   Transvaginal ultrasound of the uterus demonstrating a normal trilami-
                    nar appearance to the endometrium (arrows).

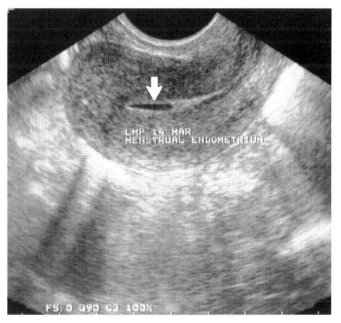

Figure 3-8   Transvaginal ultrasound 2 days after the start of a menstrual cycle,
                    demonstrating collapse of the endometrium (arrow) and a sonolucency
                    in the cavity consistent with blood. The cervix is to the right.

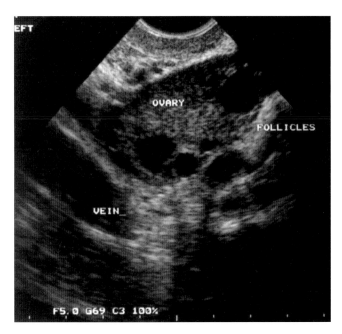

Figure 3-9   Transvaginal ultrasound examination of the ovary demonstrating multiple follicles of varying diameters.

structure is noted. All cysts are measured and their internal echogenicity described (Figure 3-10 A and B). The presence and degree of any follicular activity should be correlated with the timing of the scan to the menstrual cycle. The fallopian tubes are not imaged consistently even with higher frequency probes. Visualization may be facilitated by the presence of fluid in the pelvis. The fallopian tube may also be imaged when cystic dilation is present, as occurs with a hydrosalpinx. In one series, a single fallopian tube could be visualized in only 15% of patients.[45]

Three-dimensional (3-D) ultrasound imaging as a diagnostic tool in reproductive medicine has added, quite literally, another dimension to the two-dimensional images possible by transvaginal and transabdominal ultrasound (Figure 3-11).[49,50] Three-dimensional ultrasound imaging involves 3-D scanners and software to process the data obtained with each dimensional sweep. The procedure incorporates 2-D ultrasound imaging and a third imaging process in which several transverse sections are sequentially taken and stored in a computer file. The three planes measured are the frontal section, median sagittal section, and horizontal section. Three-dimensional images are generated when these three planes for any section are integrated and displayed on the monitor. Any plane of volume may be rotated and translated so that a variety of images of the pelvic anatomy may be presented. Depending on the structure of interest, different 3-D modes can be generated. For example, a surface reconstruction mode permits the evaluation of the outer contour of the uterus; this has particular importance in ruling out congenital

(A)

(B)

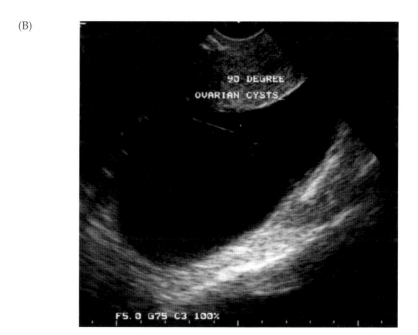

Figure 3-10   Transvaginal ultrasound examination of the ovary demonstrating sonolucent cysts. (A) A 120° scanning angle increases the field of view and the uterus is clearly demonstrated in the left-hand portion of the image (arrows). (B) The uterus is not evident on the 90° image.

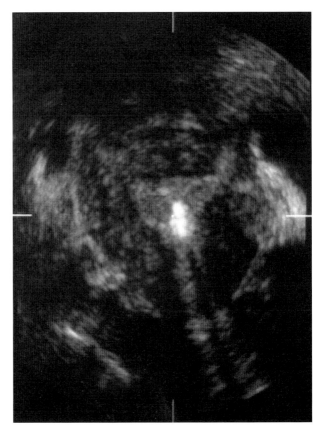

Figure 3-11   Three-dimensional coronal view of uterine cavity prior to injection during sonohysterogram. Note catheter at lower segment.

uterine abnormalities. A transparent maximum–minimum mode delineates the endometrial cavity with high echodense signals. Volume and surface renderings may be acquired in a single automated sweep. Datasets can be generated, stored and recalled for retrospective review. Software enables reconstruction of specific "slices" of anatomy for analysis. The exact role that 3–D imaging has awaits further, more detailed studies, including comparative studies of transvaginal ultrasound and 3–D ultrasound to rule out uterine abnormalities.

Intraoperative Ultrasound Imaging

Transabdominal imaging provides an added dimension to complex intrauterine hysteroscopic surgery. This technique enables precise identification of the tip of the hysteroscope and instruments (Figure 3-12).[51] Laparoscopic grayscale ultrasound imaging with a semi-flexible ultrasound probe extends imaging capabilities into the operating room (Figures 3-13 and 3-14).[51,52] The probe is 9.6 mm in diameter and 35 cm long (Figure 3-15). It has

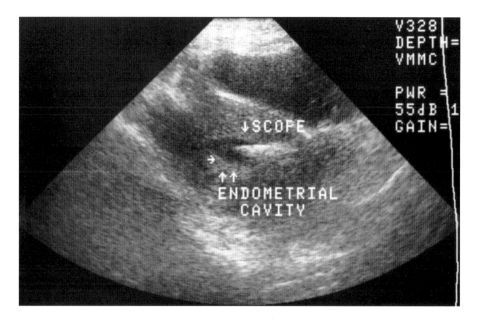

Figure 3-12   Intraoperative sonohysterogram showing distension of uterine cavity and tip of operating hysteroscope.

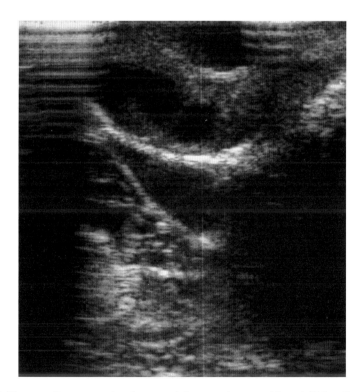

Figure 3-13   Laparoscopic ultrasound image of ovary. Note follicles. Interference lines are noted to either side of ovary.

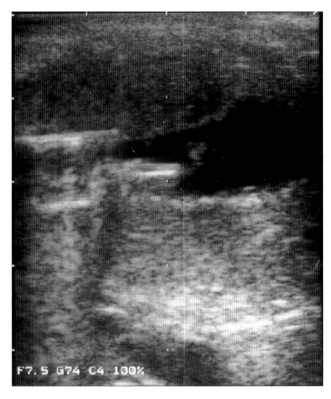

Figure 3-14   Laparosopic intraoperative sonohysterogram demonstrating resecto-scope and operative loop.

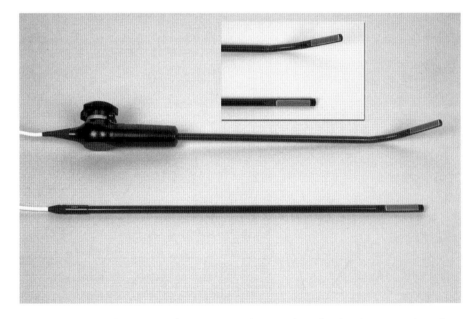

Figure 3-15   A 7.0-MHz laparoscopic ultrasound probe for intraoperative ultra-sound. Note panels in inset.

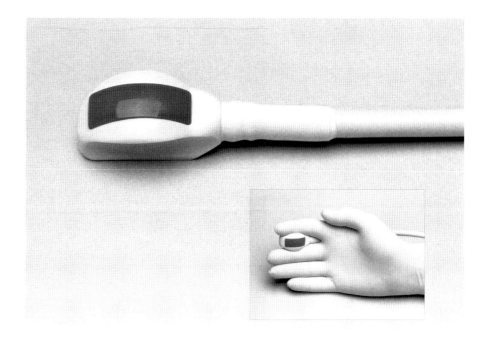

Figure 3-16   A 3.5-MHz finger-grip probe for intraoperative ultrasound. Note position in inset.

multifrequency capability (5.0, 6.5, and 7.5 MHz) and employs a complex array transducer with maximal penetration of 13 cm and a sector scanning angle of 60°. The flexible nature of this ultrasound probe enables it to pass through a 10-mm diameter trocar. It is useful to differentiate vascular from nonvascular structures (the Doppler mode) and the presence of masses within a variety of abdominal and pelvic organs.[52,53] A 3.5-mHz finger grip probe has also been described for intra-abdominal reproductive surgery.[54] This probe is useful in defining anatomy at surgical sites, such as the uterus or ovary, prior to incision (Figure 3-16). Ultrasound guidance provides information of internal architecture and is of benefit to guide dissections. For example, intraoperative ultrasound of an ovarian endometrioma may enable a more precise and limited incision avoiding normal ovarian architecture.

Sonohysterography

The spectrum for transvaginal imaging was expanded with the demonstration that the infusion of fluid into the endometrial cavity enhances the image quality of the cavity. Indications for sonohysterography include irregular bleeding, the evaluation for suspected submucous myomata on standard transvaginal or transabdominal screening (because the instillation of saline better determines the exact location of the fibroid), and postmenopausal

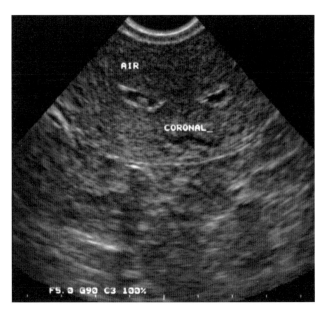

Figure 3-17   Coronal uterine image of sonohysterogram demonstrating two cavities of a septate uterus.

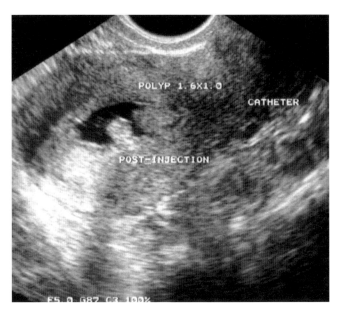

Figure 3-18   Postinjection sonohysterogram demonstrating distension of the endometrial cavity (sonolucency) and a pedunculated polyp partially filling the cavity in the fundal region.

bleeding (Figures 3-17 and 3-18). This procedure is especially useful in assessing for polyps, submucous fibroids, or, in patients receiving tamoxifen to detect, "tamoxifen-induced" changes. In circumstances in which transvaginal imaging of the endometrium or HSG suggest an intracavitary abnormality, saline injected into the uterine cavity and imaging with a high-resolution endovaginal probe in 2-D or 3-D provide a sensitive and specific assessment of the endometrial cavity. The procedure may be interposed between transvaginal scanning or HSG as screening procedures to detect uterine abnormalities and the more invasive and expensive hysteroscopy for definitive diagnosis. Sonohysterography may eliminate the need for diagnostic hysteroscopy in a large percentage of patients. Sonohysterography is an inexpensive, simple, and well-tolerated office procedure. Sonohysterography or fluid enhanced endovaginal scanning aids primarily in evaluation of the endometrial cavity. The procedure takes advantage of the well-known enhancement of ultrasound imaging when fluid–solid interfaces are present. The most common indication to perform this procedure is irregular bleeding. The second-most-common indication is as part of an infertility evaluation to further evaluate the abnormal findings on HSG. The technique, however, is nonspecific for evaluating the fallopian tubes. Fluid in the cul-de-sac is often seen with this technique and indicates at least unilateral tubal patency. However, a specific tubal outline as seen on HSG may not be consistently imaged.

There is marked agreement in findings between sonohysterography and HSG. Sonohysterography and HSG findings for uterine and tubal assessment were similar in 82% and 72% of women, respectively.[55–58] However, contrast-enhanced materials or color-flow Doppler ultrasound equipment may improve this technique for tubal assessment. Sonographic hydrotubation as a simple office procedure may be considered as a preliminary assessment of the uterine cavity and fallopian tubes.

Technique

Sonohysterography is performed under sterile conditions. Timing should be in the follicular phase in a patient with regular menstrual cycles to avoid both intrauterine debris and the possibility of pregnancy or at any time in a patient in whom pregnancy can be reliably ruled out. A rapid pregnancy test is sufficient for this purpose. Prophylactic antibiotics are recommended under the same circumstances as HSG. Any small-caliber, flexible catheter such as an intrauterine insemination catheter or Tefcat catheter (Cook Ob/Gyn, Spencer, IN) may be used for this purpose. Balloon catheters are also available for this purpose (Ackrad Labs. Co., Cranford, NJ). A catheter is advanced into the endometrial cavity and attached to an IV extension tubing and a 10-mL syringe containing sterile saline. A baseline ultrasound examination is performed before injection. An initial scanning image prior to injection of the fluid is essential to note any fluid in the cul-de-sac. The appearance or expansion of any fluid collection in the cul-de-sac at the conclusion of the procedure could indicate tubal patency. The uterus and catheter tip are imaged, and by gentle thumb pressure, a small amount of saline is instilled into the endometrial cavity. Under direct visualization, the saline can be seen to fill the cavity, defining the endometrial architecture. Imaging should be performed from cornua to cornua in the longitudinal plane and from lower uterine segment to fundus in the coronal plane. Close attention is paid to the adnexa to determine the flow of any fluid in this region. The cul-de-sac is subsequently inspected for the collection or expansion of any fluid. These procedures are well tolerated and seldom require analgesics prior to their performance. Other contrast media, such as bubbles stabilized in a galactose matrix or in an albumin matrix have been investigated. Hysterosalpingo-contrast sonography (HyCoSy) also provides enhanced images using a combination of air and saline.[59] Sonohysterography may also be used intraoperatively to monitor the precise location of instruments during intrauterine surgery. The cavity may be imaged intraoperatively using transabdominal, laparoscopic, or finger-grip probes.

Other Techniques to Assess Tubal Patency

Radionuclide HSG with technetium-99 pertechnetate has been described and shown to be an efficient means of assessing tubal patency.[60] When compared with conventional HSG, this technique showed an 85% rate of accuracy with the advantage of a decrease in the amount of radiation to the ovaries. Hysterosalpingography remains the standard. Color-flow Doppler ultrasonography is a technique to evaluate tubal patency using real-time, simultaneous-display curve mapping, along with ultrasound with high-resolution tissue detail. Color ultrasound HSG was shown to have a high correlation to conventional HSG results. These studies are primarily descriptive. The role that these techniques will play in the assessment of pelvic anatomy awaits further prospective study. These techniques fall outside of mainstream, standard care but provide possible alternatives in select cases.

Magnetic Resonance Imaging

The magnetic properties of matter form the underlying basis of magnetic resonance imaging (MRI). MRI produces images via the interaction between static magnetic fields, radio waves, and atomic nuclei.[61,62] MRI provides high-contrast resolution and multiplanar views of female pelvic anatomy.[63,64] The detail and the thin sections available through MRI are not possible by the conventional transabdominal and transvaginal ultrasound imaging techniques. MRI is a process that involves stimulating a tissue sample with a radiofrequency pulse and detecting the emitted radiofrequency energy from the stimulated tissue. For a specific radiofrequency transmitted to the tissue, the nuclei of the tissues realign in a particular fashion. The radiofrequency to the tissue determines the rate of energy transfer, which may occur in two ways. The two parameters are designated T1 and T2. The first parameter, T1, is sometimes called the longitudinal relaxation time with a time constant that describes the return of tissue magnetization to its original orientation, the so-called spin lattice relaxation time. The second parameter, T2, is the transverse relaxation time, so-called spin–spin relaxation time. Any image can be weighted toward either T1 or T2, depending on the times chosen for a particular sequence and the anatomy of interest. The images that result from manipulating the variables of the magnetic field, the pulse sequence, and the relaxation times are displayed on the final images as points of relative brightness or darkness and represent a display of spatially localized signal intensities. MRI offers an ability to detail anatomic subdivisions of the pelvic organs, especially the uterus and cervix. The ability to differentiate subtle tissue types offers an advantage to conventional radiography or ultrasound.

The superb soft-tissue contrast of MRI provides a unique characterization of zonal anatomy in the pelvic organs, enabling the different types of tissues contained within a single organ, for example the uterus, to be differentiated (Table 3-1). In addition, the absence of motion within the pelvis yields excellent images. MRI also provides an ability to differentiate vascular from nonvascular structures, thus minimizing the need for IV contrast media.

T1-weighted images in the pelvis are of medium signal intensity for the uterus and cervix.[65] T1-weighted images are best for the detection of lymphadenopathy and extensions of pelvic neoplasms into the adjacent fat. On T1-weighted studies, the pelvic fat serves as a bright background for the dark blood vessels, pelvic musculature, and lymph nodes. MRI is ideally suited to gynecologic imaging because of its ability to differentiate the zonal anatomy of the uterus, cervix, and vagina in T2-weighted images. Uterine images are divided into three parts. The endometrium appears as a high-signal central stripe. The inner myometrium, that is, the junctional zone, produces a surrounding low-to-medium signal band. The outer myometrium is typically shown as a band of intermediate intensity (Figure 3-19 A and B). In an analogous manner, the cervical canal is represented by a high-density signal in the central zone and the adjacent stroma by a lower signal contiguous with the junctional zone and cervical stroma. The vaginal canal is similarly demarcated by the adjacent muscular wall. T2-weighted images are best for the endometrium and endocervical canal and are hyperintense in character. Leiomyomas, for example, are low-signal intensity because of the large amount of fibrous tissue in the myoma itself. The signals for different tissue regions diminish at different rates, resulting in the two specific signal-decay processes. Varying the pulse sequences and delay times yields spin density images, T1- or T2-weighted images.

Interpretation of images of the ovary and tube are more difficult with MRI than of the uterus or cervix. The ovary is a medium signal on T1 and has high signal intensity on T2. MRI imaging is sensitive to the presence of blood. However, it cannot differentiate sources of blood; specifically, it

(A)

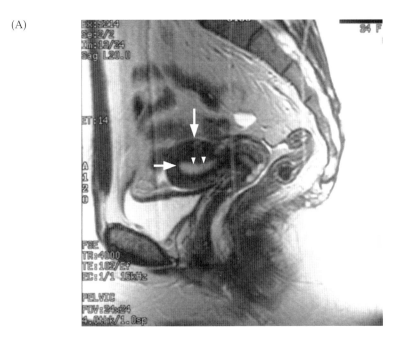

(B)

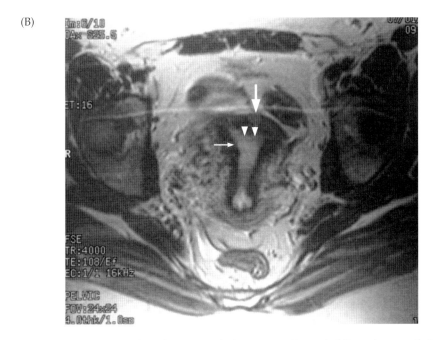

Figure 3-19   Zonal architecture of the uterus. Sagittal (A) and coronal (B) T2-
                   weighted image demonstrating normal uterus (large arrow) junctional
                   zone (small arrow) and endometrium (arrowheads).

	Table 3-1.	
Signal Characteristics of Normal Pelvic Anatomy with Magnetic Resonance Imaging		
Structure	**T1-Weighted Images**	**T2-Weighted Images**
Uterus	Homogeneous, low signal	Central, high signal intensity stripe (endometrium)
		Low-density band surrounding the endometrium (junctional zone)
		Outer signal of moderate intensity (myometrium)
Cervix	Hypointense signal intensity	Central high signal intensity (canal)
		Hyperintense intensity surrounding the canal (stroma)
Vagina	Hypointense signal intensity	Hyperintense outer core (vaginal wall)
		Hypointense central core (canal)
		High signal intensity at the perimeter (venous plexus)
Ovary	Homogeneous and hypointense	Isointense (stroma) Hyperintense (follicles)

cannot differentiate a benign from a malignant process. On MRI, the blood in an endometrioma may very well appear identical to the blood in a corpus luteum.[16] The differential diagnosis is frequently inclusive in these circumstances with additional imaging acquired. Variable tissue densities will be detected as distinct structures within an otherwise homogeneous signal field.

Imaging of the uterus may be influenced by timing in the menstrual cycle. There is a slight increase in the myometrial diameter at the midsecretory phase and in patients who are using oral contraceptives. There are no changes in the junctional zone, which measures approximately 5 mm regardless of cycle day. The endometrium on MRI measures 6 mm during the follicular phase and 10–12 mm during the secretory phase. Slight changes in the cervical length have been noted, but are of uncertain clinical significance. The length measures 2.7 and 2.9 cm in the follicular and luteal phases, respectively. The vagina has no changes that are menstrually related. The ovary can change markedly, depending on whether it is premenarchal or postmenopausal and when in the menstrual cycle the image is taken.

MRI has found application in a variety of circumstances in reproductive medicine. In evaluating for anatomic abnormalities, the absence of any respiratory motion within the pelvis, which has been so problematic in other imaging techniques, creates an ideal imaging environment. MRI has been useful in imaging the uterus to rule out congenital abnormalities.

T2-weighted images are useful in conjunction with ultrasound and laparoscopy in defining congenital uterine abnormalities such as bicornuate and septate uteri.[67,68] MRI has been particularly helpful for the former because as a noninvasive means for determining the need for and type of surgical therapy.[69] In the evaluation of the cervix, a potential role for MRI is the assessment of the incompetent cervix. MRI of the vagina is particularly useful in the adolescent population, in which both uterine and adnexal anatomy may be simultaneously demonstrated. The noninvasive nature of MRI (like ultrasound) is especially important as it may preclude the need for a clinical examination in this sensitive population. When either obstruction or congenital absence of the vagina is suspected as the etiology of primary amenorrhea, MRI can define pelvic anatomy, determine the presence of a uterus and position of the ovaries. MRI of the ovary, especially with gadolinium-enhanced imaging and fat saturation, has provided a sensitive means to assess the character of ovarian cysts such as hemorrhagic cysts, endometriomas, and dermoid cysts.

Endoscopic Techniques

Hysteroscopy

Office hysteroscopy in conjunction with sonohysterography has an increasing role in the assessment of the endometrial cavity using rigid and flexible hysteroscopes. The technique has rightfully settled into clinical decision making as a simple, outpatient diagnostic tool and as a follow-up, next-step examination to sonohysterography. It is a definitive study in assessing submucous polyps, uterine synechiae, and mullerian fusion defects when these abnormalities are suggested on HSG, ultrasound or MRI.[71,72] Several studies suggest increased sensitivity and specificity to HSG in the assessment of uterine cavity abnormalities.[70] The false-negative and false-positive rate for intrauterine defects associated with HSG make diagnostic office hysteroscopy a useful adjunct to HSG and sonohysterography. For example, only 55% of intrauterine adhesions suggested by HSG are confirmed by hysteroscopy.[73] However, HSG remains the most important screening procedure for the diagnosis of normal or abnormal uterine cavities. Hysteroscopy should be reserved for the confirmation and treatment of intrauterine anomalies discovered by HSG and sonohysterography.[74] In some settings, hysteroscopy is a definitive and essential evaluation of the endometrial cavity prior to ART. These techniques are complementary and should follow each other sequentially.

Hysteroscopy allows direct visualization of the endometrial cavity and tubal ostia. It is performed to make or corroborate a diagnosis. Indications for hysteroscopy include further assessment of abnormalities detected on HSG, such as intrauterine adhesions, septate uteri, or to further evaluate irregular bleeding and rule out endometrial polyps or uterine fibroids.[72] A flexible catheter and cytobrush enables sampling of proximal tubal mucosa in cases where chlamydial and tubal damage are suspected.[75] Sample tissue may be used for chlamydial testing by both cell culture and polymerase chain reaction. Contraindications are similar to those for HSG. A recent history of PID or adnexal tenderness are also contraindications.

There are several different types of hysteroscopes, ranging from rigid to flexible to contact hysteroscopes. Rigid scopes have variable or fixed focus with varying diameters. Hysteroscopes have outer diameters from 2.7 to 4 mm. The viewing angle may range from 0° to oblique lenses providing views of 12°, 15°, 25°, or 30° from the horizontal. For diagnostic purposes, all hysteroscopes provide excellent visualization of the endometrial cavity. The choice of hysteroscope is largely one of personal preference and ease of use.

Distension media range from gas such as CO_2, which affords a wider field of view and lower magnification than a liquid medium, to electrolyte-containing solutions such as normal saline and Ringer's lactate, to non-electrolyte solutions such as glycine and sorbitol. CO_2 is the only gas used as a distending medium. It is used through an insufflator with a maximal flow of 100 ml per minute and maximal pressure of 200 mmHg. Fluid contrast media are of two types, depending on their viscosity. Low-viscosity agents include 5% glucose in water, normal saline, Ringer's lactate, 3.3% sorbitol, or 1.5% glycine. One high-viscosity agent is Hyskon (32% dextran 70 and 10% dextrose in water; Pharmacia, Inc., Piscataway, NJ). Hyskon has the advantage of maintaining clear visualization of the endometrial cavity in spite of the blood or debris that can enter the field of view (it is nonmiscible with blood). It is a viscous solution and flows slowly, permitting steady distension while using minimal amounts. It does have the disadvantage of being slippery and cumbersome to use.

The low-viscosity and high-viscosity agents may be used in combination. For example, normal saline and Hyskon can be combined in one-to-one mixtures. This solution uses the optical qualities of Hyskon as a distending medium, but reduces messiness by mixing it with the low-viscosity saline. Nonelectrolyte solutions such as 1.5% glycine, 3% sorbitol, and mannitol are used for both diagnostic and operative procedures. The osmolality of the nonelectrolyte solutions (sorbitol and glycine) make these media ideal for intrauterine surgery requiring electrosurgery, such as a resectoscopic myomectomy. In contrast to electrolyte-containing distending media, these solutions do not conduct electrical current and can be used safely with electrosurgery.

Technique

The procedure is best performed in the early follicular phase in patients with normal menstrual cycles or after withdrawal of medroxyprogesterone acetate in patients with irregular bleeding. Precautions to rule out pregnancy should be taken using a rapid and sensitive urinary pregnancy test. Preoperative analgesics such as nonsteroidal anti-inflammatory drugs

(NSAIDs) may be helpful in some patients. NSAIDs are most effective when used 1 to 2 hours before the procedure. Given the narrow diameters of the diagnostic hysteroscopes, cervical priming is usually not necessary. However, if cervical stenosis is present, pre-medication with intravaginal misoprostol or laminaria placement may be helpful. The procedure is performed after a sterile vaginal prep and a paracervical block of 1% lidocaine. The need for and degree of anesthesia, analgesia, or both depends on the patient preference, tolerance and cooperation. Adequate counseling before the procedure may reduce the need for medication. With video monitoring, observation by the patient is possible, enhancing any post-procedural explanation. The more comfortable the patient is during the procedure, the easier it is for her to view the monitor.

After a sterile prep of the vault, the cervix is gently dilated approximately to the diameter of the hysteroscope to be used. The hysteroscope is gently advanced under direct visualization. The endocervical canal is closely inspected, and the scope advanced to the internal os. A careful panoramic inspection of the endometrial cavity from the vantage point of the internal os should be made. The scope is slowly advanced into the cavity. Close attention is directed to the fundus to rule out any midline septal defects. Lateral walls of the cavity should be inspected closely. The scope should be advanced and the cornual regions evaluated. These can usually be visualized by angling the scope laterally, almost against the thigh of the patient's opposite side.

Complications of hysteroscopy are extremely low at a rate of less than 1%. Diagnostic procedures have the lowest rate at 0.13% with operative procedures at 0.95%. The most common complication is perforation, which may occur either during dilatation of the cervix or during the insertion of the hysteroscope (incidence, 0.76%). Other complications may be related to the medium used and the type of procedure performed. For more extensive operative hysteroscopic procedures, such as resectoscopic myomectomies or endometrial ablations, the complications may be related to fluid overload with nonelectrolyte solutions such as sorbitol or glycine. Anaphylactic reactions and pulmonary edema with the Hyskon have been described.[76]

Laparoscopy

In-Hospital Outpatient Procedures

The role of diagnostic laparoscopy has changed considerably in the recent past. Once considered an integral part of the evaluation for any infertility patient, it is increasingly applied in select circumstances in patients who are at risk either for pelvic adhesive disease or endometriosis/ endometriomas. Its role is primarily in patients who are less than 35 who are interested in conservative options for management, i.e., intrauterine inseminations and are unwilling to consider IVF. In this circumstance, it may be useful in detecting early stages of endometriosis and pelvic adhesions amenable to laparoscopic intervention. After the procedure follow-up therapies with ovarian stimulation using either Clomiphene or gonadotropins and intrauterine inseminations are appropriate. However, in patients over 35 for whom in vitro fertilization is an option, patients may be better advised to move directly to in vitro fertilization rather than undergoing diagnostic and operative laparoscopy. This is appropriate when there are no other conditions present such as pelvic pain, the history is negative for PID or prior unsuccessful attempts at pregnancy. The threshold for recommending laparoscopy should rise or fall based on the patient's history.

Of all diagnostic procedures available, diagnostic laparoscopy is one of the most sensitive and specific in the evaluation of patients with suspected structural abnormalities and reproductive problems.[77–79] In exchange for the intensive and invasive nature of the procedure, the clinician is given definitive information through direct visualization of the reproductive anatomy. No inferences are needed. This procedure found a resurgence in the late 1960s and early 1970s after a series of publications suggested that clinically significant and relevant information that could markedly alter management of infertility patients could be obtained.[79] Laparoscopy in conjunction with HSG is both a diagnostic and therapeutic modality and essential for select cases for the evaluation of pelvic anatomy.[77,80] With increasing use of assisted reproductive technologies earlier in the evaluation and treatment of infertility, the role of laparoscopy has changed.[81] There is a growing tendency to bypass laparoscopy and opt for more aggressive ART when the HSG is normal and history is negative. Care is required in patient selection. Any recommendation for laparoscopy should consider the age of the female partner and the ultimate role ART may play in their reproductive plans. In some cases, it is appropriate to delay or bypass entirely laparoscopy.[82]

Laparoscopic instrumentation includes tools needed for both diagnosis and operative laparoscopy.[83] The skills of the diagnostic laparoscopist must be the same as those of the operative laparoscopist. Diagnostic laparoscopy should always be immediately convertible into an operative procedure. Hence, appropriately trained personnel and all instruments should be readily available. In particular, techniques for cutting and coagulating should be accessible. To this end, skill and equipment for electrosurgery, laser surgery, and basic instruments for stapling and suturing are essential (Table 3-2).

Electrosurgery represents the convergence of the sciences of electrical engineering and surgical practice. Fundamental to electrosurgery is an understanding of the basic aspects of electrocautery. Electrosurgery involves the application of a current of electricity at a specific point, for example body tissue, to generate a desired effect, such as coagulation or cutting, with the exit of the current through a larger surface area in another part of the body.

Table 3-2. Endoscopic Hemostatic Techniques		
Method	**Technique**	**Device**
Electrocoagulation	Electrical energy in a dampened wave form; coagulum forms at 45–60°C	Needle-tip or spatula and solid-state electrical generator (various manufacturers)
Laser	Various modes to deliver energy to surgical site	COZ, ND:YAG, KTP
Thermocoagulation	Electrical current to heat an electrode to 100–120°C and transmit to the tissue by convection	Endocoagulator (Wysap Co.)
Suturing techniques		
Loop ligatures	Suture loop with pre-tied knot available as 0 chromic, 0 plain cat gut, 0 Vicryl, and 0 PDS	Endoloop (Ethicon, Summerville, NJ)
Extracorporeal suturing and knot tying	Suture placement laparoscopically and knot tying. Extracorporeally	Endosutures of 0 chromic and 0 Vicryl (Ethicon, Summerville, NJ)
Intra-abdominal suturing and knot tying	Suturing technique using 4-0 graspers and needle	Various sutures and needles available from 0 to 4-0
Clipping techniques	Titanium and stainless steel permanent and absorbable clips are available to achieve hemostasis on isolated vessels or small pedicles	PDS Ligating Clips (Ethicon, Summerville, NJ)
Linear stapling device	Two or three rows of parallel titanium staples are applied	Endo-GIA (Autosuture Co.) Endo-Cutter (Ethicon, Summerville, NJ)

Electrosurgical generators are designed to produce an alternating current of electricity that provides tissue desiccation but does not stimulate muscle activity. Three basic wave forms that are used in electrosurgery are coagulating wave forms (interrupted, varied, modulated, or damped output); cutting wave forms (continuous, simple, unmodulated, or undamped output); and a blended wave form, which is literally a combination of undamped and damped wave forms.

Electrosurgical techniques vary in their tissue effects and consequently the clinical circumstances in which their use is appropriate. The application and effects of electrical energy to a specific tissue point depend on several factors such as the size and shape of the instrument applying the current, the frequency and wave modulation (coagulating versus cutting), the peak voltage and current, the speed of the motion and device, the pressure on the device, and the degree of contact between the electrode and the tissue. For example, electrocoagulation may be done by fulguration or by desiccation. Fulguration occurs when no tissue contact occurs between the electrode and the tissue and the peak voltage is sufficiently high to result in an arc to the tissue to create surface-only necrosis. With desiccation, the tissue effect is influenced by the size and shape of an electrode in direct contact with the tissue. Electrosurgery using a unipolar technique consists of a current that passes from an electrode at the tip of the instrument to the tissue being cut or cauterized. In this technique, the flow moves from the electrode through the tissue and passes out through a grounding pad that is usually attached over a large surface area, such as a thigh or buttock. The advantage to this technique is that it can be used for both cutting and coagulating.[84] The potential danger, however, is damage to an adjacent organ as a result of the broad flow. Electrosurgery using a bipolar technique limits the area of damage and minimizes the potential for unintentional damage to adjacent structures. In a bipolar technique, there is no return plate, and the current passes through an adjacent electrode immediately at the instrument tip. In this regard, the current flows only between the active electrode and the return electrode immediately adjacent to the active one.

Laser techniques are a second method to cut and coagulate during operative laparoscopy. While electrosurgery generates its tissue effect with electricity (the movement of electrons), the laser produces a tissue effect by the conversion of photons of light energy into heat.[85] The biologic effect (coagulation or cutting) at the tissue is achieved secondary to the heat generated by the conversion. In gynecology, the CO_2 (with a 10.6 μm wavelength) laser was one of the first investigated for widespread clinical use. This laser provided excellent cutting and vaporization abilities but had poor hemostatic abilities. In addition, the unit was mechanically cumbersome to use. The articulating arms limited maneuverability, and the mirrors in the articulating arm required absolute and frequent alignment for proper use.

Although the CO_2 laser is applicable to a variety of clinical scenarios and is still widely used, other solid-state laser systems such as potassium-titanyl-phosphate (KTP) and neodymium:yttrium-aluminum-garnet (Nd:YAG) lasers provide a degree of convenience not available with the CO_2 laser. In these systems, the energy is transmitted via fiberoptics. The energy at this wavelength also is transmissible through fluid, thus making it usable through a hysteroscope. These units offer the ability for cutting, coagulating, and vaporization. The fiber can be used in a contact mode for cutting, a near-contact mode for vaporization, and a noncontact mode for coagulation. Hence, by varying the distance between the beam and the tissue of interest, variable effects can be achieved, a degree of versatility not present in other, older systems. The primary advantage, however, remains the ease of use of these systems because of the flexible fiber. The fiber is narrow enough that it can be placed through a variety of channels including the aspirating channel of a tissue irrigator and the operating channel of a laparoscope. The energy of the KTP and Nd:YAG can be delivered through flexible 400- or 600-μm fibers. The primary effects are coagulation or vaporization when contact or near-contact occurs with the tissue and the fiber. Advantages include the ability to achieve hemostasis, vaporization, and coagulation with a single system, and the shorter depth of penetration, thus obviating the need for a backstop.

Lasers may be fired using four different modes. A single pulse mode releases one burst of energy for a set interval of time. Each burst of energy requires triggering the foot pedal by the operator. The intervals may last from 0.05 to 0.5 seconds. A repeat pulse mode releases a continuous fixed burst of energy for a specified length of time as long as the operator triggers the foot pedal. Continuous wave mode releases continuous laser energy as long as the pedal remains depressed. A super pulse mode characteristic of a CO_2 laser releases the laser energy in rapid bursts, creating less heat build up and reducing the potential for adjacent tissue injury.

There are no clear-cut advantages of a laser, regardless of type, to electro-cautery; it is a matter of personal choice of the operating surgeon. Of the lasers that are available, the CO_2, argon, KTP-535, and Nd:YAG are clinically useful for reproductive reconstructive surgery, the fulguration of endometriosis, and coagulation and dissection. Each has a particular advantage and disadvantage. Outcome measures for laparoscopic and hystero-scopic procedures performed with electrosurgery and laser surgery are similar.

The harmonic scalpel is a third technique for simultaneous cutting and coag-ulating. This tool converts electrical energy into ultrasonic mechanical vibra-tions. The scalpel utilizes an acoustic transducer that converts electrical power into the mechanical vibrations of the scalpel tip. It vibrates longitudi-nally at 55,500 cycles per second with minimal thermal effect transmitted. The concept behind the harmonic scalpel is vibration of the surgical tip gen-erating a low level of heat as a result of the ultrasonic energy. This vibration causes the coagulation effect at the tip. The scalpel is designed for use in soft tissue and provides adequate hemostasis with minimal thermal injury to adjacent tissue and no smoke production. This instrument has proven to be exceptionally safe, but damage to adjacent structures has been described.

Technique

Laparoscopy is best performed with the patient under general anesthesia, though under select circumstances, it may be performed with use of spinal or epidural anesthesia. The procedure is best performed with the patient in a low lithotomy position. Both arms may be tucked at the patient's side to provide operators with maximal access and position options during surgery, and the least discomfort to the patient. The procedure may be performed at any time in the menstrual cycle, provided that adequate safeguards to rule out pregnancy have been taken. In anticipating any laparoscopic procedure, consideration should be made for converting the procedure from a strictly diagnostic to a full operative procedure. To this end, careful selection of the placement of the trocars is essential. The usual point of entry of the laparascope is at an infraumbilical site, although this may be varied depending on the clinical circumstances.

The standard placement of the laparoscope for gynecologic procedures is infraumbilical using a 5- to 10-mm incision depending on scope diameter. Debate centers on the method of trocar placement: direct insertion of the larger trocar followed by insufflation or initial placement of a Verres needle followed by insufflation and then placement of the larger 10-mm trocar. Both have proven to be safe with exceedingly low complication rates in cases where there is no history of abdominal surgery. Neither direct insertion nor pre-insufflation after Verres needle placement has proven to be complication-free. The choice of technique should be made on the surgeon's degree of comfort and familiarity. To facilitate trocar placement and increase safety, disposable trocars may be used. These trocars have extremely sharp tips and the tips are designed to immediately retract upon entry into the abdominal cavity. In addition to this, direct visualization trocars are also available for select circumstances providing a limited view of the tissue at the tip. These instruments add to the cost of the procedure and have not conclusively been shown to reduce complications significantly. Cases with prior abdominal surgery require a more considered approach. Primary concern is bowel damage after trocar insertion secondary to anterior abdominal wall adhesions. These adhesions occur with a frequency ranging from 5 to 35%. Open laparoscopy with laparoscope placement through a Hasson cannula is the most cautious and advisable route. In this technique, a 2–3-cm incision is made and the abdominal cavity entered under direct visualization. A cannula is then sutured into place and the laparoscope inserted. However, even with this approach, bowel injuries may occur in the setting of previous abdominal surgery. One study suggested that an open insertion may be no safer than direct trocar insertion. An alternative approach is to place a 3- or 5-mm laparoscope at a site removed from the prior incision, usually at a lateral position. Any adhesions may be lysed and a site cleared for placement of the primary laparoscope. Adequate preoperative counseling regarding the possibility of bowel damage and need for immediate repair is essential.

If other probes are necessary, care should be taken in placing them to avoid the inferior epigastric vessels, especially when placing the lateral probes. Complications may be reduced (but not necessarily eliminated) by transilluminating the abdominal wall and identifying the vessels. Two to three additional punctures may be necessary. The placement of the punctures should be determined after visualization of the pelvic anatomy and assessment of the extent and type of surgery required. It may be necessary to place two probes more laterally if extensive dissection on a particular side is required. Occasionally, and depending on the clinical circumstances, all probes may be placed in the midline. After placement of the scope and the ancillary probes, a panoramic inspection of the pelvic organs should be made, then an assessment of the uterus – its size, shape, position, and mobility. The tubal architecture, tubal mobility, and character of the fimbriated ends should then be noted. The ovaries should be closely inspected next, and any evidence of ovulation noted. Chromotubation is essential to any laparoscopic procedure. A variety of agents including methylene blue and indigo carmine have been used in this regard. During chromotubation, the fimbriated ends of the tubes should be carefully observed. The dye should flow easily and spill readily. Distension of the tube proximal to the fimbriae and delayed but eventual spill suggests a phimosis and requires careful evaluation. If there is no fill of the tubes, proximal tubal obstruction should be suspected only after verification that the injection system is well applied to the cervix. There should be no reflux of the dye into the vagina. If the system is sealed, gentle pulsing thumb pressure should result in easily observed distension of the uterus.

Major complication rates for diagnostic and operative laparoscopy are extremely low at 0.22%. The incidence is nearly equal for operative procedures than for diagnostic. The complications arise with equal frequency from Verres needle and trocar placement as from the operative procedure itself. These complications include damage to bowel and bladder either through the use of cautery or laser or through trocar insertion, vascular injuries usually occurring after the placement of the 5-mm trocars in the lower abdomen.

Transvaginal Hydrolaparoscopy (THL)

Transvaginal hydrolaparoscopy is a safe and well-tolerated method for investigating pelvic anatomy.[86–88] It has been shown to be more sensitive than HSG for the diagnosis of pelvic adhesions. Transvaginal hydrolaparascopy combines the classic colposcopic approach for scope insertion with advanced microendoscopic technology. Small diameter optic, high-intensity light source endoscopes are used to evaluate the pelvis. In transvaginal hydrolaparascopy, the ovaries, distal fallopian tubes, pelvic sidewalls, and cul-de-sac is clearly visualized. Access into the cul-de-sac is successful in 95% of patients attempted. It may be performed in an office setting under local anesthesia. It may also be combined with mini-hysteroscopy and chromotubation for a single endoscopic evaluation for infertility.

Office Laparoscopy

The availability of microlaparoscopes has brought diagnostic laparoscopy from the operating room into the office.[89,90] A variety of procedures may be performed in office settings, including diagnostic laparoscopy and chromotubation for infertility, endometriosis, and pelvic pain.[91] In select cases, more aggressive operative procedures such as lysis of adhesions and tubal ligations may be performed.

The procedure is performed using miniaturized 2-mm laparoscopes, and either intravenous sedation or local anesthesia and paracervical block can be used. The degree of anesthesia used depends in part on the indication for the procedure and in part on the tolerance and cooperation of the patient. In some settings (for example, chronic pelvic pain), minimal anesthesia may enhance the ability of the patient to identify areas of maximal pain intensity. The patient should be in the low lithotomy position and a system for transcervical chromotubation, either with a flexible catheter system or a more standard rigid cannula, should be incorporated. Insufflation is carefully and slowly carried out. A frequent limiting factor is the tolerance for progressive abdominal distension. The amount of insufflation can be actively varied in the course of the procedure or maintained at extremely low levels just sufficient to enable visualization of the pelvic organs. Different gases for insufflation, such as nitrous oxide, can reduce the discomfort of insufflation. Inspection of anatomy and any operative procedures are carried out in a conventional fashion. Because of the size of the punctures (i.e., 2 mm) no stitches are required. Miniaturized scissors and grasping instruments are available for lysis of adhesions, fulguration of endometriosis, and transfer of gametes for any gamete intrafallopian transfer (GIFT) procedure in very select circumstances.

The primary advantages of office laparoscopies are lowered costs (as great as 60% reductions; especially important in an infertility population for which third-party payment can vary tremendously) and reduced hospitalization. Initially met with considerable enthusiasm, this procedure has not been as widely accepted and embraced in all centers. Its exact role in diagnostics and therapeutics in reproductive surgery awaits further study and evaluation.

Optical Catheters

The 1.8-mm outer diameter of optical catheters provides an easy means of accessing the abdominal cavity.[92] The rigid catheters give excellent optics of the pelvis without the need for general anesthesia. A small, 18-mm-outer-diameter optical catheter has been developed by Medical Dynamics (Englewood, CO) and a 1.8-mm Pixie microendoscope by Origin Med Systems, Inc. (Palo Alto, CA). The catheters contain a bundle of image fibers 6 μm in diameter. These catheters have been used to further investigate the pelvis, and offer an alternative to laparoscopy using a 2-mm laparoscope. Indications, techniques, and costs are similar with either system. As with office laparoscopy, the field of view may be limited.

Falloposcopy

The most common method of assessing tubal pathology is the indirect method of HSG and chromotubation under laparoscopic observation. Miniaturized optical systems directed through the proximal tube from the proximal to distal into the fallopian tube itself has enabled direct inspection of the tubal lumen and epithelium.[93,94] Falloposcopy provides a visual means of scoring endotubal disease and may also be therapeutic for dislodging intra-luminal debris and breaking down film adhesions in the normal minimally diseased tubes. A falloposcopic classification and scoring system has been developed to characterize and quantitate the site, type, and severity of endo-tubal disease and to correlate this scoring system with surgical results and pregnancy outcomes.[95,96] Distal salpingostomy is possible with all restrictions and cautions attendant to this procedure. Severe tubal disease is a contraindi-cation for endotuboplasty as reflected by poor pregnancy outcome. Such women should be referred for in vitro fertilization.

Molecular Approaches to Infertility

With the sequencing of mammalian genomes, a catalogue of expression pat-terns of all transcription units is now possible.[97] The challenge is to deter-mine the function of the genes regarding normal physiology, health and well-being and their malfunction in disease. This new discipline – *functional genomics* – describes these patterns. The detection may be accomplished in part through *microarray technology*. The development of microarray techno-logy has provided a method to analyze the expression of thousands of genes in a single assay (Figure 3-20). Microarrays are powerful methods of assess-ing gene expression via complementary DNA (cDNA) or RNA analysis. This technology enables the analysis of a wide range of biomolecules such as DNA, RNA, protein, carbohydrates, and lipids. Microarrays provide a

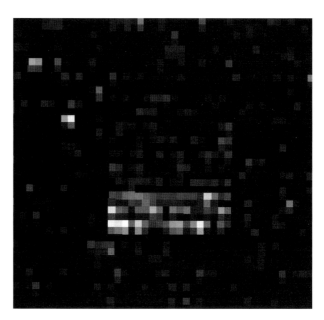

Figure 3-20   Surface of an expression chip hybridized with biotinylated cRNA and stained with streptavidin-phycoerythrin.

method to simultaneously measure where and when thousands of genes are expressed. In studying disease-related changes in gene expression, microarray technology may provide insight in the first step in a long process in the translation of genomic research to clinical application.[98-100]

A microarray or "gene chip" measures the expression level of a gene by determining the amount of mRNA that is present (sometimes referred to as mRNA abundance). (The term "gene chip" is a registered trademark GeneChip of the company Affymetrix. In common parlance, the term "gene chip" is generally applied to microarray technology.) Microarray technology offers the ability to analyze large numbers of genes. In a conventional Northern blot, analysis of one tube and up to 20 mRNAs may take place. With microarray technology, simultaneous analysis of the expression levels of tens of thousands of genes is possible in a single study. Contemporary chip technology provides up to 450,000 loci for analysis of as many as 20,000 genes and gene sequences on a single glass slide. This technology provides for quantitative measurement of concentrations of mRNA and thus a method of assessing gene expression.

Microarray technology is used in three circumstances: (1) gene expression profiling; (2) genotyping; and (3) DNA sequencing. In gene expression profiling, mRNA is extracted from a biologic sample. In genotyping, DNA is extracted from the specimen and amplified by a polymerase chain reaction. The resultant product is then applied to the microarray assay. In this circumstance, hundreds and up to thousands of genetic markers can be determined in a single study. In DNA sequencing, DNA is again extracted from a specimen, amplified, and applied to specific "sequencing microarrays". In this setting, the scope for precise molecular diagnosis in a single gene is enhanced considerably.

A critical aspect of microarray technology is the selection of the probe to be printed on the array. Gene databases provide the most frequently used selections. There are two platforms to generate microarrays (Table 3-3): cDNA

Table 3-3. Microarray Platforms
cDNA Arrays
• Requires a collection of gene sequences as PCR products ranging from 100 to 2000 bp derived from cDNA • DNA probes (i.e., PCR products) of cDNA of specific genes spotted onto a glass slide • Sample RNA is converted to target using reverse transcription
Oligonucleotides Arrays
• Requires synthesis of single stranded probes based on sequence information from databases • Target is hybridized to probe (purified mRNA from sample) • Amount of inbound or nonspecifically bound target is calculated

array technology uses DNA probes (that is, PCR products representing the complementary DNA code of specific genes that are spotted onto a glass slide). The second type is called oligonucleotide array technology. In this technology, all the nucleotides are synthesized onto a silica slide by a process known as photolithography. The target consists of purified mRNA from the specimen (either blood or tissue, for example). This is labeled by fluorescence or radioactivity and then hybridized to the microarray. mRNA consists of a sequence built of four different oligonucleotides (thymidine, guanine, cytosine, and uracil) that is specific for each gene. Hybridization occurs between the target of the nucleotides or the nucleotide sequences and the spot oligonucleotide sequences. By analyzing large numbers of genes and gene products, microarray technology generates huge databases. For example, a single microarray experiment can produce between 100,000 and 1,000,000 data points in a typical experiment. The best statistical analysis for this data is yet to be defined. The Microarray Gene Expression Database Consortium has the goal of developing common standards of annotation, data representation, and data analysis.

Microarrays may have their most powerful application in four specific areas: disease susceptibility definition; enhancement of sensitivity in early disease diagnosis; prognostic markers; and assessment of individual treatment patterns. In reproductive medicine and infertility, these technologies may apply to a broad range of processes. The most recently evaluated processes have been endometriosis, and polycystic ovarian syndrome.

Microarray technology for endometriosis may provide a method to gain further insight into the pathophysiology of endometriosis and as a possible diagnostic test.[102,103] Endometrial biopsies have been used for the histologic dating of the endometrium since the early descriptions in the mid-1950s. In the classic sense, any discrepancy between the chronologic timing of the menstrual cycle by history and appearance of the endometrial biopsy suggested a *luteal phase defect*. Microarray technologies offer an analysis beyond histologic evaluations. Several recent studies suggest that, in patients with endometriosis, the endometrium may be histologically normal but biochemically abnormal during the window of implantation. Several genes or gene products in the endometrium may be aberrantly expressed during this window as part of the spectrum of endometriosis or at other times during the cycle. This aberrant gene expression may find its clinical expression in either failure of implantation or contribute to the establishment and growth of endometriotic cells in areas other than within the endometrial cavity. Thus compromised fertility in patients with endometriosis may be related to functional abnormalities in the endometrium or aberrant gene expression during the time of implantation. Microarray technology to assess endometrial gene expression may provide insight regarding the etiology of infertility in these patients and more targeted and specific therapy for these abnormalities. In its fullest possibilities, this technology may enable a simple diagnostic tool, the endometrial biopsy, as a sensitive test for endometriosis.

A hallmark of polycystic ovarian syndrome is hyperandrogenism, probably related to excessive stromal cell androgen secretion. Both quantitative linkage analysis and candidate gene approaches are options to study polycystic ovary syndrome.[104] These studies may reveal that polycystic ovary syndrome is composed of a variety of subtypes influenced by one or more dominant gene causes. Although the mode of inheritance is unclear, various genes have been suggested as candidates for polycystic ovary syndrome. By using microarray technology, stromal cells in patients with polycystic ovarian syndrome appear to have a gene expression profile that is different from those patients with regular ovulatory cycles. This technology may provide further understanding of the functional changes that accompany the well-defined structural changes in ovarian morphology.

Summary and Recommendations

The evaluation for structural abnormalities in reproductive surgery has progressed from simple radiographic techniques as the sole means of assessing the reproductive tract to noninvasive, precise, and sensitive techniques such as MRI. The advent of microlaparoscopes and miniaturized trocars and optical fibers may remove diagnostic laparoscopy from the hospital and operating room and place it as a convenient, quickly performed, in-office procedure. In this circumstance, the procedure would provide rapid, low-cost direct visualization of the anatomy imaged by MRI or ultrasound, though these techniques are preferred by some clinicians, widespread acceptance has been slow. In spite of a large amount of data regarding imaging techniques and microlaparoscopic procedures, contemporary evaluation of structural abnormalities still relies on conventional laparoscopy and hysteroscopy. In addition, because of the in-hospital setting and use of general anesthesia, they are quickly and easily convertible to operative procedures. Microarray technology is a method to assess function and a complementary technique to structural evaluations gained through imaging and direct visualization. Future infertility evaluations will incorporate all three (imaging, endoscopy and microarray analyses) techniques to provide insight into structure and function, and guide therapy along either direction.

References

1. Rubin IC. The nonoperative determination of patency of Fallopian tubes. JAMA 1920;75:661–665.

2. Siegler AM. Hysterosalpingography. Fertil Steril 1983;40:139–158.

3. Heuser C. Lipiodol in the diagnosis of pregnancy. Lancet 1925;i:1111.

4. Binkovitz LA, King BF, Corfman RS. Advances in gynecologic imaging and intervention. Mayo Clin Proc 1991;66:1133–1151.

5. Montoya JM, Bernal A, Borrero C. Diagnostics in assisted human reproduction. Reprod Biomed Online 2002;5:198–210.

6.   Musich JR, Behrman SJ. Infertility laparoscopy in perspective: review of five hundred cases. Am J Obstet Gynecol 1982;143:293–303.

7.   Glatstein IZ, Harlow BL, Hornstein MD. Practice patterns among reproductive endocrinologists: further aspects of the infertility evaluation. Fertil Steril 1998;70:263–269.

8.   Watrelot A, Nisolle M, Chelli H, Hocke C, Rongieres C, Racinet C; International Group for Fertiloscopy Evaluation. Is laparoscopy still the gold standard in infertility assessment? A comparison of fertiloscopy versus laparoscopy in infertility. Results of an international multicentre prospective trial: the 'FLY' (Fertiloscopy-LaparoscopY) study. Hum Reprod 2003;18:834–839.

9.   Fatum M, Laufer N, Simon A. Investigation of the infertile couple: should diagnostic laparoscopy be performed after normal hysterosalpingography in treating infertility suspected to be of unknown origin? Hum Reprod 2002;17:1–3.

10.   Yoder IC, Hall DA. Hysterosalpingography in the 1990s. Am J Roentgenol 1991;157:675–683.

11.   Philips Z, Barraza-Llorens M, Posnett J. Evaluation of the relative cost-effectiveness of treatments for infertility in the UK. Hum Reprod 2000;15:95–106.

12.   Mackey RA, Glass RH, Olson LE, Vaidya R. Pregnancy following hysterosalpingography with oil and water soluble dye. Fertil Steril 1971;22:504–507.

13.   Mol BW, Collins JA, Van Der Veen F, Bossuyt PM. Cost-effectiveness of hysterosalpingography, laparoscopy, and *Chlamydia* antibody testing in subfertile couples. Fertil Steril 2001;75:571–580.

14.   Horbach JG, Maathuis JB, van Hall EV. Factors influencing the pregnancy rate following hysterosalpingography and their prognostic significance. Fertil Steril 1973;24:15–18.

15.   Alper MM, Garner PR, Spence JE, Quarrington AM. Pregnancy rates after hysterosalpingography with oil- and water-soluble contrast media. Obstet Gynecol 1986;68:6–9.

16.   Johnson NP, Farquhar CM, Harden WE, et al. The FLUSH-trial: flushing with lipoidal for unexplained subfertility by HSG: Randomized trial. Human Reprod 2004;19:2043–2051.

17.   Watson A, Vandekerckhove P, Lilford R, et al. A meta-analysis of the therapeutic role of oil soluble contrast media at hysterosalpingography: a surprising result? Fertil Steril 1994;61:470–477.

18.   Letterie GS, Rose GS. Pregnancy rates after the use of oil-based and water-based contrast media to evaluate tubal patency. South Med J 1990;83:1402–1403.

19.   Rasmussen F, Lindequist S, Larsen C, Justesen P. Therapeutic effect of hysterosalpingography: oil- versus water-soluble contrast media–a randomized prospective study. J Radiol 1991;179:75–78.

20.   Lindequist S, Justesen P, Larsen C, Rasmussen F. Diagnostic quality and complications of hysterosalpingography: oil versus water soluble contrast media–a randomized, prospective study. J Radiol 1991;179:69–74.

21.   Steiner AZ, Meyer WR, Clark RL, Hartmann KE. Oil-soluble contrast during hysterosalpingography in women with proven tubal patency. Obstet Gynecol 2003;101:109–113.

22.   Goodman SB, Rein MS, Hill JA. Hysterosalpingography contrast media and chromotubation dye inhibit peritoneal lymphocyte and macrophage function in vitro: a potential mechanism for fertility enhancement. Fertil Steril 1993;59:1022–1027.

23.   Johnson JV, Montoya IA, Olive DL. Ethiodol oil contrast medium inhibits macrophage phagocytosis and adherence by altering membrane electronegativity and microviscosity. Fertil Steril 1992;58:511–517.

24.   Vandekerckhove P, Watson A, Lilford R, et al. Oil-soluble versus water-soluble media for assessing tubal patency with hysterosalpingography or laparoscopy in subfertile women. Cochrane Database Syst Rev 2000;(2):CD000092.

25.   Opsahl MS, Miller B, Klein TA. The predictive value of hysterosalpingography for tubal and peritoneal infertility factors. Fertil Steril 1993;60:444–448.

26.   Swart P, Mol BW, van der Veen F, et al. The accuracy of hysterosalpingography in the diagnosis of tubal pathology: a meta-analysis. Fertil Steril 1995;64:486–491.

27.   Letterie GS, Haggerty MF, Fellows DW. Sensitivity of hysterosalpingography after tubal surgery. Arch Gynecol Obstet 1992;251:175–180.

28.   Wadin K, Lonnemark M, Rasmussen C, Magnusson A. Frequency of proximal tubal obstruction in patients undergoing infertility evaluation. Acta Radiol 1994;35:357–360.

29.   Lang EK. Organic vs functional obstruction of the fallopian tubes: differentiation with prostaglandin antagonist- and beta 2-agonist-mediated hysterosalpingography and selective ostial salpingography. Am J Roentgenol 1991;157:77–80.

30.   Gerlock AJ, Hooser CW. Oviduct response to glucagon during hysterosalpingography. Radiology 1976;119:272–278.

31.   Lang EK, Dunaway HE, Roniger WE. Selective osteal salpingography and transvaginal catheter dilatation in the diagnosis and treatment of fallopian tube obstruction. Am J Roentgenol 1990;154:735–740.

32.   Glatstein IZ, Sleeper LA, Lavy Y, et al. Observer variability in the diagnosis and management of the hysterosalpingogram. Fertil Steril 1997;67:233–237.

33.   Renbaum L, Ufberg D, Sammel M, et al. Reliability of clinicians versus radiologists for detecting abnormalities on hysterosalpingogram films. Fertil Steril 2002;78:614–618.

34.   Thurmond AS, Jones MK, Matteri R. Using the uterine push-pull technique to outline the fundal contour on hysterosalpingography. Am J Roentgenol 2000;175:359–361.

35.   Pittaway DE, Winfield AC, Maxson W, et al. Prevention of acute pelvic inflammatory disease after hysterosalpingography: efficacy of doxycycline prophylaxis. Am J Obstet Gynecol 1983;147:623–626.

36.   Stumpf PG, March CM. Febrile morbidity following hysterosalpingography: identification of risk factors and recommendations for prophylaxis. Fertil Steril 1980;33:487–492.

37.   Dabekausen YA, Evers JL, Land JA, Stals FS. *Chlamydia trachomatis* antibody testing is more accurate than hysterosalpingography in predicting tubal factor infertility. Fertil Steril 1994;61:833–837.

38.   Nunley WC Jr, Bateman BG, Kitchin JD 3rd, Pope TL Jr. Intravasation during hysterosalpingography using oil-base contrast medium–a second look. Obstet Gynecol 1987;70:309–312.

39.   Perisinakas K, Damilakis J. Radiogenic risks from hysterosalpingography. Eur Radiol 2003;13: 1522–1528.

40.   Committee on the Biological Effects of Ionizing Radiation. The effect on populations of exposure to low levels of ionizing radiation: genetic effects of radiation. Washington, DC: National Academic, 1990.

41.   Karande VC, Pratt DE, Balin MS, et al. What is the radiation exposure to patients during a gynecoradiologic procedure? Fertil Steril 1997;67:401–403.

42.   Cheung GW, Lok IN, Wong A, Yip SK. Unsuspected pregnancy at hysterosalpingography: A report of three cases with different outcomes. Human Reprod 2003;18:2608–2609.

43.   Dijkhuizen FP, Brolmann HA, Potters AE, et al. The accuracy of transvaginal ultrasonography in the diagnosis of endometrial abnormalities. Obstet Gynecol 1996;87:345–349.

44.   Sheih CP, Li YW, Liao YJ, et al. Early detection of unilateral occlusion of duplicated mullerian ducts: the use of serial pelvic sonography for girls with renal agenesis. J Urol 1994;151:708–710.

45.   Friberg B, Joergensen C. Tubal patency study by ultrasonography. A pilot study. Acta Obstet Gynecol Scand 1994;73:53–55.

46.   Atri M, Tran CN, Bret PM, et al. Accuracy of endovaginal sonography for the detection of fallopian tube blockage. J Ultrasound Med 1994;13:429–434.

47.   Kupesic S, Kurjak A, Skenderovic S, Bjelos D. Screening for uterine abnormalities by three-dimensional ultrasound improves perinatal outcome. J Perinat Med 2002;30:9–17.

48.   Kupesic S, Kurjak A. Predictors of IVF outcome by three-dimensional ultrasound. Hum Reprod 2002;17:950–955.

49.   Pretorius DH, Nelson TR. Three-dimensional ultrasound. Ultrasound Obstet Gynecol 1995;5:219–221.

50.   Wu MH, Hsu CC, Huang KE. Detection of congenital mullerian duct anomalies using three-dimensional ultrasound. J Clin Ultrasound 1997;25:487–492.

51.   Letterie GS. Ultrasound guidance during endoscopic procedures. Obstet Gynecol Clin North Am 1999;26:63–82.

52.   Hurst BS, Tucker KE, Awoniyi CA, Schlaff WD. Endoscopic ultrasound. A new instrument for laparoscopic surgery. J Reprod Med 1996;41:67–70.

53.   Letterie GS, Catherino WH. A 7.5-MHz finger-grip ultrasound probe for real-time intraoperative guidance during complex reproductive surgical procedures. Am J Obstet Gynecol 2002;187:1588–1590.

54.   Letterie GS, Marshall L. Evaluation of real-time imaging using a laparoscopic ultrasound probe during operative endoscopic procedures. Ultrasound Obstet Gynecol 2000;16:63–67.

55.   Deichert U, Schlief R, van de Sandt M, Daume E. Transvaginal hysterosalpingo-contrast sonography for the assessment of tubal patency with gray scale imaging and additional use of pulsed wave Doppler. Fertil Steril 1992;57:62–67.

56.   Mitri FF, Andronikou AD, Perpinyal S, et al. A clinical comparison of sonographic hydrotubation and hysterosalpingography. Br J Obstet Gynaecol 1991;98:1031–1036.

57.   Gaucherand P, Piacenza JM, Salle B, Rudigoz RC. Sonohysterography of the uterine cavity: preliminary investigations. J Clin Ultrasound 1995;23:339–348.

58. Goldstein SR. Use of ultrasonohysterography for triage of perimenopausal patients with unexplained uterine bleeding. Am J Obstet Gynecol 1994;170:565–570.

59. Exacoustos C, Zupi E, Carusotti C, et al. Hysterosalpingo-contrast sonography compared with hysterosalpingography and laparoscopic dye pertubation in evaluating tubal patency. J Am Assoc Gynecol Laparosc 2003;10:367–372.

60. Jacobson A, Uszler JM. A simplified technique for radionuclide hysterosalpingography. J Assist Reprod Genet 1993;10:4–10.

61. Council on Scientific Affairs. Magnetic resonance imaging. Prologue. JAMA 1987;258:3283–3285.

62. Council on Scientific Affairs. Fundamentals of magnetic resonance imaging. JAMA 1987;258:3417–3423.

63. Imaoka I, Wada A, Matsuo M, et al. MR imaging or disorders associated with female infertility: use in diagnosis, treatment and management. Radiographics 2003;23:1401–1421.

64. Council on Scientific Affairs. Magnetic resonance imaging of the abdomen and pelvis. JAMA 1989;261:420–433.

65. McCarthy S. MR imaging of the uterus. Radiology 1989;171:321–322.

66. Komatsu T, Konishi I, Mandai M, et al. Adnexal masses: transvaginal US and gadolinium-enhanced MR imaging assessment of intratumoral structure. Radiology 1996;198:109–115.

67. Letterie GS, Haggerty M, Lindee G. A comparison of pelvic ultrasound and magnetic resonance imaging as diagnostic studies for mullerian tract abnormalities. Int J Fertil 1995;40:34–38.

68. Minto CL, Hollings N, Hall-Craggs M, Creighton S. Magnetic resonance imaging in the assessment of complex Mullerian anomalies. Br J Obstst Gynaecol 2001;108:791–797.

69. Marten K, Vosshenrich R, Funke M, Obenauer S, Baum F, Grabbe E. MRI in the evaluation of mullerian duct anomalies. Clin Imaging 2003;27:346–350.

70. de Jong P, Doel F, Falconer A. Outpatient diagnostic hysteroscopy. Br J Obstet Gynaecol 1990;97:299–303.

71. Jansen FW, Vredevoogd CB, van Ulzen K, Hermans J, Trimbos JB, Trimbos-Kemper TC. Complications of hysteroscopy: a prospective, multicenter study. Obstet Gynecol 2000;96:266–270.

72. Nagele F, O'Connor H, Davies A, et al. 2500 Outpatient diagnostic hysteroscopies. Obstet Gynecol 1996;88:87–92.

73. Oliveira FG, Abdelmassih VG, Diamond MP, et al. Uterine cavity findings and hysteroscopic interventions. Fertil Steril 2003;80:1371–1375.

74. Fayez JA, Mutie G, Schneider PJ. The diagnostic value of hysterosalpingography and hysteroscopy in infertility investigation. Am J Obstet Gynecol 1987;156:558–560.

75. Haeusler G, Tempfer C, Lehner R, et al. Fallopian tissue sampling with a cytobrush during hysteroscopy: a new approach for detecting tubal infection. Fertil Steril 1997;67:580–582.

76. McLucas B. Hyskon complications in hysteroscopic surgery. Obstet Gynecol Surv 1991;46:196–200.

77. Duff DE, Fried AM, Wilson EA, Haack DG. Hysterosalpingography and laparoscopy: a comparative study. Am J Roentgenol 1983;141:761–763.

78. Tanahatoe S, Hompes PG, Lambalk CB. Accuracy of diagnostic laparoscopy in the infertility work-up before intrauterine insemination. Fertil Steril 2003;79:361–366.

79. Lavy Y, Lev-Sagie A, Holtzer H, et al. Should laparoscopy be a mandatory component of the infertility evaluation in infertile women with normal HSG and suspected unilateral distal tubal pathology? Eur J Obstet Gynecol Reprod Biol 2004;11:64–68.

80. Tanahatoe S, Hompes PG, Lambalk CB. Accuracy of diagnostic laparoscopy in the infertility work-up before intrauterine insemination. Fertil Steril 2003;79:361–366.

81. Brosens I, Campo R, Puttemans P, Gordts S. One-stop endoscopy-based infertility clinic. Curr Opin Obstet Gynecol 2002;14:397–400.

82. Tanahatoe SJ, Hompes PG, Lambalk CB. Investigation of the infertile couple: should diagnostic laparoscopy be performed in the infertility work up programme in patients undergoing intrauterine insemination? Human Reprod 2003;18:8–11.

83. Manyonda IT. Gynaecological Endoscopic Surgery, 16th–17th March 1993: Conference Report. Br J Obstet Gynaecol 1993;100:856–858.

84. Grosskinsky CM, Hulka JF. Unipolar electrosurgery in operative laparoscopy. Capacitance as a potential source of injury. J Reprod Med 1995;40:549–552.

85. Bhatta N, Isaacson K, Bhatta KM, et al. Comparative study of different laser systems. Fertil Steril 1994;61:581–591.

86. De Wilde RL, Verhoeven HC, Keith LG. Transvaginal hydrolaparoscopy. J Am Assoc Gynecol Laparosc 2000;7:599–600.

87. Jonsdottir K, Lundorff P. Transvaginal hydrolaparoscopy: a new diagnostic tool in infertility investigation. Acta Obstet Gynecol Scand 2002;81:882–885.

88. Moore ML, Cohen M. Diagnostic and operative transvaginal hydrolaparoscopy for infertility and pelvic pain. J Am Assoc Gynecol Laparosc 2001;8:393–397.

89. Childers JM, Hatch KD, Surwit EA. Office laparoscopy and biopsy for evaluation of patients with intraperitoneal carcinomatosis using a new optical catheter. Gynecol Oncol 1992;47:337–342.

90. Haeusler G, Lehner R, Hanzal E, Kainz C. Diagnostic accuracy of 2 mm microlaparoscopy. Acta Obstet Gynecol Scand 1996;75:672–675.

91. Downing BG, Wood C. Initial experience with a new microlaparoscope 2 mm in external diameter. Aust NZ J Obstet Gynaecol 1995;35:202–204.

92. Dorsey JH, Tabb CR. Mini-laparoscopy and fiber-optic lasers. Obstet Gynecol Clin North Am 1991;18:613–617.

93. De Bruyne F, Puttemans P, Boeckx W, Brosens I. The clinical value of salpingoscopy in tubal infertility. Fertil Steril 1989;51:339–340.

94. Scudamore IW, Dunphy BC, Cooke ID. Outpatient falloposcopy: intra-luminal imaging of the fallopian tube by trans-uterine fibre-optic endoscopy as an outpatient procedure. Br J Obstet Gynaecol 1992;99:829–835.

95. Kerin JF, Williams DB, San Roman GA, et al. Falloposcopic classification and treatment of fallopian tube lumen disease. Fertil Steril 1992;57:731–741.

96. Surrey ES, Adamson GD, Nagel TC, et al. Multicenter feasibility study of a new coaxial falloposcopy system. J Am Assoc Gynecol Laparosc 1997;4:473–478.

97. Jordan B. Historical background and anticipated developments. Ann N Y Acad Sci 2002;975:24–32.

98. Cutler P. Protein arrays: the current state-of-the-art. Proteomics 2003;3:3–18.

99. Petricoin EF 3rd, Hackett JL, Lesko LJ, et al. Medical applications of microarray technologies: a regulatory science perspective. Nat Genet 2002;32 Suppl:474–479.

100. Forster T, Roy D, Ghazal P. Experiments using microarray technology: limitations and standard operating procedures. J Endocrinol 2003;178:195–204.

101. Grody WW. Ethical issues raised by genetic testing with oligonucleotide microarrays. Mol Biotechnol 2003;23:127–138.

102. Bischoff FZ, Simpson JL. Heritability and molecular genetic studies of endometriosis. Hum Reprod Update 2000;6:37–44.

103. Giudice LC. Elucidating endometrial function in the post-genomic era. Hum Reprod Update 2003;9:223–235.

104. Wood JR, Nelson VL, Ho C, et al. The molecular phenotype of polycystic ovary syndrome (PCOS) theca cells and new candidate PCOS genes defined by microarray analysis. J Biol Chem 2003;278:26380–26390.

4 Vaginal Agenesis

By blunt dissection, a free space was created between the bladder and rectum to a depth of five inches
— Robert Abbe, 1898

Vaginal agenesis is a rare condition diagnosed most commonly at the time of puberty or early adolescence in the course of an evaluation for amenorrhea or pelvic pain. The earliest references to vaginal agenesis and a proposed therapy can be found in Hippocrates' work, *On the Nature of Women*. He alluded to a "membranous obstruction" of the vagina that was amenable to the persistent insertion of a pessary to lengthen the vagina. The first descriptions recorded in the medical literature were by Engle in an autopsy report and the surgical correction by Dupuytren in 1817.

Early proposals for reconstruction included bougie dilators as a conservative option and interposition of flap pedicles as a surgical therapy.[1] Split-thickness skin grafts (a common method for surgical reconstruction today) were initially described in 1898 by Robert Abbe of New York City.[1] The procedure involved harvesting a split-thickness skin graft and placing it over a balsa wood mold. Graft and mold were then inserted into the space between the bladder and rectum that had been bluntly dissected. In addition to the description of surgical reconstruction, Dr. Abbe also described a well-known but infrequent complication, graft contracture, and the need for continuous dilatation to avoid shrinkage. The procedure gained acceptability when McIndoe described a series emphasizing the "ease of performance, low morbidity, excellent end results, and absence of mortality", a bold endorsement even by contemporary standards.[2] At approximately the same time, Baldwin described success using intestinal transposition as a means of constructing an artificial vagina.[3] These early reports focused on vaginal agenesis as a single clinical entity requiring a specific surgical therapy. The spectrum of associated abnormalities had been described in other isolated reports but the full spectrum not appreciated. Subsequent to descriptions of surgical repair, other investigators described abnormalities in additional systems associated with vaginal agenesis.

The description of congenital absence of the vagina and incompletely developed uterine remnants or completely absent uterus as a *specific syndrome* can be traced to the work of four individuals whose names are now commonly attached to this entity.[4] In 1829, Mayer described congenital absence of the vagina with a rudimentary uterus in stillborn infants as only one of several multiple-system abnormalities. In 1838 and in 1910, Rokitansky and

Küster, respectively, described an entity of congenital absence of the vagina, rudimentary uterine structures, normal ovaries, and renal and skeletal abnormalities. In a series of publications in the German literature between 1961 and 1973, Hauser described the most extended series, including a citation of the frequency of the disorder and the full spectrum of abnormalities associated with congenital absence of the vagina. Hence, the term, *Mayer-Rokitansky-Küster-Hauser syndrome* has come to be applied not only to congenital absence of the vagina but also to a variety of other system defects that most prominently include skeletal and renal abnormalities. The terms Mayer-Rokitansky-Küster-Hauser syndrome and vaginal agenesis are used interchangeably.

Various systems and classifications for management have been proposed but are of questionable clinical utility.[5,6] This chapter reviews the etiology of vaginal agenesis, a diagnostic and therapeutic plan, the surgical and nonsurgical methods of correction, and techniques to achieve reproductive potential in these patients through ART.

Etiology

The incidence of vaginal agenesis varies from 1 in 4000 to 1 in 10,000 female births, depending on the clinical population studied, and 1 in 40,000 to 1 in 72,000 in the general population.[7] As an etiology of primary amenorrhea in an adolescent population, congenital absence of the vagina is the second-most-common cause after gonadal dysgenesis (45 X or 45 XO/XX). It must be differentiated from the 46,XY androgen insensitive syndrome and transverse vaginal septum.

The exact etiology of absence of the uterus and vagina is unknown. The frequent association of renal (34%) and skeletal (12%) anomalies suggests that the basis of the condition lies in a broad teratogenic disorder of mesoderm development at the 11 to 12-mm stage during the fifth to sixth week of development. Failure of caudal progression of the paramesonephric duct toward urovaginal sinus may explain in part the rudimentary development or absence of the uterus. Failure to initiate upward growth of the vagina may explain complete inhibition of vaginal embryogenesis. A genetic cause is suggested (as in other congenital reproductive abnormalities) by cases in which siblings have isolated vaginal, skeletal, or ureterorenal anomalies. Discordance for these disorders among monozygotic twins, however, complicates these proposed modes of inheritance. In three cases, a patient with vaginal agenesis and an unaffected monozygote twin have been described. The equal birth weight of the twins in these cases suggests no gross discrepancy in intrauterine environment.[8] Discordance of vaginal agenesis in this setting makes an exclusively genetic etiology unlikely.

Familial clustering is noted for these abnormalities, and a polygenic multifactorial inheritance has also been hypothesized. No specific gene/s have been identified. Of patients with primary amenorrhea, 23% have vaginal agenesis, and of these patients, 7% have abnormal karyotypes when studied using conventional chromosomal analysis.[7] The abnormalities include Turner's mosaicism, 46,XX t (10q1;12q2); 46,XX del (15)(p11); 46,Xi(xq); 46,XX t (12;14) (14q,13q); 45,X46; XX47,XXX.[10] In one series, 10 of 13 families with one affected member had another relative with vaginal agenesis. Most commonly, an affected paternal relative was identified, suggesting the possibility of a female-linked autosomal dominant pattern. Analysis of data from offspring of patients with vaginal agenesis conceived through assisted reproductive technologies suggest that if the condition is genetically transmitted it is not inherited in a dominant fashion.[11]

Environmental causation has been demonstrated in laboratory animals by dietary administration of teratogens and supported in humans by a case in a series associated with fetal alcohol syndrome.[9] However, there appears to be no relationship of vaginal agenesis to diet, work environment, chemical exposure, drugs, radiation, or infections.

Clinical Correlates

Vaginal agenesis is a result of arrested development of the mullerian ducts. The external genitalia have a normal appearance. A small depression or dimple may be present where the vaginal opening should be. Vaginal agenesis is diagnosed by the presence of a blind vaginal pouch and is seldom connected with any forms of intersexuality. The principal clinical features of the syndrome are primary amenorrhea,[12] a 46,XX karyotype, variable development of rudimentary uterine and tubal remnants, normal ovarian function, normal female habitus with normal pubertal landmarks, and the frequent association of renal, skeletal, and other congenital anomalies. Congenital absence of the vagina is consistently associated with amenorrhea (100% of patients) and a broad spectrum of other variable clinical findings. In one series, palpable uterine remnants were described in 25% of patients.[13] In this series, 75% of the patients had total agenesis; 11% had partial agenesis; 7% had hematometra; 75% were found to have normal ovaries to inspection. On further evaluation of those ovaries with an abnormal or streak-like appearance, 92% had histologically normal ovaries and normal ovarian function. Depending on the presence or absence of uterine remnants and any functional endometrium, recurrent cyclic pelvic pain has been described in 20% of patients, and when present the fallopian tubes were normal in 32% and rudimentary in 46%.

Congenital absence of the vagina may exist as an isolated finding or in association with uterine and tubal remnants and a more generalized condition involving several other additional systems. Associated abnormalities, primarily renal and skeletal, are present in 30% to 40% of patients. Renal abnormalities include unilateral horseshoe and pelvic kidneys and minor abnormalities such as malrotation in the collecting system and double collecting systems. There is a 12% incidence of skeletal abnormalities primarily spinal in the cervical and lumbar vertebrae.[14] These include wedge vertebrae, fusion defects, rudimentary vertebral bodies, and spinal asymmetry such as kyphosis and scoliosis. Abnormalities of the skeletal structures of the hand, including radial and scaphoid hypoplasia, abnormally formed and positioned trapezium, and slender first metacarpal may also be present.[15]

The association of congenital absence of the vagina with other system abnormalities has led to the description of two separate entities, referred to as typical and atypical forms of the syndrome.[14,16,17] This distinction offers a clinically useful approach to differentiate those patients with vaginal agenesis as a sole problem from those most likely to have multiple system involvement in addition to vaginal agenesis. The cornerstone of this differentiation is the symmetry or asymmetry of any additional mullerian structures. The typical form of the syndrome is characterized by symmetrical abnormalities, such as small uterine buds and remnants or completely developed fallopian tubes, and accounts for 46% of patients. The atypical form of the syndrome includes patients with asymmetric pelvic abnormalities and accounts for 54% of patients. These asymmetric abnormalities include unilateral uterine remnants and fallopian tubes. Abnormalities in other systems, whether skeletal, renal, or ovarian, are found almost exclusively in patients with asymmetric pelvic abnormalities. These other system involvements include spinal abnormalities, especially Klippel-Feil syndrome and variants of the more expanded syndrome of mullerian hypoplasia/aplasia, renal agenesis, cervicothoracic somite dysplasia (MURCS).[18] A variation of the MURCS syndrome is an association of vaginal agenesis with renal agenesis, ectopia, and cervicospinal dysplasia.[19] This association occurs in as many as 20% of patients with poorly developed or absent fallopian tubes and asymmetric bud development.

The symmetry or asymmetry of mullerian structures can be used as a guide to determine which patients require extensive evaluations. (In some studies, the designations type A and type B vaginal agenesis are used for typical and atypical forms.) Table 4-1 summarizes the main clinical features of vaginal agenesis.

Diagnostic Studies

Clinical examination and pelvic imaging are the cornerstones of diagnosis. Care must be exercised for adolescent patients suspected of having vaginal agenesis. For many of these patients, this evaluation may be their first encounter with a provider of women's health care and perhaps their first need for a gynecologic examination. A caring and thoughtful attitude is

Table 4-1. Principal Clinical Features of Vaginal Agenesis
• Primary amenorrhea associated with congenital absence of the vagina 46,XX karyotype
• Uterus that varies from symmetric or asymmetric rudimentary uterus buds to complete absence
• Normal ovarian function and normal ovulation
• Normal female breast development, body proportions, and body hair
• Frequent association of renal, skeletal, and other congenital anomalies (depending on type A or type B)
• Gestational surrogacy to fulfill reproductive potential

essential in approaching any patient in this category. This diagnosis will have far-reaching implications for the patient regarding identity, sexuality, self-image and reproduction. The initial appointment should be used to establish trust and solid lines of communication. Several options for counseling exist. For some patients, a discussion beforehand with the patient's family, suggesting that the family review with the patient what will take place during the examination, may be helpful. In other circumstances, direct discussion with the adolescent patient may be best. Regardless of the attempts to prepare the patient, in some circumstances a clinical examination will be extremely difficult, if not impossible. In these circumstances, little will be gained subjecting the patient to an uncomfortable and threatening examination. In such circumstances, it is more appropriate to proceed with transabdominal ultrasound or magnetic resonance imaging (MRI) to define pelvic anatomy in as noninvasive and nonthreatening a fashion as possible.[20–22] Most patients will fall into this category. For this group, the initial visit(s) should focus on discussion and establishing trust. If appropriate, counseling may be suggested as an option as the evaluation progresses.

Transabdominal ultrasound to assess the presence or absence of a uterus or uterine remnants in a patient suspected of having congenital obstructive lesions of the vagina is essential.[23] The procedure is especially important for children and early adolescents. Even in circumstances in which clinical examination can be successfully performed, differentiation between a transverse vaginal septum, vaginal agenesis, or congenital absence of the cervix cannot be made solely by clinical examination.[24] In this regard, transabdominal ultrasound provides important information on which to plan therapy. This technique for patients with obstructed uterovaginal anomalies has provided a sensitive and specific means of assessing the presence or absence of the uterus, uterine remnants, or functioning endometrium in identified remnants. In patients for whom equivocal findings are noted on transabdominal ultrasound examination, MRI may be informative.[25] MRI may provide more details and be useful in demonstrating the presence or absence of uterine remnants and any functioning endometrium. MRI will detect uterine remnants in 50% of cases. Smaller remnants may require laparoscopy for detection.[25] MRI may also assist in classification of the abnormality as type A or type B by noninvasively demonstrating the details of the pelvic anatomy, the morphologic characteristics and symmetry of the uterine remnants (if any), and location of the ovaries.[26] When findings are suggestive of an atypical form, such as asymmetric uterine remnants, further evaluation for other abnormalities should be undertaken.[14,16]

Diagnostic laparoscopy may be required for patients in whom imaging techniques provide incomplete information about uterine remnants and ovarian location.[18] Operative laparoscopy in patients who have functioning endometrium within the remnants (an infrequent finding) may also enable removal of the remnants and in select cases to reconstruct the vagina with the Vecchietti procedure. As a prerequisite to any laparoscopy, ultrasound or MRI is essential to assess the presence or absence of uterine remnants and to plan for their possible removal if present.

One of the most important aspects in the evaluation of patients with vaginal agenesis is an assessment of the psychological impact it may have on both the patient and the family (Table 4-2). This assessment is essential at the time of diagnosis, well in advance of any planned therapy. Both the patient and her family present with concerns because of failure to undergo menarche. Expectations are usually focused on reversible causes and medical therapies. The discovery that the etiology is in fact anatomic and irreversible can cause an immense shock. The patient and her family must confront dual concerns regarding both sexual function *and* fulfillment of reproductive potential. A common reaction may be a request to proceed immediately with a surgical

---

Table 4-2.
Vaginal Agenesis: Key Points in Counseling

- Consultation to discuss congenital absence of the vagina apart from any clinical examination. The first evaluation upon referral should focus on the diagnostic possibilities and emphasize that reproductive potential and sexual function may be achieved

- Focus on discussion regarding imaging; i.e., transabdominal ultrasound or magnetic resonance imaging for assessment of pelvic anatomy

- Emphasis on broader clinical definition of sexuality

- Encourage ongoing dialogue of family and patient with a counselor

- Long-term follow-up both with clinical visits and periodic phone consultations

- Assurance that suicide is not considered after diagnosis (given limited case series describing this event)

procedure in hopes of establishing "normalcy". This route is precisely what should be avoided. Immediate surgical intervention may compromise more detailed discussion regarding nonsurgical and less invasive therapies and can jeopardize postoperative compliance. Psychological assessment and appropriate counseling and intervention are absolutely essential prior to considering any management, especially surgical. The patient should be evaluated by a professional trained in psychosocial and sexual adolescent development prior to any therapy.[27,28] This not only will make plans for surgery easier, but with better understanding and insight, also will ensure compliance with the use of dilators in the postoperative period.

Ongoing psychosocial support is essential for these patients after initial evaluation and throughout treatment.[29,30] In one series, 23 patients were interviewed; 22 of them had undergone creation of a neovagina.[31] A consistent finding was diminished self-esteem when a diagnosis of vaginal agenesis was made. Five patients indicated that they felt suicidal. How well the patient accepted the anomaly and therapy appeared to depend on family interactions and physician support. Acceptance did not appear to be related to socioeconomic status. Nineteen of the women reported an increase in self-esteem and good psychosocial function following vaginal reconstruction. Four patients with poor adjustment were described as having poor interpersonal interactions prior to the discovery of the anomaly. These same four patients also experienced various degrees of treatment failure, in part because of lack of compliance with postoperative dilator use. Since all procedures for vaginal reconstruction require strict patient compliance the type of procedure, that is, whether surgical or nonsurgical, may not be as important as the establishment of a stable psychosocial environment in which the treatment takes place. *The need to establish a sound psychological basis before proceeding with any therapy cannot be overemphasized. The potential for fulfillment of both sexual and reproductive potential must be emphasized.*[32]

In most circumstances, congenital absence of the vagina does not present a surgical emergency. No immediate operation is necessary, and a conservative, slow-paced approach is possible. At times, the patient can decide on the timing of the surgery on the basis of how well she has progressed in accepting the congenital abnormality. It may require 12 to 18 months to adjust emotionally and to pursue appropriate counseling in a nonpressured circumstance. Corrective surgery for patients opting for a surgical approach may often be scheduled during summer vacation or other time that avoids conflict with an academic or professional schedule.

Management

The key decisions in the management of congenital absence of the vagina are threefold: assessment of the degree of need for psychosocial support, adequate counseling regarding options and outcomes (as noted above), and the selection of the appropriate approach (surgical or nonsurgical) for an individual patient.[33-35]

In counseling patients at an initial consultation, it is convenient to divide the discussion between the psychological, social, and sexual aspects and the surgical aspects. Patients should be encouraged to seek regular consultation with counselors regarding the former. For some patients, explanations and discussions at clinical evaluations are sufficient. The issues of sexuality and reproduction should be addressed at the very outset. Assurances must be given that both are attainable. Studies describing outcomes of sexual activity in patients with vaginal agenesis as comparable to those of a normal population should be emphasized.[36-40] Gestational surrogacy outcomes are excellent and provide viable options for achieving reproductive potential.[41] A gentle and caring approach in describing the surgical procedure should be undertaken. Balance should be struck between an accurate clinical description and using language acceptable to the patient. The patient should be made to feel as normal as possible; the use of terms such as "artificial vagina" or expressions such as "we can create a vagina" should be avoided.

Contemporary therapy for vaginal agenesis may be nonsurgical (using techniques of self-dilatation) or surgical (using operative laparoscopy or split-thickness skin grafts). An excellent functional result can be achieved by progressive self-dilatation technique or by surgical cavitation using laparoscopy or with skin grafting, although histologic and steroid receptor properties of surgical cavitation are less physiologic than are those of self-dilatation. The previously described techniques of intestinal transposition and labioperineal pouch construction are no longer used as primary treatment. They are secondary considerations for patients in whom the above options are not viable or in whom both nonoperative and operative techniques have failed.

Laparoscopic Technique for Formation of a Neovagina (Vecchietti Procedure)

The goal of the procedure is to establish a vaginal depth of 6–8 cm, adequate for satisfactory intercourse. Laparoscopy is performed in a standard fashion, placing the laparoscope through an infraumbilical puncture.[42-45] Inspection of the pelvic anatomy should identify the exact location of the ovaries in anticipation of IVF and any mullerian remnant not detected during imaging preoperatively. Excision of any remnants may also be undertaken at this time. The apex of the vaginal vault is defined using gentle upward vaginal pressure with a dilator. The Vecchietti needle is passed through the anterior abdominal wall well away from the ureter to the area just above the peritoneum and threaded inferiorly in the subperitoneal space. The needle tip is readily identifiable. The needle is then brought out into the vaginal vault just inferior to the bladder. Care should be exercised in placing the needle precisely below the bladder and just above the rectum. In this location, the vaginal sutures may then be hooked through the Vecchietti needle and drawn subperitoneally to the anterior abdominal wall. The suture is then

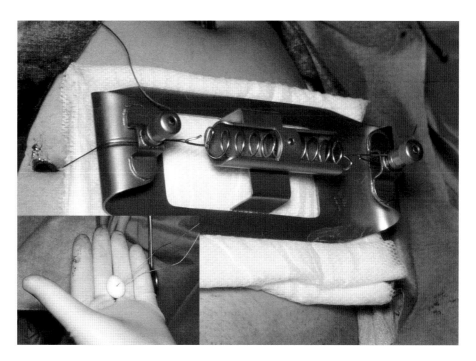

Figure 4-1   Traction device in place on anterior abdominal wall after Vecchietti procedure. Inset: Teflon olive with sutures prior to placement.

passed through an acrylic olive held against the vaginal vault. (Figure 4-1). The procedure is again performed on the opposite side. The sutures passed through the olive are secured suspending the olive against the vaginal dimple by the subperitoneal sutures. The needles are then drawn cephalad retracing their subperitoneal path. The needle and attached sutures are then drawn onto the anterior abdominal wall. The two free ends of the suture on the anterior abdominal wall are then passed through the Vecchietti traction device. The device is placed upon a gauze pad for protection of the underlying skin. The suture ends are then engaged within the device. Adequate traction is then placed on the sutures, snugging the acrylic olive against the apex of the vaginal vault. Adequate traction on the olive should draw the olive snugly against the vaginal dimple yet allow approximately 0.5 to 1.0 cm of movement.

Postoperatively, gradual increments of traction should be empiric: adequate to extend the vagina, prevent mucosal necrosis, and well-tolerated by the patient.[46–49] A schedule to incrementally increase tension should be outlined after surgery, but patient compliance should be the top-most priority. If progress is being made, no change in management is required. If pain or non-compliance are inhibiting progress, the plan should be revised. One gauge of adequacy is the degree of tension on the two springs of the device. The degree of spring traction is typically at a mid-point between minimum and maximum tension. Adjustments of the traction sutures should be made at 48-hour intervals. Periodic inspection of the vaginal vault is required to evaluate the vaginal mucosa. Any areas of pressure or excoriation should prompt relaxation of the sutures until healing is achieved. The traction device and dilating olive may be removed after the neovagina has lengthened to 8 cm. Vaginal dilators are used regularly for approximately three months afterwards.

Vaginal Approach (McIndoe) for Formation Of Neovagina

The McIndoe technique consists of the introduction of a form or stent wrapped in a mesh of split-thickness skin graft or biodegradable membrane such as Interceed® (Johnson and Johnson). The stent is designed to conform exactly to a newly created neovaginal space. Adequate preoperative bowel preparation and prophylactic antibiotics are essential. The procedure is performed in two parts, sequentially, at the same operative setting: harvest of a split-thickness skin graft and creation of a peritoneal space between the bladder and rectum. Appropriate consultation for harvest of the skin graft with plastic surgery may be necessary, depending on an individual surgeon's preference and institutional guidelines.

A split-thickness skin graft can be taken from an area in the gluteal region located within the "bikini line". One method of ensuring that the graft site will be covered by a bathing suit is to have the patient wear a one- or two-piece bathing suit to the operating room and use a skin marker to outline the panty line. This will provide a means of defining the limits in which the graft may be taken. With the patient in the lateral recumbent position, a skin graft of 9 x 15 x 0.02 cm may be taken from the buttock, using a Reese or Brown dermatome.

Once the mesh graft has been harvested, it is sutured around a stent with the raw edge outward. A variety of stents have been described. An inflatable vaginal stent, and a precut (10 x 20 to 25 cm) sponge, plastic or foam-rubber stent have all been used successfully. The most commonly used mold is a foam-rubber mold covered with a condom to minimize pressure and necrosis of the grafted skin.[50] Sponge or foam rubber is inexpensive, easy to tailor to the neovaginal space, and exerts even, gentle pressure in all directions. The foam may be cut with scissors, compressed, and covered by a condom. A trial insertion may be undertaken and the foam stent altered if necessary to better conform to the space after expansion. An additional condom is placed over the form and tied securely. The graft is then sutured to the mold with dermal surface outward, before it is placed in the neovaginal space (Figure 4–2A, B and C). In select cases, an inflatable vaginal stent can be used instead of foam. This appliance can be inflated to variable diameters to fit the size of the neovagina. With this device, the graft and mold are inserted into the vagina and the stent inflated.

After the graft has been sutured to the mold, the patient is placed in the lithotomy position. A Foley catheter is introduced into the bladder. Labia majores may be separated and, only if absolutely necessary, sutured laterally to avoid repeated trauma. The apical point of vaginal depression that will be the site of the future vagina is identified (Figure 4-3), and a horizontal incision is

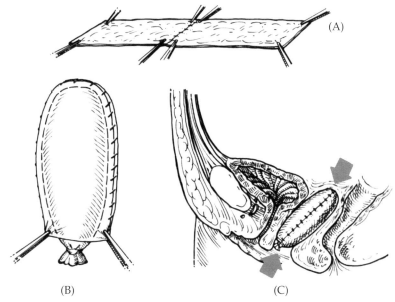

Figure 4-2   A split-thickness skin graft taken from the buttock should measure approximately 10 to 12 by 20 to 35 cm (A) and should be stitched to a suitable mold created from foam rubber and covered by a condom (B). The stent itself may be created from a variety of materials. (C) Cross-section showing the stent in place and its relationship to the bladder anteriorly and rectum posteriorly.

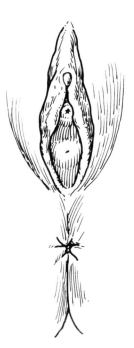

Figure 4-3   Vaginal agenesis. A dimple may be noted upon close inspection of the introitus and provides a point for initiating the dissection.

made at the dimple or depression between the urethral meatus and the anus. Care must be taken to avoid the urethra above and rectum below. The vaginal space is dissected to a depth of 6 to 8 cm by simple blunt digital dissection (Figure 4–4 A and B) as far as the peritoneal vesicorectal reflection between the urethra and bladder at the front and rectal ampulla at the rear (Figure 4–5). After creation of an adequate neovaginal space, the graft and

(A)

(B)

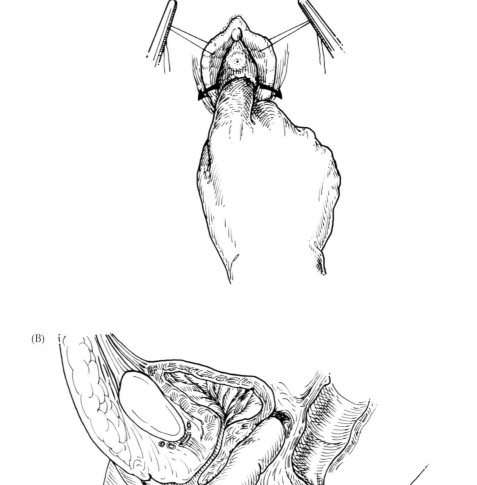

Figure 4-4   By blunt digital dissection, a potential space between the bladder and rectum is developed (A) and the dissection carried to a depth of approximately 6 to 8 cm; (B, lateral view).

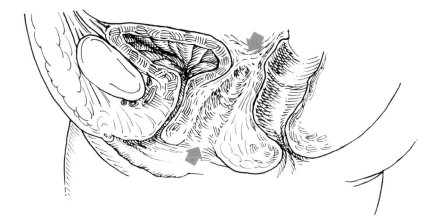

Figure 4-5   At the completion of the dissection, the cavitation should extend from
the introitus at the start to the peritoneum at the apex (arrows).

stent may then be gently inserted into the vagina and the introitus sutured to prevent expulsion.

The stent should be removed in the operating room after approximately 5 or 6 days. After verification that the graft has taken place, a second, soft vaginal stent is inserted and left in place for periodic removal every 2 to 3 days for cleansing during the next 2 to 3 weeks. This stent can be constructed with an inner core of styrofoam and an outer cover of soft foam rubber. The inner core of styrofoam can be molded to a specific size and provides a degree of rigidity to facilitate insertion. This core can then be covered by a layer of soft foam rubber for comfort and compliance. This unit is encased in two condoms. The outer condom can be changed frequently without altering the shape of the stent. Since McIndoe's original description, several modifications of the procedure have been described, each with acceptable results.[46,50] Modifications have included a shorter interval from the initial placement to the first mold removal, prophylactic antibiotics to prevent infections, and a variety of different forms on which to make the graft.

Dilators should be used for 4 to 6 months after the procedure. Longer intervals without any stent may then be instituted. Intercourse may be attempted when examination reveals complete healing of the graft site and supple vaginal walls. One gauge of the adequacy of the vaginal vault is the ease of insertion of the stent and lack of dyspareunia. The interval without the stent may be gradually increased, provided that reinsertion is without difficulty and there is no dyspareunia. Should the patient experience difficulty in reinserting the stent or if dyspareunia occurs, evaluation is warranted. Graft contracture may be occurring. Prolonged (not shorter) wearing of the stent may be necessary in this circumstance. The patient may then change to any one of a variety of other vaginal dilators, such as lucite and soft rubber vaginal dilators, for dilatation and maintenance of the patency and caliber of the vagina (Figures 4-6 and 4-7). These dilators are easier to use and care for and are intended for periodic use. Lucite and soft rubber vaginal dilators are available in sizes ranging from 1 to 2 cm in diameter and in various lengths. Since the goal is a vaginal length of 6 to 8 cm, a stent of 8 to 13 cm can be used. The dilator should be clearly labeled to identify a distance of 8 cm to guide this self-dilation. Continued, gentle, and regular dilatation after surgical reconstruction has increased the functional success rate and lack of dyspareunia.

Intraoperative or early postoperative complications include distal urethrotomy, infected hematoma and subsequent graft failure, expulsion of the vaginal stent and active bleeding necessitating reoperation, perforation of the bladder and rectum, and rectovaginal fistula.[7,32,36] Postoperative vaginal and urinary tract infections, rectovaginal, vesicovaginal, and urethrovaginal fistula formation, infection of the graft donor site, keloid of the graft donor site, and granulation tissue requiring reoperation have also been described.[52,55] Graft contracture may occur in patients who do not use some form of continuous, periodic dilation. The contracture may be overcome by constant and conscientious use of a medium-sized, semi-rigid stent. Alternate ways of dealing with contracture are surgical and involve placement of lateral incisions (at the 3 and 9 o'clock positions), dilation of the vagina, and placement of a stent.

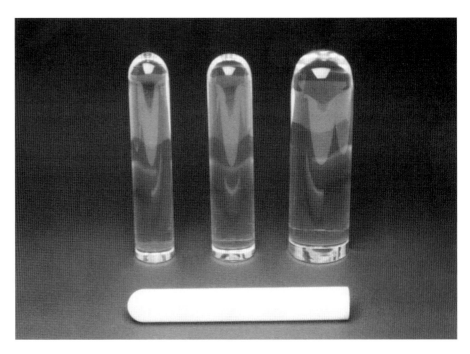

Figure 4-6   Graduated rigid vaginal dilators. Rigid dilators of lucite (background) and polyethylene (foreground), ranging from 1.0 to 3.0 cm in diameter and 8.0 to 12.0 cm in length.

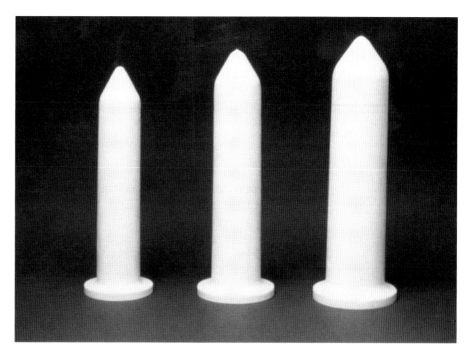

Figure 4-7   Graduated flexible vaginal dilators. Flexible vaginal dilators of silicone, ranging from 2.5 to 3.5 cm in diameter and 12.0 to 14.0 cm in length.

When uterine remnants with functioning endometrial tissue are present, and the clinical history is significant for recurrent abdominal or pelvic pain, laparoscopic removal of the uterine remnants may be performed. As noted above, laparoscopy may be performed as part of the McIndoe procedure as a separate procedure at the time of removal of the stent. Removal of the remnants may be accomplished using the same technique described in Chapter 5 for removal of rudimentary uterine horns.[56–58]

McIndoe vaginoplasty using a split-thickness skin graft is one option for surgical therapy. Several additional techniques have been described.[59–63] An INTERCEED (Johnson & Johnson, Arlington, TX) barrier may be used instead of the skin graft with complete epithelialization in three to six months.[64] A full-thickness skin graft, Z-plasty, and tissue expanders have all had limited trials with satisfactory results, both in terms of surgical ease and coital satisfaction.[65–70]

Nonoperative Management

The Frank procedure of progressive self-dilatation is a nonoperative approach.[71] Success rates vary greatly from 0 to 40%. Failure of the technique may be a result of noncompliance with the recommendations for progressive self-dilatation and because of an inability of the patient to push aggressively enough for adequate duration. The need for absolute compliance and adherence to a rigid schedule of self-dilatation has limited the applicability of the Frank technique. With this technique, vaginal dilation can be carried out at home by the patient. A variety of dilators made of lucite or soft rubber are available as described above. Selection of size should be guided by the diameter and length of the vaginal opening and the attitude of the patient regarding her aggressiveness and comfort level. A graduated series of cylindrical dilators ranging in size from 4 to 5 cm in length and 1 to 1.5 cm in diameter to 8 to 10 cm in length and 2 to 3 cm in diameter can be used.

To assure familiarity and compliance the patient should be instructed carefully in the techniques of using the dilators. The dilator should be lubricated with any vaginal cream. It can be passed into the vaginal dimple with the patient in the supine position, advancing it upward. Patients should advance the dilator to the apex of the vaginal vault, pressing it firmly to achieve slight discomfort. Two daily sessions of 10 to 15 minutes per session are initially required. Clinical follow-up should be at one- to two-month intervals. This frequency may be determined by the patient's need for contact with the medical team, her comfort and compliance level, and her need for encouragement. Clinical examination at each follow-up session should involve an estimation of the vaginal size, measurement of the depth and diameter, and of ease of passage of a dilator. Depending on comfort, a speculum examination may be performed to assess the vaginal mucosa. Periodic consultation with the patient's counselors provides continuity of care and is as essential as clinical examination.

After achievement of a normally sized vagina (6–8 cm) and satisfactory intercourse, periodic dilator use two to three times per week may be all that is required to maintain the caliber and suppleness of the vaginal walls. The most sensitive indicator of the adequacy of vaginal size is satisfactory intercourse. Once this point is reached, follow-up is on an as-needed basis.

To reduce the need for self-dilatation, the Frank technique was translated by Ingram from one requiring active participation to a more passive regimen.[72] This approach in common clinical parlance is sometimes referred to as "the bicycle technique". The four essential components of this technique are a bicycle seat stool, specially designed lucite vaginal dilators, an undergarment to hold the dilators in place, and appropriate support personnel. In some circumstances, an ergonomically designed office chair with a saddle seat and chest support can be used as a substitute for the bicycle seat. The technique involves holding a vaginal dilator in place for a total of 2 hours a day divided into 2 or 3 sessions. The patient sits on a firm bicycle seat and, using her body weight, gentle upward pressure on the dilator is exerted by perineal positioning. The pressure of the dilator against the vaginal apex should be sufficient to cause some discomfort. The greatest advantage is that the patient may carry out daily activities and routines that are possible in a sitting position – the need for a fixed period of time dedicated solely to self-dilatation is eliminated.

The Ingram modification method of the Frank technique has a 75% success rate, and most importantly, no complications. Isolated reports suggest that vaginal prolapse may rarely occur after this method because of the lack of endopelvic support.[73] This complication has not been reported in one series with as long as 54 months of follow-up in some patients.[72] An alternate non-surgical approach involves a technique of interfemoral intercourse. In a series of 33 patients, 24 patients achieved a vaginal depth of 8 cm.[74]

Assisted Reproductive Technologies

Potential for pregnancy in this population is achieved through gestational surrogacy. This option should be presented early in the evaluation to provide a complete profile of reproductive options.

Ovarian responsiveness for assisted reproductive technologies is similar to patients with normal pelvic anatomy. There is no suggestion of diminished ovarian reserve. Number of oocytes, fertilization rates, and clinical pregnancy rates are similar to an age-matched group undergoing IVF for tubal obstruction. Pregnancy outcome using gestational carriers is comparable to outcomes for other patients using carriers.[75] Clinical management of the IVF cycle is conducted in an identical manner to that of any other patient. A few aspects of management are noteworthy. The surgical creation of a neovagina may make transvaginal retrieval more difficult and in some cases impossible. Hence, laparoscopy or transabdominal oocyte retrieval may be more appropriate in this group of patients. Careful assessment of the vaginal walls and depth are essential prior to planning the approach for oocyte retrieval. Precise location of both ovaries is essential prior to IVF. Any abnormally located ovary should prompt laparoscopic retrieval (Table 4-3).

Table 4-3. Evaluation Prior to ART: Vaginal Agenesis
• Clinical assessment of vaginal vault: Depth, suppleness of vaginal walls on examination and ease of access to ovaries on ultrasound
• Monitoring of ovarian responsiveness by transvaginal ultrasound (TVS) examination: Depth and length of vagina must easily accommodate the transvaginal ultrasound imaging
• Transabdominal imaging if TVS not possible
• Consideration of laparoscopic retrieval depending on vaginal anatomy
• Identify location of ovaries to rule out an abdominal ovary and need for transabdominal ultrasound monitoring and laparoscopic retrieval of oocytes from the abdominal site

Outcomes Analysis

Endpoints for success are ill defined in many studies of operative and nonoperative correction of vaginal agenesis. The depth and diameter of the neovagina often may be less than normal anatomically but functionally sufficient. Vaginal length may range from 4 to 8 cm and be adequate for intercourse and sexual responsiveness. The functional results are more important than anatomic approximation of a normal vagina. The key determinant of success is sexual fulfillment. Functional results are difficult to evaluate and quantify because the primary mode of assessment is usually by questionnaire, a technique that has limitations and potential bias.

Overall, the functional success rate with the McIndoe and similar procedures is greater than 80%. Significant complications, for example, fistulas or complete vaginal contraction, is less than 3%.[76,77] In one series, 79 cases were reported with a 100% functional success rate. Sixty patients had 100% success of the graft. Two patients lost the graft because of hematoma and infection; however, they were able to obtain a functional vagina with continued mold placement. In addition, 25% of the patients had contractures of less than 30% of the graft area. No fistulas were reported. In this series, success was attributed to antibiotics, to careful aseptic and hemostatic techniques, to suprapubic catheter drainage of the bladder postoperatively, and to the soft mold.

Long-term follow-up of patients after a vaginoplasty (using as main outcome measures coital adequacy and long-term satisfaction) showed 80% of respondents with good functional satisfaction and 90% stating that the reconstruction had a positive effect on their lives.[32,39,40] In another survey series done by mail, with a follow-up interval of 6.5 years, two rectovaginal fistulas and one graft failure were reported, and 5 of 50 patients required additional reconstructive procedures. Operative vaginoplasty was considered functionally successful by 40 of 47 (85%) of the patients who responded to the survey, yet only 36% of the 40 had remained coitally active by the time of the survey.[52]

Summary and Recommendations

The management of vaginal agenesis has progressed from a variety of surgical techniques using intestinal transposition and amnion in very early cases to the more commonly used Vecchietti procedure and split-thickness skin grafts in select circumstances. Operative laparoscopy using the Vecchietti procedure offers a conservative surgical option without the need for skin grafts. The nonsurgical options include the classic technique described by Frank to Ingram's method of dilatation using a bicycle seat. The technique used for the creation of a neovagina should be tempered in part by the anatomic findings and in part by the patient's interests and ability to comply with techniques of self-dilatation. Follow-up of patients undergoing these procedures is extensive, both by interview and questionnaire. The results are satisfactory from the standpoint of anatomic adequacy and functional satisfaction. Recommendations for the management of vaginal agenesis include the following:

- The presence or absence of any functioning uterine remnants and symptoms of pelvic pain may dictate the need and timing of intervention. In the presence of both, attention should be directed to acute management. Laparoscopy may be undertaken for diagnostic purposes and possible removal of uterine remnants. Operative laparoscopy may also be used for creation of a neovagina. Depending on the acuteness of the circumstances this may best be addressed at a later time.
- Ongoing counseling particularly during the early stages is essential.
- If there is no functioning uterus or nonfunctioning remnants, care should proceed through initial psychological assessment and psychosocial counseling and support.
- Conservative approaches using the dilatation method of Frank or a bicycle-seat tube invagination as described by Ingram may then be attempted.
- If these methods fail, consideration may be given to surgical intervention.
- Fertility potential can be realized through assisted reproductive technology using a gestational carrier.
- Evaluation of other systems may be required and guided by the presence and location of uterine remnants.

References

1. Goldwyn RM. History of attempts to form a vagina. Plast Reconstr Surg 1977;59:319–329.

2. McIndoe AH. An operation for the cure of congenital absence of the vagina. J Obstet Gynaecol Br Commonw 1938;45:490–494.

3. Baldwin JF. The formation of an artificial vagina by intestinal transplantation. Ann Surg 1904;40:398–400.

4. Griffin JE, Edwards C, Madden JD, et al. Congenital absences of the vagina: The Mayer-Rokitansky-Küster-Hauser syndrome. Ann Intern Med 1976;85:224–236.

5. American Fertility Society. The American Fertility Society classifications of adnexal adhesions, distal tubal occlusion, tubal occlusion secondary to tubal ligation, tubal pregnancies, mullerian abnormalities, and intrauterine adhesions. Fertil Steril 1988;49:944–955.

6. Cordeiro P, Pusic A, Disa J. A classification system and reconstructive algorithm for acquired vaginal defects. Plast Reconstr Surg 2002;110:1058–1065.

7. Buttram VC Jr. Mullerian anomalies and their management. Fertil Steril 1983;40:159–163.

8. Lischke JH, Curtis CH, Lamb EJ. Discordance of vaginal agenesis in monozygotic twins. Obstet Gynecol 1973;41:920–924.

9.   Templeman CL, Lam AM, Hertweck SP. Surgical management of vaginal agenesis. Obstet Gynecol Surv 1999;54:583–591.

10.   Jaffe SB, Loucopoulos A, Jewelewicz R. Cytogenetics of mullerian agenesis. A case report. J Reprod Med 1992;37:242–246.

11.   Petrozza JC, Gray MR, David AJ, Reindollar RH. Congenital absence of the uterus and vagina is not commonly transmitted as a dominant genetic trait: outcomes of surrogate pregnancies. Fertil Steril 1997;67:387–389.

12.   Edmonds DK. Vaginal and uterine anomalies in the paediatric and adolescent patient. Curr Opin Obstet Gynecol 2001;13:463–467.

13.   Cali RW, Pratt JH. Congenital absence of the vagina. Long-term results of vaginal reconstruction in 175 cases. Am J Obstet Gynecol 1968;100:752–763.

14.   Strubbe EH, Lemmens JA, Thijn CJ, et al. Spinal abnormalities and the atypical form of the Mayer-Rokitansky-Küster-Hauser syndrome. Skeletal Radiol 1992;21:459–462.

15.   Strubbe EH, Thijn CJP, Willemsen WNP, Lappohn R. Evaluation of radiographic abnormalities of the hand in patients with Mayer-Rokitansky-Küster-Hauser syndrome. Skeletal Radiol 1987;16:227–231.

16.   Strubbe EH, Willemsen WN, Lemmens JA, et al. Mayer-Rokitansky-Küster-Hauser syndrome: distinction between two forms based on excretory urographic, sonographic, and laparoscopic findings. Am J Roentgenol 1993;160:331–334.

17.   Strubbe EH, Cremers CW, Willemsen WN, et al. The Mayer-Rokitansky-Küster-Hauser (MRKH) syndrome without and with associated features: two separate entities? Clin Dysmorphol 1994;3:192–199.

18.   Mahajan P, Kher A, Khungar A, et al. MURCS association—a review of 7 cases. J Postgrad Med 1992;38:109–111.

19.   Duncan PA, Shapiro LR, Stangel JJ, et al. The MURCS Association: Mullerian duct aplasia, renal aplasia, and cervicothoracic somite dysplasia. J Pediatr 1979;95:399–402.

20.   Economy KE, Barnewolt C, Laufer MR. A comparison of MRI and laparoscopy in detecting pelvic structures in cases of vaginal agenesis. J Pediatr Adolesc Gynecol 2002;15:101–104.

21.   Burgis J. Obstructive Mullerian anomalies: case report, diagnosis, and management. Am J Obstet Gynecol 2001;185:338–344.

22.   Minto CL, Hollings N, Hall-Craggs M, Creighton S. Magnetic resonance imaging in the assessment of complex Mullerian anomalies. BJOG 2001;108:791–797.

23.   Paniel BJ, Haddad B, el Medjadji M, Vincent Y. Value of ultrasonography in utero-vaginal aplasia. J Gynecol Obstet Biol Reprod (Paris) 1996;25:128–130.

24.   Blask AR, Sanders RC, Rock JA. Obstructed uterovaginal anomalies: demonstration with sonography. Part II. Teenagers. Radiology 1991;179:84–88.

25. Togashi K, Nishimura K, Itoh K, et al. Vaginal agenesis: classification by MR imaging. Radiology 1987;162:675–677.

26. Barach B, Falces E, Benzian SR. Magnetic resonance imaging for diagnosis and preoperative planning in agenesis of the distal vagina. Ann Plast Surg 1987;19:192–194.

27. Coney PJ. Effects of vaginal agenesis on the adolescent: prognosis for normal sexual and psychological adjustment. Adolesc Pediatr Gynecol 1992;5:8–12.

28. Poland ML, Evans TN. Psychologic aspects of vaginal agenesis. J Reprod Med 1985;30:340–344.

29. Evans TN, Poland ML, Boving RL. Vaginal malformations. Am J Obstet Gynecol 1981;141:910–920.

30. Edmonds R. Malformations of the vagina. Semin Reprod Endocrinol 1988;6:89–98.

31. Strickland JL, Cameron WJ, Krantz KE. Long-term satisfaction of adults undergoing McIndoe vaginoplasty as adolescents. Adolesc Pediatr Gynecol 1993;6:135–137.

32. Selvaggi G, Monstrey S, Depypere H, et al. Creation of a neovagina with use of a pudendal thigh fasciocutaneous flap and restoration of uterovaginal continuity. Fertil Steril 2003;80:607–611.

33. Laufer MR. Congenital absence of the vagina: in search of the perfect solution. When, and by what technique, should a vagina be created? Curr Opin Obstet Gynecol 2002;14:441–444.

34. Robson S, Oliver GD. Management of vaginal agenesis: review of 10 years practice at a tertiary referral centre. Aust NZ J Obstet Gynaecol 2000;40:430–433.

35. Roberts CP, Haber MJ, Rock JA. Vaginal creation for mullerian agenesis. Am J Obstet Gynecol 2001;185:1349–1352.

36. Hecker BR, McGuire LS. Psychosocial function in women treated for vaginal agenesis. Am J Obstet Gynecol 1977;129:543–547.

37. Raboch J, Horejsi J. Sexual life of women with Küster-Rokitansky syndrome. Arch Sex Behav 1982;11:215–220.

38. Goerzen JL, Gidwani GP. Outcome of surgical reconstructive procedures for the treatment of vaginal anomalies. Adolesc Pediatr Gynecol 1994;7:76–80.

39. Klingele CJ, Gebhart JB, Croak AJ, et al. McIndoe procedure for vaginal agenesis: long-term outcome and effect on quality of life. Am J Obstet Gynecol 2003;189:1569–1573.

40. Communal PH, Chevret-Measson M, Golfier F, Raudrant D. Sexuality after sigmoid colpopoiesis in patients with Mayer-Rokitansky-Küster-Hauser Syndrome. Fertil Steril 2003;80:600–606.

41. Batzer FR, Corson SL, Gocial B, et al. Genetic offspring in patients with vaginal agenesis: specific medical and legal issues. Am J Obstet Gynecol 1992;167:1288–1292.

42. Borruto F, Chasen ST, Chervenak FA, Fedele L. The Vecchietti procedure for surgical treatment of vaginal agenesis: comparison of laparoscopy and laparotomy. Int J Gynaecol Obstet 1999;64:153–158.

43. Fedele L, Bianchi S, Zanconato G, Raffaelli R. Laparoscopic creation of a neovagina in patients with Rokitansky syndrome: analysis of 52 cases. Fertil Steril 2000;74:384–389.

44. Vecchietti G. Neovagina della sindrome di Rokitansky-Küster-Hauser. Annu Ostet Gunecol 1965;11:131–147.

45. Veronikis DK, McClure GB, Nichols DH. The Vecchietti operation for constructing a neovagina: indications, instrumentation, and techniques. Obstet Gynecol 1997;90:301–304.

46. Rock JA, Jones HW Jr. Vaginal forms for dilatation and/or to maintain vaginal patency. Fertil Steril 1981;12:187 190.

47. Busacca M, Perino A, Venezia R. Laparoscopic-ultrasonographic combined technique for the creation of a neovagina in Mayer-Rokitansky-Küster-Hauser syndrome. Fertil Steril 1996;66:1039–1041.

48. Laffargue F, Giaclone PL, Boulot P, et al. A laparoscopic procedure for the treatment of vaginal aplasia. Br J Obstet Gynaecol 1995;102:565–567.

49. Vecchietti, G. Le néovagin dans le syndrome de Rokitansky-Küster-Hauser. Rev Med Suisse Romande 1979;99:593–601.

50. Ozek C, Gurler T, Alper M, et al. Modified McIndoe procedure for vaginal agenesis. Ann Plast Surg 1999;43:393–396.

51. Graziano K, Teitelbaum DH, Hirschl RB, Coran AG. Vaginal reconstruction for ambiguous genitalia and congenital absence of the vagina: a 27-year experience. J Pediatr Surg 2002;37:955–960.

52. Buss JG, Lee RA. McIndoe procedure for vaginal agenesis: results and complications. Mayo Clin Proc 1989;64:758–761.

53. Smith MR. Vaginal aplasia: therapeutic options. Am J Obstet Gynecol 1983;146:488–494.

54. Hojsgaard A, Villadsen I. McIndoe procedure for congenital vaginal agenesis: complications and results. Br J Plast Surg 1995;48:97–102.

55. Bryans FE. Management of congenital absence of the vagina. Am J Obstet Gynecol 1981;139:281–284.

56. Casthely S, Maheswaran C, Levy J. Laparoscopy: an important tool in the diagnosis of Rokitansky-Küster-Hauser syndrome. Am J Obstet Gynecol 1974;119:571–572.

57. Chapron C, Morice P, La Tour MD, et al. Laparoscopic management of asymmetric Mayer-Rokitansky-Küster-Hauser syndrome. Hum Reprod 1995;10:369–371.

58. Yeko TR, Parsons AK, Marshall R, Maroulis G. Laparoscopic removal of mullerian remnants in a woman with congenital absence of the vagina. Fertil Steril 1992;57:218–220.

59. Giraldo F. Cutaneous neovaginoplasty using the Malaga flap (vulvoperineal fasciocutaneous flap): a 12-year follow-up. Plast Reconstr Surg 2003;111:1249–1256.

60. Fliegner JR. Long-term satisfaction with Sheares vaginoplasty for congenital absence of the vagina. Aust NZ J Obstet Gynaecol 1996;36:202–204.

61. Wierrani F, Grunberger W. Vaginoplasty using deepithelialized vulvar transposition flaps: the Grunberger method. J Am Coll Surg 2003;196:159–162.

62. Parsons JK, Gearhart SL, Gearhart JP. Vaginal reconstruction utilizing sigmoid colon: Complications and long-term results. J Pediatr Surg 2002;37:629–633.

63. Seccia A, Salgarello M, Sturla M, et al. Neovaginal reconstruction with the modified McIndoe technique: a review of 32 cases. Ann Plast Surg 2002;49:379–384.

64. Jackson ND, Rosenblatt PL. Use of Interceed absorbable barrier for vaginoplasty. Obstet Gynecol 1994;84:1048–1050.

65. Darai E, Soriano D, Thoury A, Bouillot JL. Neovagina construction by combined laparoscopic-perineal sigmoid colpoplasty in a patient with Rokitansky syndrome. J Am Assoc Gynecol Laparosc 2002;9:204–208.

66. Creatsas G, Deligeoroglou E, Makrakis E, et al. Creation of a neovagina following Williams vaginoplasty and the Creatsas modification in 111 patients with Mayer-Rokitansky-Küster-Hauser syndrome. Fertil Steril 2001;76:1036–1040.

67. Chudacoff RM, Alexander J, Alvero R, Segars JH. Tissue expansion vaginoplasty for treatment of congenital vaginal agenesis. Obstet Gynecol 1996;87:865–868.

68. Chen YB, Cheng TJ, Lin HH, Yang YS. Spatial W-plasty full-thickness skin graft for neovaginal reconstruction. Plast Reconstr Surg 1994;94:727–731.

69. Chudacoff RM, Alexander J, Alvero R, Segars JH. Tissue expansion vaginoplasty for treatment of congenital vaginal agenesis. Obstet Gynecol 1996;87:865–868.

70. Serra JM, Sanz J, Ballesteros A, et al. Surgical treatment for congenital absence of the vagina using tissue expansion. Surg Gynecol Obstet 1993;177:158–162.

71. Frank RT. The formation of an artificial vagina without operation. Am J Obstet Gynecol 1938;35:1053–1055.

72. Ingram JM. The bicycle seat stool in the treatment of vaginal agenesis and stenosis: a preliminary report. Am J Obstet Gynecol 1981;140:867–873.

73. Roberts CD, Haber MJ, Rock JA. Vaginal creation for mullerian agenesis. Amer J Obstet Gynecol 2001;185:1349–1353.

74. Lappohn RE. Congenital absence of the vagina—results of conservative treatment. Eur J Obstet Gynecol Reprod Biol 1995;59:183–186.

75. Wood EG, Batzer FR, Corson SL. Ovarian response to gonadotropins, optimal method for oocyte retrieval and pregnancy outcome in patients with vaginal agenesis. Hum Reprod 1999;14:1178–1181.

76. Rock JA, Reeves LA, Retto H, et al. Success following vaginal creation for Mullerian agenesis. Fertil Steril 1983;39:809–813.

77. Rock JA. Anomalous development of the vagina. Semin Reprod Endocrinol 1986;4:13–20.

5 Unicornuate Uterus and Rudimentary Uterine Horn

Labour may be normal in every respect but premature onset ... and complications are frequent ....
— Braxton Hicks, 1881

Among the earliest descriptions of congenital uterine malformations were reports of rudimentary uterine horns. These cases came to clinical attention because of their dramatic presentations. In one of the earliest reports in 1699, Mauriceau described a case of maternal death secondary to a ruptured pregnancy in a rudimentary horn.[1] The early literature focused on the obstetric difficulties and the attendant morbidity and mortality secondary to the catastrophic outcomes associated with these abnormalities. Maternal mortality was high, and it was unusual for the diagnosis to be made prior to a complicated obstetric event.[2] A retrospective collection of 84 cases from the literature published up to 1900 suggested that a noncommunicating rudimentary horn was the most common uterine abnormality and accounted for 78% of cases reported.[3] A mortality of 47% was described in this series. The frequency of this observation reflected a reporting bias. Disasters came to clinical attention. More prevalent but clinically silent abnormalities simply went unnoticed. The clinical entities described in many of these early reports were a combination of a unicornuate uterus with an obstructed rudimentary horn that usually ended in catastrophic events.

With an increased awareness of their clinical significance, interest grew to find a reliable method for earlier diagnosis. The symptom of unilateral dysmenorrhea was considered a reliable symptom of an obstructed horn secondary to retained menstrual products. Hay in 1958 systematized this approach and suggested 10 criteria for the diagnosis of uterine abnormalities including, among others, persistent breech presentation, prematurity, and unilateral pelvic pain.[4] A lower threshold to evaluate suspected abnormalities with HSG and ultrasound led to a more accurate diagnosis and assessment of prevalence of the unicornuate uterus and rudimentary uterine horns among other more common uterine anomalies.

The anatomic abnormalities associated with a unicornuate uterus are a diverse group with several subtle but distinct variations. The utility of a classification system arises as a method to sort and stratify the various subtypes. The unicornuate uterus may be divided into four clinical categories (types II A through D) depending on the presence of a rudimentary horn and the

may be attached to the unicornuate uterus by shared midline myometrium or it may be held in place with fibrous tissue or a thin band of peritoneum. Communicating horns present with less threatening circumstances and term deliveries are possible. Rupture is a potential problem. Their presence, however, should require prompt removal if detected in the non-pregnant state.

Types II-A, II-B, and II-C mullerian anomalies present paired uterine systems differing either in the presence or absence of a functioning endometrium or in the presence or absence of communicating tracts to the adjacent hemi-uterus. A pregnancy in an intact hemi-uterus (the unicornuate uterus) may progress appropriately with spontaneous labor and delivery at term and respond to oxytocin agents when administered.[20] A pregnancy in the rudimentary horn may present with obstetric complications, including intrauterine fetal demise, and rupture of the horn, depending on whether the horn communicates with the vagina. Isolated case reports describe live births.

Of the four types of unicornuate uterus, the presence of a noncommunicating functional rudimentary horn has the most significant implications for obstetric management and perinatal outcome. Pregnancies in noncommunicating rudimentary horns may present as catastrophic events with rupture and hemorrhage. Outcomes are less favorable than for communicating horns and include rupture prior to viability and intrauterine fetal demise necessitating hysterectomy. With early ultrasound monitoring, suspicion may be aroused based on intrauterine growth restriction, malpresentation, or failure to demonstrate continuity between the cervix and lower uterine segment. These findings should prompt more detailed imaging with 3-D ultrasound or MRI. Early diagnosis and better operative intervention when rupture occurs have eliminated maternal mortality in these cases.

The management of a noncommunicating uterine horn depends on the circumstances at diagnosis. If diagnosis is made prior to conception, the horn should be removed. Unfortunately, this abnormality may not be detected until the advanced stages of a pregnancy. Obstetric events in this setting seldom end with spontaneous labor and concerted efforts to induce labor frequently fail. Prior cases of failed induction have used both oxytocin and prostaglandin.[23] One possible explanation for this clinical observation may be the lack of communication between the cervix and lower uterine segment and the role these structures play in integrating labor induction and maintenance. The concept that events at a cervical level are responsible for uterine contractions at parturition was initially put forth in 1941 when Ferguson suggested that mechanical stretching of the cervix enhanced uterine contractions.[24] Prostaglandins from the cervix may act locally to effect dilation and at a higher anatomic level of the myometrium to initiate and sustain regular uterine contractions both through direct action and disruption of uterine decidua.[25] The clinical behavior of a noncommunicating horn appears to further support the concept that all anatomic levels are required to integrate and coordinate labor.

A pregnancy in the intact unicornuate uterus (regardless of associated structures) may progress, with spontaneous labor and delivery at term, and respond to oxytocic agents. A pregnancy in a communicating rudimentary horn is an intermediate circumstance that requires careful ultrasound imaging and monitoring of fetal growth. Term delivery is possible. Care should be individualized. A pregnancy in the rudimentary noncommunicating horn (as noted above) is a complex problem ultimately requiring surgical intervention. Presentation may be variable and the diagnosis not made until the pregnancy is advanced. Ultrasound examination may reveal the absence of a cervix and the presence of an adjacent unicornuate uterus or the pregnancy may progress to an advanced state and end with a failure to initiate spontaneous labor and a resistance to induction with both oxytocin and prostaglandins. The lack of communication between cervical and uterine structures may contribute to the failure in this clinical setting.

Diagnostic Studies

A unicornuate uterus is usually discovered as part of an evaluation for infertility when hysterosalpingography is performed (Figure 5-1).[26] If a hemi-uterus is detected on HSG, the most probable diagnosis is a unicornuate uterus. However, a concerted clinical exam should be undertaken to search for a second cervical os. Bicornuate, bicollis uteri will image as a hemi-uterus if one cervical opening is overlooked. The abnormality may be discovered at

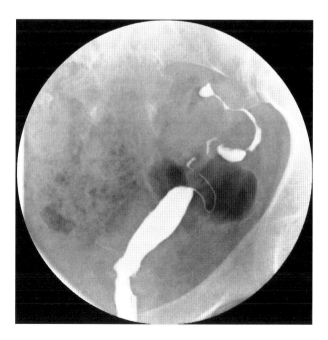

Figure 5-1   Hysterosalpingogram demonstrating left unicornuate uterus with unilateral tubal patency.

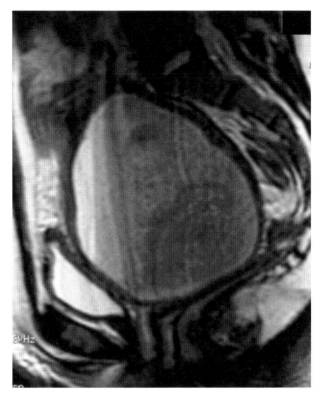

Figure 5-3   MRI image of massive hematometra within an obstructed uterine horn.

demonstrate idiopathic or unexplained infertility, assisted reproductive technologies are an excellent option. In a small series of patients, a pregnancy rate of 90% was described when human menopausal gonadotropins were used to enhance fertility.[34] In one case, triplets were delivered by cesarean section at 33 weeks after such therapy.[35]

The presence of a rudimentary horn does not influence pregnancy outcome when the pregnancy is in the hemi-unicornuate uterus. Management of the rudimentary horn depends on the presence or absence of functioning endometrium within the horn. Conventional teaching held that a rudimentary horn, with or without functioning endometrium, should be removed because of an adverse influence on pregnancy outcomes when the pregnancy occurred in the normal hemi-uterus.[36] Assessment of outcomes from larger series has not substantiated this view.[16,17] Excision of the rudimentary horn without functioning endometrium attached to the unicornuate uterus merely to enhance obstetric outcomes is not warranted. When no functioning endometrium is demonstrated, no intervention is required. When functioning endometrium is present, excision should be considered. In this circumstance, the risk of a pregnancy within the horn, hematometrium and associated abnormalities make a compelling case for surgery (Figure 5-4).

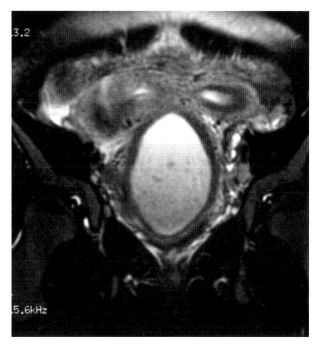

Figure 5-4   Magnetic resonance image of hematocolpos in a patient with an obstructed uterine horn and fistulization of the horn into a blind vaginal pouch. Note endometrial stripes of both normal hemi-uterus (right) and obstructed horn (left).

Reported series suggest that 13% of patients with a noncommunicating rudimentary horn had a pregnancy in the horn probably secondary to transmigration of sperm.[36,38] The possibility of pregnancy in the horn and subsequent rupture warrants removal, especially with endoscopic removal. The diagnosis of a noncommunicating horn is at times made only after the diagnosis of the demise and after attempts at labor induction are unsuccessful. One case report described the diagnosis at the time of an unsuccessful induction using extremely high doses of oxytocin and prostaglandins.[23] A missed abortion or intrauterine fetal demise in the noncommunicating rudimentary horn presents a difficult clinical problem requiring excision of the horn containing the pregnancy.

Management of the tube of the rudimentary horn is controversial. Pregnancies after transposition of the tube from the side of the rudimentary horn to the normal hemi-uterus in circumstances in which the tube of the normal hemi-uterus had been removed after an ectopic pregnancy suggest a possible role for conservation of the tube.[37] The ovary should be left in situ regardless of location with the prospect of future in vitro fertilization. Given success rates of ART, contemporary management should include removal of the tube and conservation of ovary.

Role of Cervical Cerclage

Cervical cerclages is indicated in the management of cervical incompetence. Cervical incompetence has been described in association with any uterine anomaly and may be a contributory cause of poor obstetric outcomes. Cervical incompetence has been described in 15 to 40% of patients with mullerian abnormalities.[39] A cerclage in patients with a unicornuate uterus and repeated loss may improve obstetric outcome.[40] Its exact role is extremely controversial. There are no prospective, randomized trials to support it. The available series are observational, use patients as their own controls and compare reproductive performance prior to and after intervention. Despite these limitations, cerclage placement has a role in patients with the dual problem of cervical incompetence and a unicornuate uterus.

On the basis of this hypothesis, suggestions have been made to place a cervical cerclage as an attempt to prevent first-trimester loss or preterm labor and delivery. The success rate for term deliveries improved in one series to 85% (with a history in the same group of only 22% achieving term deliveries prior to intervention).[41] In another series using a more rigid definition of cervical incompetence, the survival rate increased from 57 to 92%.[42] Cerclage in any anomalous uterus with cervical incompetence may improve both the term-delivery rate and the mean birth weight. A multicenter trial of cervical cerclage in this setting supports the efficacy of cervical cerclage placement for uterine anomalies, regardless of type.[43] Because of the frequency distribution of the types of uterine anomalies, the placement of the cerclage has been most frequent for the bicornuate-unicollis-type uteri. Outcomes are similar for either McDonald or Shirodkar cerclage.

Transabdominal Excision of Obstructed Uterine Horn

Careful discussion and counseling with the patient and the patient's family, depending on age, is necessary in planning whether or not to perform a hemi-hysterectomy. In rare and unusual circumstances there is communication between the horns of sufficient size to consider anastomosis. In general, however, the obstructed horn should be removed. The patient should be carefully counseled regarding possible findings of endometriosis and its impact on reproductive outcome. Management options for endometriosis include fulguration or excision. Management of the tube, i.e., excision or leaving in situ on the obstructed side should be part of the counseling. With the advent of ART, the tube should be removed. A preoperative IVP is essential to identify the precise location of the kidneys and ureters if present on the involved side.

Examination under anesthesia should be undertaken with palpation of the vaginal walls, particularly on the obstructed side, to rule out hematocolpos. An intrauterine catheter system should be placed transcervically for intrauterine chromotubation to verify tubal patency of the normal hemi-uterus before, during, and after surgery.

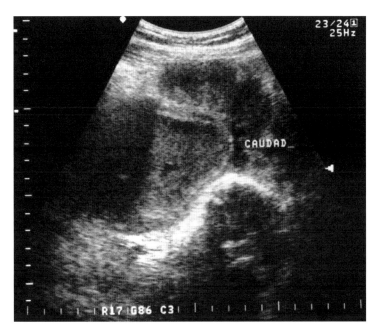

Figure 5-5   Intraoperative ultrasound image of lower segment of obstructed, dilated uterine horn.

A transabdominal approach is necessary in cases when the obstructed horn is dilated (see below for laparoscopic management in circumstances where the uterine horn is small, nondilated, and marginally attached by thin serosal tissues to the contralateral normal hemi-uterus). Depending on circumstances, individual skills and interests, laparoscopy *may* be attempted in this setting. Extreme care is required in patient selection. At the time of surgery, clear definition of the fundus, tube, and ovary on the unaffected side is essential. In cases of a massively dilated rudimentary horn, the anatomy on the contralateral side may be distorted. The obstructed horn may be 3 to 5 times the diameter of the normal hemi-uterus (Figure 5-5). Extreme care is necessary to preserve the architecture on the unaffected side. Chromotubation should reveal a patent tube on that side. Periodic chromotubation during the procedure is suggested to verify continued patency of the uninvolved side.

On the affected side, depending on size, and if dilatation of the horn obscures anatomy, the obstructed horn should be opened and drained. In cases of hematometra, characteristic chocolate fluid is usually contained within the obstructed horn. Occasionally, this will be mixed with mucopurulent fluid suggestive of an occult infection. In extreme circumstances, the myometrial walls and cervical canal will become markedly dilated and thinned, particularly in the lateral portions. The lowermost or caudad portion of the obstructed hemi-uterus may extend well into the ipsilateral paravaginal space (Figure 5-6). Careful dissection into the paravaginal space is often required for excision of the cervical portion of the obstructed horn,

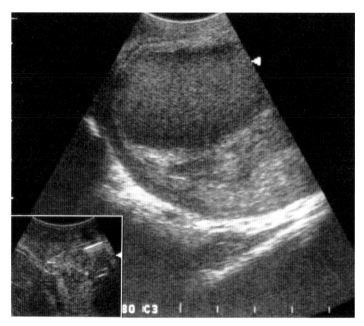

Figure 5-6   Intraoperative ultrasound image using 7.5 MHz finger-grip probe
                    showing hematoma adjacent to normal myometrium. Insert: Image
                    prior to incision and drainage. Note scalpel at upper right of image.

i.e., that area corresponding to the cervix, and beyond the cervix on the contralateral unaffected side. The area of dissection in the paravaginal space will require reapproximation and closure of the dead space after excision.

After opening and draining the obstructed side and defining the anatomy on the contralateral unaffected side, the shared myometrial tissue in the midline is then infiltrated with a dilute vasopressin solution. This tissue can be of variable thickness, from a few millimeters to 1 to 2 cm of myometrium. The line of incision should be as far away from the unaffected side as possible, making certain to remove all viable endometrial tissue from the obstructed side. The uterine vessels are frequently variable in location. Care is required to isolate them and ligate them to minimize blood loss. Identification of the ureter is essential. However, in most cases of obstructed uterine horns the ureter on the affected side is absent secondary to congenital renal agenesis. After excision of the obstructed horn, the incision line is then reapproximated using #0 to 2-0 Vicryl suture. The anatomic end result should be a normal hemi-uterus. After excision of the obstructed horn, attention should then be directed to managing any endometriosis present. Care should be taken to use appropriate techniques to reduce or prevent any possible adhesion formation.

Laparoscopic Technique for Excision of Rudimentary Uterine Horn

Laparoscopic resection of a noncommunicating uterine horn, whether cavitary or noncavitary, may be accomplished using a simple variation of techniques described for laparoscopically assisted hysterectomy.[29,44–50] This approach is restricted to small non dilated uterine remnants and is applicable to a minority of cases. However, depending on surgical skills and interest, this approach may be appropriate in select cases of enlarged horns. Using a four puncture technique, the round ligament should be identified, elevated, cauterized, and divided. A bladder flap should then be created by dissecting the peritoneum from the lower-most portion of the uterine horn and extending the flap just beyond the midline from the cut end of the round ligament medially. The proximal fallopian tube should then be identified, grasped, elevated, and coagulated. This will isolate the rudimentary horn on the lateral aspect. The uterine ovarian pedicle should then be identified. By use of traction and counter-traction and rotating the horn to the midline, the uterine artery may be identified. In some circumstances, the uterine artery may not be present and vasculature to the horn may be aberrant. Care should be taken to identify the ureter (if present). The uterine artery should then be ligated and cut using a linear stapling device or cautery. The dissection should be taken down to the most inferior portion of the horn. By use of counter-traction, the rudimentary horn may then be rotated laterally to expose the fibrous tissue at the medial insertion. The horn may then be resected from its medial attachment to the adjacent hemi-uterus. The specimen may then be removed by morcellation by placing the morcellator through an 11-mm channel in the lower abdomen.[46] The tube may then be excised using a stapler or cautery for resection from the mesosalpinx. Any areas of endometriosis should be coagulated using cautery or laser. A combined laparoscopic-hysteroscopic approach has also been described.[46]

Specific System Defects Associated with Mullerian Anomalies

Abnormalities in the renal and skeletal systems, and to a lesser extent, in the alimentary, cardiovascular, and auditory systems, ovarian malposition, and endometriosis are associated with mullerian abnormalities.

Renal

The association of renal and mullerian tract abnormalities is well known.[45,46] Because of more obvious clinical manifestations, renal tract abnormalities were initially described in several large series and their association with uterine abnormalities was subsequently appreciated.[51,52] The earliest series of congenital genitourinary abnormalities was published in 1932 describing 581 cases of congenital solitary kidney.[52] This study described anomalies of the genital tract in 70% of patients with congenital solitary kidney. The association between mullerian and renal abnormalities ranges from 15 to 30% of the cases of uterine abnormalities.[53,54] Ipsilateral renal agenesis and pelvic kidney have been described in 67 and 15%, respectively (Figure 5-7).[55,56]

Renal cysts, abnormal renal morphology (e.g., horseshoe kidney), and ureteral abnormalities, such as duplication and a bifid collecting system, are

Table 5-1.
Reproductive Outcomes for Unicornuate Uterus

	First and Second Spontaneous Abortion	Preterm Delivery	Term Delivery	Living Children
Pregnancy Rate	49%	13%	41%	49%
	(43,56)	(8,17)	(34,48)	(42,56)

95% confidence intervals in parentheses
References: 13, 16, 17, 18, 19, 22, 32, 21, 33, 81, 82

in situ and 11% without (no statistical difference).[77] In a series of 240 cases, there was an increased incidence of premature rupture of the membranes (89%) between 18 and 35 weeks' gestation, and 11% progressed to fetal viability. In addition, a 50% incidence of breech presentation and IUGR were also described.[17] In another series, delivery was by cesarean section in 80% of patients because of breech presentation, IUGR, and previous cesarean birth. The need for a cervical cerclage for cervical incompetence was 13%.[19]

Pregnancies in rudimentary horns are a complex clinical circumstance influencing both management and outcome. In one review of the literature, 300 cases of rudimentary horn gestations were described; 90% of the cases had horns that were noncommunicating.[36] When pregnancy occurs on the rudimentary side that communicates with the cervix, labor may ensue normally. Labor induction or augmentation may be successfully carried out in these patients. Patients who have a pregnancy in a rudimentary noncommunicating horn and approach term may not go into labor spontaneously and attempts to induce labor suggest oxytocin may fail.[21,23] Ruptures occurred in the second trimester in 89% of these patients, accounting for a high mortality rate. Contemporary descriptions of obstetric outcomes in pregnancies in the rudimentary horn are influenced by early diagnosis and monitoring. Viable deliveries have been achieved in select cases by cesarean section.[79,80]

Summary and Recommendations

A unicornuate uterus is the rarest of the mullerian anomalies. Literature describing reproductive outcomes in this group of patients is primarily observational. The rarity of this abnormality precludes any large-scale comparative series. However, several guidelines for the management of patients with a unicornuate uterus with or without rudimentary horns may be made. The following recommendations are suggested:

- Expectant management of the unicornuate uterus is warranted if the patient's history is unremarkable, that is, no previous episodes of repeated pregnancy loss, second-trimester loss, preterm labor, or preterm birth have occurred.
- If pregnancy occurs, the patient should be monitored as if at risk for preterm labor, preterm rupture of the membranes, preterm dilatation, or cervical incompetence. Monitoring should include serial clinical examinations and ultrasound examinations measuring the cervical length. The patient should also be monitored for IUGR.
- If the patient has an obstetric history of poor outcomes, such as preterm births, perinatal mortality secondary to prematurity, or cervical incompetence, consideration can be given to the placement of a cerclage, though no prospective, randomized studies clearly demonstrate this procedure as advantageous.
- If a rudimentary horn is present with functioning endometrium, consideration should be given to removing the horn prior to pregnancy. If the horn is noncommunicating, it should be removed. If the horn communicates with the cervix, individualization of care is warranted. In most cases the horn will be small and the prospect of delivery low. In this setting, excision is warranted.
- If a rudimentary horn is present without functioning endometrium, no intervention is warranted.
- If infertility is the clinical problem and no other contributing factors are identified, controlled ovarian hyperstimulation with gonadotropins is indicated.
- Outcomes with IVF are favorable and an excellent option. IVF should be considered early in any patient over 35 years.
- Gestational surrogacy is an option for patients with repeated failure, a negative evaluation and a constricted/reduced uterine cavity.

References

1. Jarcho J. Malformations of the uterus. Am J Surg 1946;71:106–125.

2. Rock JA, Schlaff WD. The obstetric consequences of uterovaginal anomalies. Fertil Steril 1985;43:681–692.

3. Mulsow FW. Pregnancy in rudimentary horn of uterus. Am J Obstet Gynecol 1945;40:773–779.

4. Hay D. The diagnosis and significance of minor degrees of uterine abnormality in relation to pregnancy. J Obstet Gynaecol Br Emp 1958;65:557–582.

5. American Fertility Society. The American Fertility Society classifications of adnexal adhesions, distal tubal occlusion, tubal occlusion secondary to tubal ligation, tubal pregnancies, mullerian abnormalities, and intrauterine adhesions. Fertil Steril 1988;49:944–955.

6. Lev-Toaff AS, Kim SS, Toaff ME. Communicating septate uterus with double cervix: a rare malformation. Obstet Gynecol 1992;79:828–830.

45. Yeko TR, Parsons AK, Marshall R, Maroulas G. Laparoscopic removal of mullerian remnants in a woman with congenital absence of the vagina. Fertil Steril 1992;57:218–220.

46. Schattman GL, Grifo JA, Birnbaum S. Laparoscopic resection of a noncommunicating rudimentary uterine horn. A case report. J Reprod Med 1995;40:219–220.

47. Falcone T, Gidwani G, Paraiso M, et al. Anatomical variation in the rudimentary horns of a unicornuate uterus: implications for laparoscopic surgery. Hum Reprod 1997;12:263–265.

48. Perrotin F, Bertrand J, Body G. Laparoscopic surgery of unicornuate uterus with rudimentary uterine horn. Hum Reprod 1999;14:931–933.

49. Nisolle M, Donnez J. Laparoscopic management of a unicornuate uterus with two cavitated, non-communicating rudimentary horns. Hum Reprod 2000;15:1873–1874.

50. Kriplani A, Agarwal N. Hysteroscopic and laparoscopic guided miniaccess hemihysterectomy for non-communicating uterine horn. Archiv Obstet Gynecol 2001;265:162–164.

51. Ashley DJ, Mostofi FK. Renal agenesis and dysgenesis. J Urol 1960;83:211–230.

52. Longo JV, Thompson GJ. Congenital solitary kidney. J Urol 1952;66:63–72.

53. Schattenberg M. Right uterus unicornuate associated with renal agenesis. Am J Obstet Gynecol 1940;40:293–294.

54. Wiersma AF, Peterson LF, Justema EJ. Uterine anomalies associated with unilateral renal agenesis. Obstet Gynecol 1976;47:654–657.

55. Woolf RB, Allen WM. Concomitant malformations: the frequent, simultaneous occurrence of congenital malformations of the reproductive and urinary tracts. Obstet Gynecol 1953;2:236–265.

56. Fedele L, Bianchi S, Agnoli B, et al. Urinary tract anomalies associated with unicornuate uterus. J Urol 1996;155:847–848.

57. Vitko RJ, Cass AS, Winter RB. Anomalies of the genitourinary tract associated with congenital scoliosis and congenital kyphosis. J Urol 1972;108:655–659.

58. Eckford SD, Westgate J. Solitary crossed renal ectopia associated with unicornuate uterus, imperforate anus and congenital scoliosis. J Urol 1996;156:221.

59. Willemsen WN. Renal-skeletal-ear- and facial-anomalies in combination with Mayer-Rokitansky-Küster (MRK) syndrome. Eur J Obstet Gynecol Reprod Biol 1982;14:121–130.

60. Robin NH, Neidich JA, Bason LD, et al. Frontonasal malformation and cloacal exstrophy: a previously unreported association. Clin Genet 1980;18:417–420.

61. Meyers MA. The reno-alimentary relationships. Anatomic-roentgen study of their clinical significance. Am J Roentgenol Radium Ther Nucl Med. 1975;123:386–399.

62. Curtis JA, Sadhu V, Steiner RM. Malposition of the colon in right renal agenesis, ectopia, and anterior nephrectomy. Am J Roentgenol 1977;129:845–850.

63. Letterie GS, Venbrux A, Vaccaro J. Coexistent renal, mullerian and alimentary tract developmental defects. A case report. J Reprod Med 1987;32:153–156.

64. Hsu YR, Chuang JH, Huang CB, Changchien CC. The McKusick-Kaufman hydrometrocolpos-poly-dactyly syndrome—a case report. Changgeng Yi Xue Za Zhi 1994;17:173–177.

65. Letterie GS, Vauss N. Mullerian tract abnormalities and associated auditory defects. J Reprod Med 1991;36:765–768.

66. King LA, Sanchez-Ramos L, Talledo OE, Reindollar RH. Syndrome of genital, renal, and middle ear anomalies: a third family report and report of a pregnancy. Obstet Gynecol 1987;69:491–493.

67. Cruz OL, Pedalini ME, Caropreso CA. Sensorineural hearing loss associated to gonadal dysgenesis in sisters: Perrault's syndrome. Am J Otol 1992;13:82–83.

68. Hilson D. Malformation of ears as a sign of malformation of genito-urinary tract. Br Med J 1957;33:785–789.

69. Winter JS, Kohn G, Mellman WJ, Wagner S. A familial syndrome of renal, genital, and middle ear anomalies. J Pediatr 1968;72:88–93.

70. Pinsky L. A community of human malformation syndromes involving the Mullerian ducts, distal extremities, urinary tract, and ears. Teratology 1974;9:65–79.

71. Park IJ, Jones HW, Nager GT, et al. A new syndrome in two unrelated females: Klippel-Feil deformity, conductive deafness and absent vagina. Birth Defect 1971;7:311–317.

72. Rock JA, Parmley T, Murphy AA, Jones HW. Malposition of the ovary associated with uterine anomalies. Fertil Steril 1986;45:561–563.

73. Demarea R, Devos L. Uterus unicorne avec absence congenitale unilaterale des annexes. Ann d'Anat Pathol 1938;15:1055–1061.

74. Olive DL, Henderson DY. Endometriosis and mullerian anomalies. Obstet Gynecol 1987;69:412–415.

75. Fedele L, Bianchi S, Di Nola G, et al. Endometriosis and nonobstructive mullerian anomalies. Obstet Gynecol 1992;79:515–517.

76. Mecklenberg RS, Krueger PA. Extensive genitourinary anomalies associated with Klippel-Feil syndrome. Am J Dis Child 1974;128:92–93.

77. Liu MM. Unicornuate uterus with rudimentary horn. Int J Gynaecol Obstet 1994;44:149–153.

78. Jarrell J, Effer SB, Mohide PT. Pregnancy in a rudimentary horn with fetal salvage. Am J Obstet Gynecol 1977;127:676–677.

79. Buttram V, Gibbons WE. Mullerian anomalies: a proposed classification. Fertil Steril 1979;32:40–46.

80. Maneschi M, Maneschi F, Fuca G. Reproductive impairment of women with unicornuate uterus. Acta Eur Fertil 1988;24:273–275.

81. Stein AL, March CM. Pregnancy outcome in women with mullerian duct anomalies. J Reprod Med 1990;35:411–414.

82. Moutos DM, Damewood M, Rock JA. A comparison of the reproductive outcome between women with a unicornuate uterus and women with a didelphic uterus. Fertil Steril 1992;58:88–93.

6 *Septate, Arcuate, Bicornuate, and Didelphic Uteri*

Generally, where double uteri in their various forms are associated with infertility,
the cause is never the duplication . . . but other anomalies. . . .
— *Kussmaul, 1870*

Uterine duplication, a generic term commonly used throughout the literature, has fascinated anatomists, embryologists, and clinicians. These abnormalities provide a keyhole view of the early embryology of the female reproductive tract, prompt questions regarding structure and function and challenge clinical management. The interest is longstanding. The earliest description of a "double uterus" was in 1681 by Dionis, who published a case report describing simultaneous pregnancies in each hemi-uterus.[1] In 1859, Kussmaul described in detail a double uterus in autopsy findings of a stillbirth. In 1894, Pfannenstiel presented the first extended case series of 12 cases of uterine didelphys.[2] These early reports were merely descriptive and no more than observational case series. The first report that systematically attempted to address the impact of uterine abnormalities on reproductive potential was published by Miller in 1922,[3,4] and indicated no change in fertility with a 91% pregnancy rate. Of these pregnancies, only 61% went to term.

The understanding of these entities evolved and clinicians proposed options to improve outcomes. The concept of metroplasty for the correction of uterine duplication was initially described in 1884 by Ruge.[5] In a case report, he described the excision of a uterine septum in a patient with a history of two first-trimester losses with follow-up of a term delivery after resection. The procedure performed by Ruge consisted of a transcervical resection of the septum by passage of scissors through the endocervical canal into the uterine cavity. Transabdominal metroplasty gained notoriety after Strassmann in Germany described the procedure for bicornuate uterus in 1907 and reported a series of 17 metroplasties (a procedure that now bears his name).[6] Enthusiasm increased as additional reports suggested that the unification process would improve term deliveries in a variety of circumstances. Metroplasty became a standard for both bicornuate and septate uteri. Transabdominal metroplasties for septate uteri were described in the late 1940s and early 1950s by Tompkins and Jones.[7,8]

Surgical correction and unification for both bicornuate and septate uteri became the standard of care with variable outcomes. Differing descriptive terms and lack of clear, precise definitions regarding types of abnormalities and outcomes made comparison of data nearly impossible. The condition known as *uterine duplication* represents a broad spectrum of changes ranging from complete duplication to subtle midline septal defects. As one possible solution, Kermauner in 1912 and Jarcho in 1946 proposed methods of classification based on anatomic findings and embryologic development.[9] These classification schemes served as a crude guide for determining which patients needed surgery and for monitoring outcomes after surgery. The classifications were the first attempts to separate septate from bicornuate from didelphic uteri and to report pregnancies with the acknowledgment of potential differences in outcomes based on the type of abnormality. Thereafter, several classification systems evolved to better define patient populations that would benefit from surgical intervention. Revisions of the classifications continued and led to several systems currently in use. None has proven to be without shortcoming in part due to the extreme variability of these abnormalities across a wide spectrum. One system stratifies these abnormalities based on the degree of unification.[10] The classification includes didelphys (type III – two cervices, two cavities, external cleft), bicornuate (type IV – one cervix, two cavities, external cleft), septate uterus (type V – one uterus, smooth external contour, two cavities with deep division), and arcuate (type VI – one uterus, smooth contour, two cavities with minor division).

Conceptually, these abnormalities are best viewed as a series of subtle changes. The subtleties and variations at times defy strict categorization. All forms of duplication abnormalities may be found clinically. Not all uterine abnormalities will fit precisely into one category or another, as suggested by the number of case reports of unique variants of uterine duplication that appear each year. The more commonly encountered abnormalities may be classified into types, but others fall at different points along the spectrum of changes not captured by any classification system. The clinical approach to uterine duplication abnormalities should be broadly based, keeping in mind that failure to fuse can occur at any point in the process from completely separate systems during downward migration to complete midline fusion. The objective of this chapter is to describe the four common forms of uterine duplication and discuss diagnosis, proper selection for surgical repair, outcomes, and management prior to ART.

Etiology

The etiology of uterine duplication is unclear. A genetic basis has been suggested, possibly multifactorial and polygenic.[11,12] Several family aggregates of incomplete mullerian fusion and related system defects have been reported. Incomplete mullerian fusion may be part of several genetically determined malformation syndromes, such as hand-foot-uterus syndrome (in which a bicornuate uterus is associated with malformation of the hands and feet), Meckel syndrome, Fraser's syndrome, and Rudiger syndrome (see Chapter 3).[13–16] The ideal genetic study to sort out these subtleties would be difficult, if not impossible, to perform. Such a study would require detailed study of asymptomatic relatives by hysterosalpingography (HSG), hysteroscopy, ultrasound, or magnetic resonance imaging (MRI). Because of these difficulties, understanding of the precise genetics and mode of inheritance is limited.

A pilot study was performed that provided some insight.[17] Twenty-four patients were studied. Only 1 of 37 (2.7%) sisters had a clinically symptomatic uterine abnormality and no other relatives were affected. The 2.7% frequency of affected siblings represents the minimal number of affected relatives. Those with minor uterine abnormalities would not have been recognized by the study inclusion criteria. The relatively low frequency of first-degree female relatives with incomplete mullerian fusion is not without clinical significance. That approximately 3% of female siblings were affected remains consistent with a polygenic or multifactorial cause. The study reported two families in which mullerian abnormalities or renal agenesis appeared to be caused by an autosomal dominant gene that produces unilateral or bilateral renal agenesis and a spectrum of mullerian abnormalities.

The clinical significance of these abnormalities is ultimately their influence on reproductive outcome.[18–20] The etiology of the adverse influence of bicornuate, septate, and didelphic uterine abnormalities on obstetric outcome is unclear. The altered volume of the cavity may contribute to fetal malposition, premature rupture of the membranes, or incompetent cervix and repeated pregnancy loss. A vascular pathogenesis has been proposed as an etiology of poor obstetric outcome for these abnormalities compared with the capacity of a normal uterus.[21–23] The theory maintains that the normal uterus and endometrium are reached directly by spiral and radial arterials from the medial side and by anastomosis between the arcuate arteries of the lateral sides. In uterine duplication the medial endometrium shared by the two half-cavities is vascularized by small noncommunicating radial arteries that limit vascularization to this area of the endometrium. Poor vascular supply in the medial region may contribute to these adverse obstetric outcomes. Congenital arteriovenous malformations have also been described in association with mullerian abnormalities and may also contribute to poor outcomes.[24–26] Alterations in endometrial receptivity and functionality as part of this spectrum of change has not been evaluated.

There is a well-defined association between congenital uterine anomalies and repeated pregnancy loss and preterm labor. An association with primary infertility is more controversial. Primary infertility has been described secondary to associated malformations of the uterus. This interpretation of early literature has led to the suggestion that a metroplasty may have a role in managing infertility. No prospective, comparative data support this contention. The duration of infertility, associated conditions, and male factor infertility have been poorly controlled, making the relationships between primary infertility and the anomalous uterus controversial. Any uterine reconstruction strictly for infertility should be avoided. In addition to the increased rates of preterm delivery, enhanced first-trimester loss, and prematurity, a series of case reports describe fetal abnormalities suspected to be secondary to uterine structural abnormalities and secondary to the uterine constraint these abnormalities may pose to fetal growth. These reports have led to yet another indication for performing metroplasty.[27,28]

Clinical Correlates

The incidence of uterine duplication is broad and depends on the type of abnormality studied and the thoroughness of evaluation. In the normal fertile population, the overall incidence ranges from 1 to 3%.[29,30] The incidence for uterine didelphys ranges from 3 to 30%; for bicornuate uterus, 5 to 10%; and for septate and arcuate uteri, 5 to 37%.[31] As such, their incidental finding in the course of an evaluation for problems not related to reproductive or gynecologic problems does not warrant intervention. The need for intervention is dictated by presenting complaints and overall reproductive plans.

Even the mildest mullerian anomalies may have gynecologic and obstetric implications and may require evaluation in significant clinical settings. Minor indentations of the uterine cavity were associated with increased rates of abnormal uterine bleeding and increased first-trimester loss.[32,33] The authors of the study defined the abnormalities as a ratio between the distance from the nadir of the fundal indentation to a line connecting summits of the uterine horns and the length of this line greater than 0.15. This group had a high risk of adverse pregnancy outcomes, and about half the pregnancies (42%) in this group were judged likely to be complicated in one or more ways.

A broad range of obstetric complications have been described in association with these uterine anomalies in excess of complications for control populations.[9,18,31,34] First-trimester spontaneous loss rate is increased with ranges from 21 to 50%.[34] Placental abruption, abnormal presentation, premature rupture of membranes, preterm labor, and postpartum hemorrhage are also increased in patients with these abnormalities.[35] The term birth rate is also reduced (55 to 60% versus 85 to 90% in control populations).[18,34]

Reproductive outcomes vary, depending on the uterine abnormality studied (see Table 6-1).[36–38] The variable outcomes in earlier studies are caused mainly by a lack of precise classification techniques and poor study designs. Earlier studies with very limited numbers suggested an increase in repeated pregnancy loss and fetal anomalies.[27,28] In patients with this history, a thorough evaluation for all potential factors contributory to adverse outcomes other than the uterine abnormality is required. If none are identified, these patients may benefit from surgical intervention. Future studies of homogeneous populations may provide more definitive data to guide counseling and decisions regarding optimal circumstances for either observation or surgical intervention.

The incidence of infertility in a population with uterine abnormalities is similar to that in the control population. The etiologic relationships between primary infertility and the uterine abnormalities is unproven.[39,40]

| Table 6-1. |
| Evaluation Prior to ART: Uterine Duplication |

- Option of preoperative GnRH suppression prior to resection in patients < 35 years

- Avoidance of suppression in patients > 35 years given changes in ovarian function and possible delay in resumption of ovarian responsiveness to gonadotropin

- Postoperative evaluation of the endometrial cavity with hysterosalpingography or hysteroscopy

- Prior to IVF, ultrasound evaluation of endometrial thickness two months after resection of a uterine septum

- In bicornuate uterus assessment of endometrial thickness in each cavity, selecting the most optimal endometrial thickness and most accessible cavity for transfer

- Definition of cervical anatomy in patients with bicornuate bicollis uterus to assess ease of passage of embryo transfer catheter through each of the two endocervical canals

Nonuterine causes of infertility must be ruled out before metroplasty is considered as a last resort. No prospective data support the role of metroplasty as a treatment for infertility in this population. Difficult clinical decisions arise when a uterine abnormality such as a septum is discovered during an infertility evaluation for a patient with advanced reproductive age (age ≥ 38 years) or anticipating in vitro fertilization. In these circumstances, due to the potential impact on first trimester loss, detailed discussion with the patient is required and hysteroscopic resection may be considered.

Uterine abnormalities are frequently accompanied by a vaginal septum.[18,31] Uterus didelphys is associated with a septum in 75% of the cases, septate uteri in 25%, and bicornuate uteri in less than 5%. The vaginal septum may be limited to the apex of the vagina or extend to the introitus. Concomitant renal abnormalities are present in approximately 15% to 30% of the cases. The incidence of renal agenesis ranges from 9 to 20% (see Chapter 1).[33]

Diagnostic Studies

Hysterosalpingography

HSG remains a reliable screening procedure to evaluate uterine anatomy. Uterine abnormalities diagnosed by HSG are commonly detected in the course of evaluation for irregular bleeding, repeated pregnancy loss, fetal malpresentation, infertility, and at times, an abnormal clinical examination suspicious for uterine duplication. Radiographs typically present two cavities separated by a midline region that fails to opacify (Figures 6-1 and 6-2). Diagnostic abilities of HSG are limited to defining the number of cavities. The study does not provide sufficient detail for precise classification of the type of anomaly. With the advent of endoscopic techniques, the differentiation between septate and bicornuate uteri is essential: a septate uterus can be managed transcervically with a resectoscopic or hysteroscopic resection of

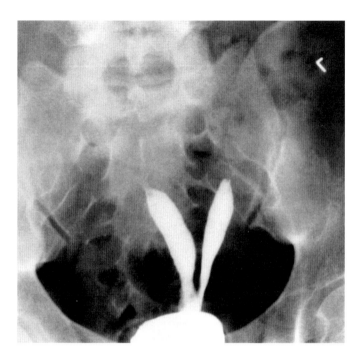

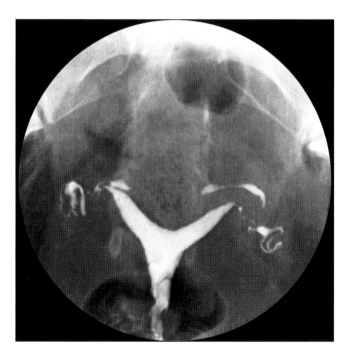

Figure 6-1   A hysterosalpingogram of a bicornuate uterus (A) and a septate uterus
                  (B). In spite of the differing appearances on hysterosalpingogram, no
                  conclusion can be made regarding the exact type of uterine abnormal-
                  ity. Definitive diagnosis requires definition of the configuration of the
                  external uterine surface.

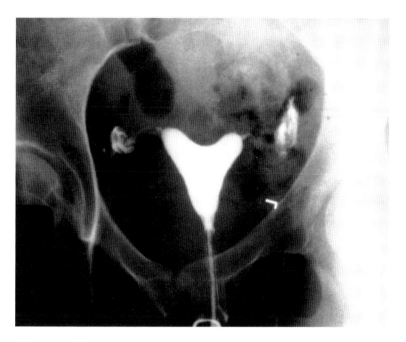

Figure 6-2   Hysterosalpingogram of an arcuate uterus.

the septum. Bicornuate uteri, if management is required, must be managed transabdominally. Definition of the fundal contour is essential for classification and deciding the necessity and type of operative approach. HSG provides information only about the interior of the uterine cavities. No differentiation between septate and bicornuate or didelphic uteri can be made. Additional studies are needed to define the external fundal contour to differentiate these two anomalies. Traditional teachings describe an angle of divergence of the two cavities less than 75° or depth of the septum as sufficient for differentiating a septate from a bicornuate uterus. However, this approach is not sufficiently sensitive to plan surgical therapy. Additional evaluation is required, as described below.

For a didelphic uterus, both cervical orifices may be difficult to visualize on speculum exam. The cervical orifice of the second hemi-uterus may be subtle and displaced to the lateral aspect of the cervix or hidden by a partial longitudinal vaginal septum. A single cervical canal may be identified, cannulated, and the contrast injected. The image may then be one of a hemi-uterus suggestive of a unicornuate uterus (Figure 6-3A). Any image of a hemi-uterus suggesting a unicornuate uterus should prompt careful inspection to locate a second cervical os. If this is found, injection of contrast will produce the second half of the didelphic system (Figure 6-3B). Hence, the differential diagnosis of a hemiuterus on HSG should always include a didelphic uterus and unicornuate uterus. These findings require clinical exam to locate a second cervical os, and if this is not found, ultrasound examination to rule out a vaginal septum occluding visualization of the contralateral os.

(A)

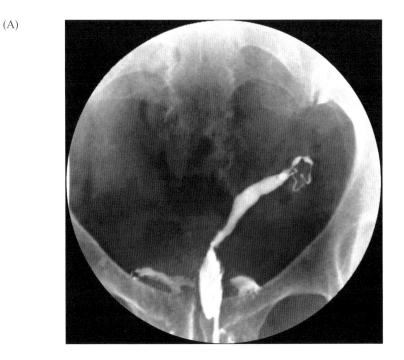

(B)

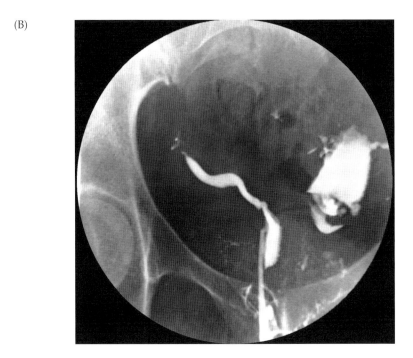

Figure 6-3   Hysterosalpingogram of didelphic uterus. Injection of contrast through left cervical os reveals normal hemi-uterus (A). Repeat injection on right reveals separate right hemi-uterus (B). Note pooled contrast at left.

Ultrasound Imaging

Both 2-D and 3-D transabdominal and transvaginal ultrasound imaging are sensitive and specific methods to assess the interior of the uterine cavity and contour of the external uterine surface.[39-41] Transvaginal ultrasound imaging has been shown to be comparable to HSG and MRI (Figure 6-4 A and B).[42]

(A)

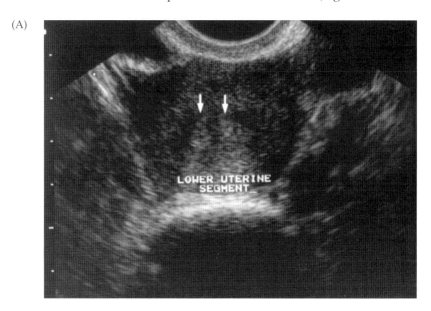

(B)

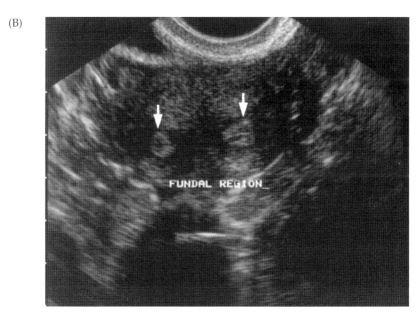

Figure 6-4   Transvaginal ultrasound image of a bicornuate uterus. Note two endometrial cavities at the lower uterine segment in close proximity (arrows) (A). The same two cavities are imaged in the fundal region laterally displaced (arrows) (B)

Transabdominal ultrasound imaging is an efficient and cost-effective preoperative screening exam to define the external contour of the uterus.[43,44] The criteria to assess the external contour and the uterine cavity and differentiate septate from bicornuate uteri include the size and contour of the uterus, the configuration of the endometrial cavity, the presence of a sagittal notch at the uterine fundus and its depth in millimeters, the width (in degrees) of the angle between the inner margins of the two endometrial cavities, and the depth of the myometrial septum (sometimes called "spur" or the lowest point in the endometrial cavity of the division between the two cavities).[45,46] A bicornuate or didelphic uterus may be separated from a septal defect when a fundal indentation greater than 10 mm or any angle between the medial margins of the two cavities not greater than 60° is noted. Transabdominal ultrasound using these criteria correctly identified 90% of the cases of didelphic and bicornuate uteri and 100% of septate uteri, the sensitivity in diagnosing bicornuate uteri was 92% and specificity was 100%.[43]

On transvaginal ultrasound imaging, a septate uterus demonstrates a convex, flat fundal contour with an echogenic mass dividing the endometrial canals. The echoes in the septum are similar to those in the adjacent myometrium. The septum may be partial (i.e., incomplete division of the uterus) or complete (i.e., extending to the endocervical canal). The distal portion of the complete septum may be somewhat hypoechoic relative to the myometrium compatible with fibrous tissue. In a bicornuate uterus, a fundal cleft larger than 1 cm may be demonstrated, with divergent uterine horns and a clearly demonstrated single cervix. The image appearance for a didelphic uterus similarly should demonstrate a large fundal cleft with divergent uterine horns and cervical duplication. A secondary consideration in ultrasound assessment in this clinical setting is the ability to assess the presence or absence and exact location of the renal structures. Ultrasound evaluation of renal anatomy does not reliably define ureteral and bladder structures, two components of the renal system likely to be affected. Intravenous pyelography should be considered for definition of these additional structures.

Three-dimensional ultrasound imaging provides details of uterine anatomy not present in conventional two-dimensional ultrasound.[47,48] The advantages of three-dimensional ultrasound include the ability to reconstruct anatomy with a precision regarding uterine structure and shape not possible in conventional two-dimensional ultrasound. In a study of 42 patients who underwent laparoscopy and HSG, uterine abnormalities were discovered by three-dimensional ultrasound in 12 patients. In 11 of these 12 (92%), correct classification and correlation with laparoscopy was made (see Chapter 3).[47] Volume and surface rendering may also provide information on fundal shape and cavity dimensions (Figure 6-5).

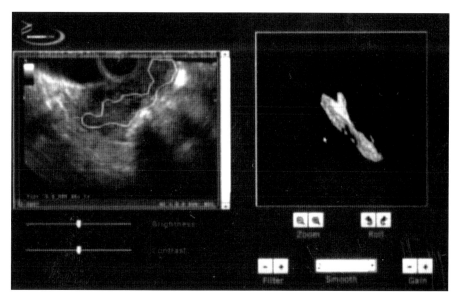

Figure 6-5   Three-dimensional reconstruction of ultrasound images of endometrial
                    cavity of a septate uterus.

Magnetic Resonance Imaging

MRI may be used to diagnose mullerian uterine abnormalities (Figures 6-6 and 6-7). It offers a noninvasive approach to potentially avoid laparoscopy to assess the external contour of the uterine cavity when two cavities have been described by HSG or pelvic ultrasonography. The method has a sensitivity of 100% and specificity of 78%. In MRI, the size and contour of the uterus and the configuration of the endometrial cavity can be analyzed. Attention should be given to detecting a sagittal notch in the uterine fundus and measuring its depth in millimeters. The width of the angle between the inner margins of the two endometrial hemicavities (in degrees) and the depth of the myometrial spur separating the two hemicavities and the level of its lower apex (uterine cavity, cervical canal) should also be measured.[50] Both T1- and T2-weighted images are useful in defining the shape of the uterus, differentiating septate from didelphic or bicornuate uterus, and assessing the thickness of a vaginal septum if present (Figure 6-8 A and B). Signal intensity characteristics of the uterus are homogeneous with medium signal intensity on T1-weighted images. On T2-weighted images, there is a differentiation of the zonal anatomy with a high signal intensity of the endometrium and myometrium separated by a linear low signal intensity of the junctional zone. The endometrial/myometrial width and ratio measurements should be made on the lateral wall and may aid in differentiating types of fusion defects.

MRI criteria for the diagnosis of didelphic, bicornuate, and septate uterus are as follows. For didelphys, a double uterus including separate cervix and

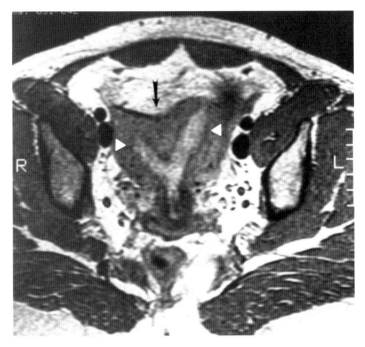

Figure 6-6   Axial T2-weighted MRI demonstrating a bicornuate uterus. Note the cleavage in the fundal region (arrow) and the two endometrial stripes in the respective horns (arrowheads).

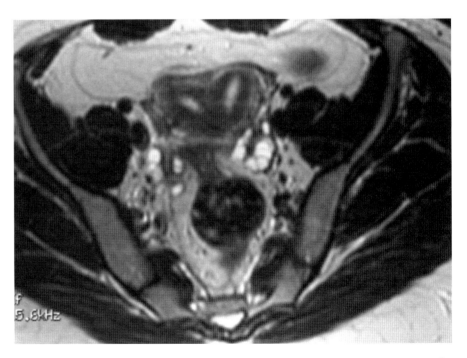

Figure 6-7   Axial T2-weighted MRI in a patient with a septate uterus. Note the smooth fundal contour and two endometrial cavities.

(A)

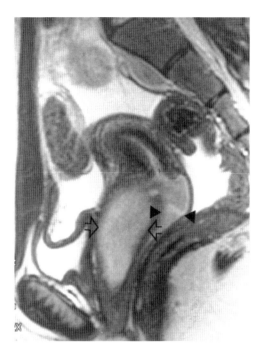

(B)

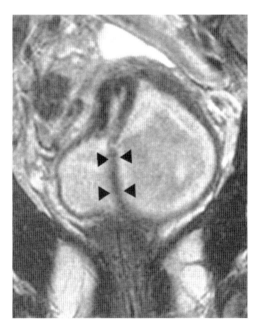

Figure 6-8   MRI of obstructive left vaginal septum in a patient with a didelphic uterus. Sagittal view to left of midline shows a left obstructed hemivagina distended with blood (arrows) and a partially obstructed right communicating hemivagina (arrowheads). Distension with hemivagina was sufficient to compress patent right (A). Coronal view demonstrates 5-mm vaginal septum (arrowheads) (B).

vagina should be demonstrated. Each uterine cavity should have an equal volume, well-demonstrated endometrium and myometrium, and a normal endometrial to myometrial ratio. In a bicornuate uterus, the uterine fundus presents a characteristic downward depression or dimple with two separate uteri clearly visualized, and an intracornual distance greater than 4 cm. In a septate uterus, the fundal convexity should protrude outward, with normal intracornual distance measuring 2 to 4 cm. There should be a high signal intensity at the uterine fundus, and the myometrium, and a low signal intensity within the fibrous tissue of the septum. Each cavity may be somewhat reduced in volume, with a normal endometrial to myometrial width and ratio and a low signal intensity on T2- and T1-weighted images.[51] Bicornuate and didelphic uteri may be differentiated from partial and complete septate uteri on MR images by the presence of a fundal indentation more than 10-mm deep and an angle between the medial margins of the hemicavities of not less than 60°.

For visualization of the uterine cavity, T2-weighted sequences are helpful to optimize contrast between the myometrium and endometrium. The endometrium has a long T2 image and the myometrium a short T2. The endometrium and myometrium have similar T1 images. The studies should be performed in the secretory phase of the cycle with almost exclusive use of frontal and transverse scans parallel to the longitudinal plane of the uterus in T2-weighted images. Oblique images of the pelvis may be necessary to optimally demonstrate fundal contour and to image the uterine fundus orthogonally. T1-weighted scans are useful in adding diagnostic specificity, particularly in the diagnosis of fatty or hemorrhagic lesions. The characteristic zonal architecture of the corpus, cervix, and vagina is clearly defined on T2-weighted scans. This definition is essential in differentiating septate and bicornuate uteri. The composition of the septum, that is, fibrous or myometrial, may be of value in differentiating septate from bicornuate or didelphic uteri, though should not be used as a sole criterion.[52] A fibrous septum is diagnosed on T1- and T2-weighted images when a uniform low signal intensity is demonstrated.

Two- and three-dimensional ultrasound and MRI are complementary techniques for determining uterine shape. Comparative studies have demonstrated nearly equal sensitivity and specificity for MRI and transvaginal ultrasound scanning.[44,53] The importance of MRI and endovaginal scanning may be in their ability to differentiate a bicornuate from a septate uterus. Imaging techniques, whether ultrasound or MRI, are intended to reduce the need for operative assessment of the fundal contour and aid better planning for resection of the septum or unification of the uterine horns. The question is of key practical importance because endoscopic approaches for the septate uterus have largely supplanted classic transabdominal metroplasty. MRI and ultrasound examination appear to fill this role, though in some studies their predictive value is low and laparoscopy may be required.[54,55]

Diagnostic Laparoscopy

In some circumstances imaging of the uterine contour is equivocal and laparoscopy is essential. Direct visualization of the uterine fundus to define its contour by laparoscopy may be required when image interpretation is questionable. This procedure is frequently used in conjunction with a hysteroscopic or resectoscopic excision of the septum to guide the intrauterine surgery. Transabdominal ultrasound-guided intrauterine surgery has reduced the absolute need for laparoscopy to guide such procedures.[56]

Evaluation Prior to ART

In cases of a septate uterus, hysteroscopic resection of the septum should be undertaken prior to any assisted reproductive technology (Table 6-1). This approach is the most cautious. Counseling regarding intervention versus observation is essential. This should be done with sensitivity to the patient's age and, in patients > 38 years, avoidance of any long-term suppression with GnRH analogs. The time invested for both endometrial suppression and resumption of menstrual cycles after the procedure may compromise outcomes with IVF in this age group. Careful assessment of the endometrial cavity after resection of the septum is essential. Hysteroscopy provides the most sensitive means of assessing both adequacy of the resection and any scarring in the area of surgery. Difficult decisions arise in differentiating an arcuate from a septate uterus and deciding which requires resection and which requires no intervention. There are no standard definitions to differentiate septate from arcuate uteri. The decision rests on clinical impression and overall distortion of the endometrial cavity.

In a bicornuate uterus careful assessment of each side for passage of an embryo transfer catheter is essential prior to in vitro fertilization. In some circumstances the anatomy favors clear and easy passage to one side over another. In this circumstance ease of passage will dictate to which side the embryos are transferred. A differential endometrial response is possible with a more favorable environment on one side. Careful monitoring of endometrial thickness in each cavity is also essential. The enhanced endometrial response will also guide decision making regarding embryo transfer. There is no evidence to suggest an advantage to splitting the embryos, placing an equal number in each side. This does have the potential disadvantage of added manipulation to the cervix and lower uterine segment and a possible compromise to outcome. In cases of a bicollis uterus, careful attention should be placed on ease of passage through the endocervical canal. The side offering the easiest passage should be chosen for transfer. Overall, outcomes are excellent. In one series, however, patients with any uterine abnormality had lower implantation and pregnancy rates regardless of surgical intervention.[57]

Management

Since Ruge first described a transcervical metroplasty for uterine unification, metroplasty has become a key aspect of management to improve outcome.[58,59] However, septate, bicornuate or didelphic uterine abnormalities do not necessarily call for surgery to improve reproductive outcome. Two key aspects to surgical planning are extreme care in patient selection and a thorough evaluation to rule out other factors contributory to infertility.

The management of didelphic, septate, and bicornuate uteri differs markedly, depending on the patient's clinical history. The types of metroplasty performed and surgical approach depends on the type of uterine abnormality. For unification of a bicornuate or didelphic uterus, a transabdominal approach is necessary. For a septate uterus, a hysteroscopic, resectoscopic, or transabdominal approach may be used. Almost without exception, no intervention is warranted for arcuate uteri.

Cervical cerclage has been advocated in select cases as a second surgical option to enhance live births though the strength of the recommendations is weak. The rationale is based on the premise that intrinsic defects in uterine musculature exist at both uterine fundus and cervix. Several reports support the efficacy of cervical cerclage as primary therapy for pregnancy wastage caused by a bicornuate uterus.[58] Success rates of 70 to 80% have been described in uncontrolled studies.[59–61] Cervical cerclage has also been used as adjunctive therapy in patients with premature cervical effacement after metroplasty, based on the assumption that patients with congenital defects of the uterus may also have defects of the internal os and cervix. The decision should be reached after consultation with perinatologists, review of history and careful patient counseling. Cerclage placement is not appropriate for patients with a negative history.

Bicornuate and Didelphic Uterus

The degree of failure of unification can be quite variable, and communication between the cavities may exist.[62,63] In patients with a history of repeated pregnancy loss or preterm labor, a unification procedure should be considered. Care is required in patient selection. In a bicornuate uterus two separate endometrial cavities and a single cervix are present. In uterine didelphys, the anomaly is characterized by two separate endometrial cavities, each with a uterine cervix that is fused in the area of the lower uterine segment. A longitudinal vaginal septum of varying length may be present (Figures 6-9 and 6-10). This septum can form an obstructed hemivagina requiring surgical excision and repair (see Figure 6-8).

No large prospective studies support surgical intervention, and metroplasty is not generally recommended for either didelphic or bicornuated uteri as

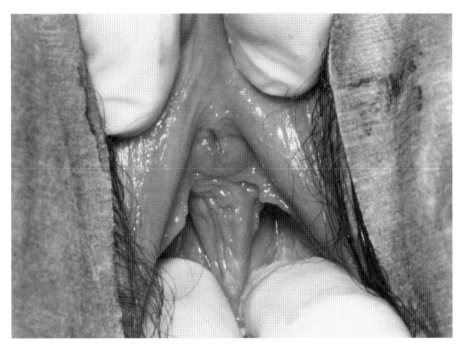

Figure 6-9   Transverse septum extending to introitus in a patient with a didelphic uterus.

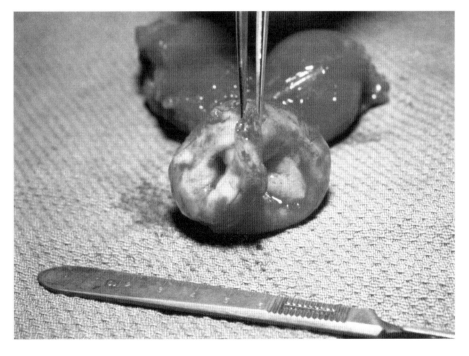

Figure 6-10   Surgical specimen of didelphic uterus showing two cervices and 2-cm vaginal septum.

first-line management. Adverse outcomes are greater with didelphic bicornuate uterii though the data are limited. Surgery must be approached cautiously. Patients with a compelling history of repeated late pregnancy losses may benefit from a metroplasty. The surgical technique to unify the uterine cavities is by a Strassmann metroplasty, which leaves the dual cervices intact in cases of bicornuate bicollis. The cervices may be united by a vaginal approach.[64] Simultaneously, a vaginal septum may be excised in some circumstances. Consideration may be given to postoperative cervical cerclage to enhance fetal survival, though extensive prospective data to support this decision are lacking.

Operative Technique

The usual corrective procedure for unification of a bicornuate or didelphic uterus is a Strassmann metroplasty (as originally described in 1907) (Figure 6-11). In this procedure, an intrauterine Foley catheter or disposable uterine manipulator is placed at the start of the procedure for chromotubation that may aid in the identification of the interior of the uterine cavity after the uterus is divided. Injection of the fundal region with a dilute vasopressin solution (20 units in 20 ml of normal saline) is used to reduce bleeding. A transverse incision is made over the uterine fundus from cornua to cornua through the midline notch, avoiding the uterotubal junctions. Care should be taken to stay at least 1.0 cm away from the insertion of the tube.

The uterine cavities are then opened by separating the uterus into anterior and posterior walls (Figure 6-11 A and B). The partition between them is split down the middle. By removing the intervening septum, both uterine cavities are converted into a single full space (Figure 6-11C). The transverse incision is converted into a vertical suture line, drawing the lateral halves of the uterus together at the midline. The incision is then closed anteriorly and posteriorly using two layers of 0 or 00 polyglactin or similar nonreactive absorbable sutures. In cases of a double vagina and double cervix, the vaginal septum may be excised. This decision should be individualized. The mere presence of a vaginal septum does not mandate excision. The septum can vary in thickness from 1 to 2 mm to as thick as 5 or 6 mm. The resection of a longitudinal septum is performed by clamping the septum at its junction with the vaginal walls using straight clamps, in a clamp-cut-tie sequence from introitus to cervix, and then repairing the vaginal mucosal defect with fine, 3-0 polyglactin sutures. Care should be taken to carefully approximate the vaginal wall under as little tension as possible. Undermining the vaginal mucosa from the bladder anteriorly or the rectum posteriorly may help mobilize the mucosa and reduce the tension. The cervices may then be split by a vaginal approach. Alternatively, the cervices may be left without unification.

(A)

(C)

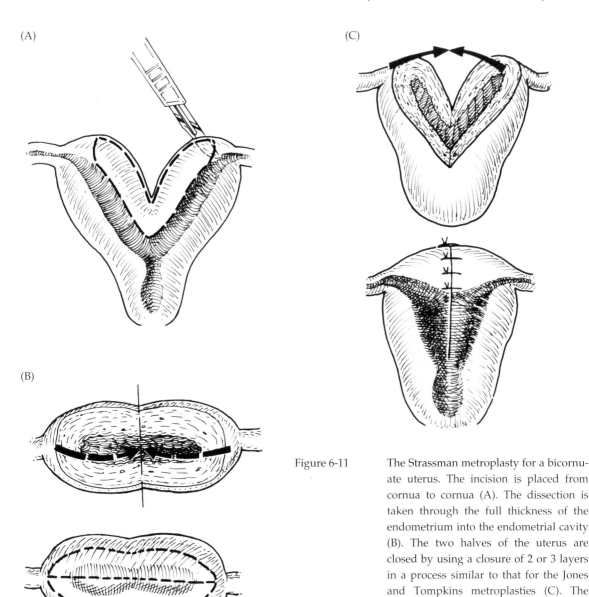

(B)

Figure 6-11   The Strassman metroplasty for a bicornuate uterus. The incision is placed from
cornua to cornua (A). The dissection is
taken through the full thickness of the
endometrium into the endometrial cavity
(B). The two halves of the uterus are
closed by using a closure of 2 or 3 layers
in a process similar to that for the Jones
and Tompkins metroplasties (C). The
Strassman technique is applicable to only
a bicornuate uterus.

Septate Uterus

Septate and arcuate uteri are characterized by a complete unification of the
exterior uterine wall with persistence of the medial segments as a septum
dividing the cavity into halves. The differentiation between septate and
arcuate is one of degree of fusion and depth of division. For the purposes of
this discussion, the term septate will be used. The length of the septum in the

midline may be quite variable, from a small dimpling occupying 1 cm in the midline of the uterine cavity to a septum extending to the level of the internal os. Regardless of length, the septum should be excised to a level even with or within 1 cm of the myometrium. This is most easily done by using a hysteroscope with microscissors or by using a resectoscope with an operating loop and transabdominal ultrasound guidance as an alternative to laparoscopic guidance. Ultrasound-guided transcervical resection reduces the need for simultaneous laparoscopy and is an excellent modality to monitor the procedure.[56] A transabdominal metroplasty may be required in 3% of cases in which complete endoscopic resection is not possible.[65,66] The procedure should be considered in patients who have repeated pregnancy loss or poor obstetric history.[67] It is extremely controversial in patients with a history of infertility and no other discernible causes. No large prospective studies support its use in this setting and care must be individualized in planning any intervention.

Hysteroscopic Operative Technique

Preoperative endometrial suppression will improve visualization and operative precision. The decision to suppress should be made with consideration of the patient's age. If used, endometrial suppression with gonadotropin-releasing hormone (depot leuprolide acetate, 3.75 mg for 2 months) prior to a procedure is adequate.[68] When suppression is not used, the procedure should be performed in the early follicular phase. Incision of the septum may be undertaken with any standard hysteroscopic scissors or resectoscope with operative loop and electrocautery.[69–71] Any of three types of scissors may be used: flexible, semirigid, or rigid, depending on the consistency and thickness of the septum. A cutting current of 30 W/s is adequate when electrocautery is used. Excision with the operating loop of the resectoscope is useful in unusual cases where the tissue is vascular and thick. However, possible damage to surrounding endometrial tissue may occur and care is required. A resectoscope or microscissors for the correction of a septate uterus have similar outcomes.[72–74]

The length of the uterine septum may vary from 1 to 5 cm and extend from the fundus to the internal cervical os. Resection starts at the apex of the septum. The incision is carried laterally on either side to produce an even, progressive division of the septum. The presence of a residual septum 0.5 to 1.0 cm in length does not adversely influence outcome.[72] During dissection the relatively fibrous, bloodless septum should give way to the myometrium. Isolated bleeding points may be encountered in the septum itself or in the myometrium and require cauterization. The septum should be excised to a level even with or within 1 cm of the myometrium. With completion of the dissection, both tubal ostia should be able to be seen clearly by moving the hysteroscope from side to side. After the septum is incised completely, the scope should be withdrawn to the level of the internal os for a panoramic view of the cavity.

Several variations on hysteroscopic or resectoscopic reduction of a uterine septum have been described.[76] One technique involves using modified Metzenbaum scissors that incorporate a rubber seal at the endocervical canal to permit an injection of contrast media into the cavity to define the uterine septum (not unlike the original description in 1884 by Ruge).[77] Under fluoroscopic control, the septum can be incised, and contrast injected periodically to assess progress. Neodymium:yttrium-aluminum-garnet (Nd:YAG) is an alternative to standard hysteroscopic microscissors or the resectoscope.[78,79] An ultrasound-guided metroplasty (without hysteroscopy) in which transabdominal ultrasound guidance is used and endoscopic scissors 4 mm in diameter are passed into the uterine cavity is a useful option in complex cases.[56] In this technique the scissors are introduced strictly under ultrasound guidance and without the use of a hysteroscope. A division and excision of the septum is documented by ultrasound assessment. The procedure was successful in all of 24 patients attempted. The advantage of this technique is that it eliminates the need for hysteroscopy or laparoscopic guidance of the procedure.

Endometrial repair after septum excision occurs through re-epithelialization of the cut surface both centripetally by the proliferation of endometrial tissue and centrifugally from the base of the remaining glands to the margin of the incisions.[80] In an evaluation of the re-epithelialization process, 19 women who underwent hysteroscopic metroplasty for a septate uterus were studied using multiple biopsies postoperatively. At 14 days after the incision, scattered epithelial cells were noted. At 1 month a thin endometrium was first noted, and at 2 months there was near complete regrowth of the epithelium and endometrium. There appears to be a progressive increase in endometrial thickness for 2 months after the time of incision.[84] Because of this, postponement of pregnancy attempts for 2 months after surgery is recommended. Traditional postoperative management using an intraoperative splint such as an intrauterine device (IUD), or high-dose conjugated estrogens, may not improve this healing process.[33,82,83] In a prospective study comparing these techniques, there was no difference in the incidence of intrauterine adhesions.[84] Intrauterine devices such as a Lippes' loop have been abandoned because of the potential for infectious complications. A soft, malleable balloon (Cooke Inc., Spencer, IN) or pediatric Foley may be placed after resection and removed 2 weeks postoperatively. Conjugated estrogen at 2.5 to 5 mg per day is used for 30 days and 10 mg of medroxyprogesterone acetate is added during the final 10 days.

Transabdominal Operative Technique

Two techniques have been described for the transabdominal unification of a septate uterus, independently by Jones and Tompkins (see Figure 6-12 A and B).[7,31] The Jones metroplasty is a technique for resection of a septum by resection of a midline en bloc wedge. Close inspection of the fundal contour of the uterus usually suggests a median raphe, and palpation of the uterus may

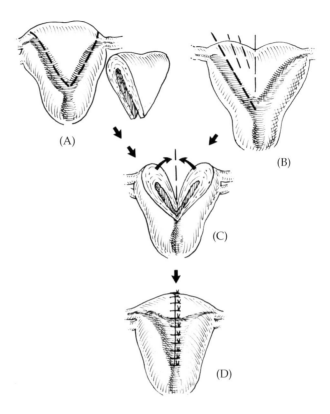

Figure 6-12   The Jones (left) and Tompkins (right) metroplasties. The Jones technique involves excision of the wedge of tissue from the midline in the
region corresponding approximately to the lateral-most portions of the
septum (A). The Thompkins technique involves a midline incision
within the region of the septum and progressive lateral dissection until
the lateral-most portions of the septum are removed (B). Both techniques employ a closure of the bivalved uterus in 2 or 3 layers (C, D).

suggest fibrous tissue at the midline. The lateral extent of the septum should
be estimated by these simple techniques as a guide to placement of the
uterine incisions. Outlining the incision with a dye or marker may be helpful
for more precise placement of the uterine incision. Intraoperative reference to
the HSG (in addition to clinical impression after intraoperative examination)
may provide further guidance for precise estimation of wedge size and
placement of the uterine incisions. For hemostasis, 20 units of pitressin
diluted in 20 ml of saline may be injected into the myometrium along the
lines of uterine incision. The incisions at the fundus may be 1.0 to 1.5 cm
from the insertion of the fallopian tubes, depending on septum width and
extend through the full thickness of the myometrium (Figure 6-12A). Care
should be taken to direct the incisions to the midline and apex of the wedge
and avoid the uterotubal junction. Closure is accomplished in two layers of

the myometrium by using 0 polyglactin sutures and 3–0 sutures on the serosa.

A Tompkins metroplasty consists of a sagittal incision in the midline of the uterine fundus extending the incision anteriorly and posteriorly to the apex of the septum. The placement of the incision may be guided by palpation of the septum and by reference to preoperative HSG. The myometrium should be infiltrated with pitressin as outlined above. The incision should be extended through the entirety of the uterus, which bivalves the uterus (Figure 6-12B). The lower-most portion of the septum may then be defined in each half of the uterine cavity. A Kelly clamp or tonsil clamp should be gently inserted into the endometrial cavity to define the upper-most portion of the cavity and lateral-most aspect of the septum in each half of the uterus. This process should guide the second and possibly third incisions on each half of the uterus to excise the septum totally. Several incisions may be required to carefully shave the septum from each half of the uterus, starting at the midline and progressing laterally. After this procedure, the two uterine halves should be unified in a fashion identical to that of the Jones procedure (Figure 6-12C and D). Appropriate measures should be undertaken to prevent adhesion formation.

Outcomes Analysis

As a general rule and particularly appropriate to remember in this setting, outcomes after repeated pregnancy loss tend to improve with each successive pregnancy, whether or not intervention is undertaken (Tables 6-2 and 6-3). Success often is determined by comparing pregnancy outcomes before and after surgical intervention.[86] As such, the study of any intervention, whether medical or surgical, in patients who have a bicornuate or septate uterus and who have had previous poor obstetric outcomes is likely to

Table 6-2. Reproductive Outcomes For Uterine Duplication				
	First and Second Spontaneous Abortion	Preterm Delivery	Term Delivery	Living Children
Uterine didelphys	42% (36,48)	36% (31,42)	32% (17,27)	56% (50,32)
Bicornuate uterus	28% (23,33)	17% (13,21)	51% (46,56)	59% (54,64)
Septate uterus	74% (70,78)	9% (6,12)	8% (6,10)	19% (16,23)

95% confidence intervals in parentheses
References: 3, 16, 31

Table 6-3.
Hysteroscopic Metroplasty for Septate Uterus*

	First and Second Spontaneous Abortion	Preterm Delivery	Term Delivery
Preoperative outcomes	90% (86,93)	6% (0,11)	12% (8,16)
Postoperative outcomes	15% (11,20)	4% (0,9)	78% (73,84)

*Pregnancy rates; 95% confidence intervals in parentheses
Data from studies with both pre- and postoperative outcome data
References: 16, 21, 33, 85

demonstrate that the intervention succeeds when the control data consist of the obstetric performance before treatment.

The literature describing outcomes after intervention is of variable quality. The majority of studies lack proper controls, randomization, or matching for other variables and follow-up that potentially contribute to outcome.[87] Two sets of data exist: a small number of studies suggesting that outcomes improve with no intervention and a second larger database supporting surgical intervention. First, the data on nonintervention will be described. In one study, data confirmed a trend in improvement with subsequent pregnancies without any intervention in patients with uterine duplication.[88] Patients had fewer spontaneous abortions and preterm deliveries after evaluation regardless of whether they had metroplasty. In a smaller series, no difference in outcome could be found when 15 patients treated with metroplasty were compared with patients who did not have surgery. The percentage of patients with living children after the diagnosis of bicornuate uterine abnormalities was 73% for the patients who underwent metroplasty and 67% for matched nonsurgical patients.[89] In a study comparing reproductive outcomes after abdominal metroplasty versus no corrective surgery for bicornuate uterus, the cumulative pregnancy rates at 12 and 24 months were 63 and 88% in patients after surgical correction and 67 and 95% in patients without surgical correction. In this study, the probability of giving birth without surgery was 30, 58, and 79% for the first, second, and third pregnancy, respectively, and after corrective surgery was 71 and 86% for the first and second pregnancy.[90] Although marked improvement in fetal salvage rates may be noted when the reproductive outcomes before and after metroplasty are compared, final obstetric outcome in these studies was similar to that of the control groups after the diagnosis was made and surgery deferred.[37,38,91–95]

In spite of encouraging data for nonintervention, surgical options are viable. When discussed with patients, most will opt for intervention. For patients with a history of repeated pregnancy loss and a didelphic or bicornuate uterus, success rates (i.e., term deliveries after abdominal metroplasty) are 93 and 84%, respectively.[96–99] Success rates for hysteroscopic metroplasty for repeated loss secondary to a septate uterus are 75% (range, 40 to 87%) (Table 6-3).[100–105] In patients undergoing a transabdominal or hysteroscopic metroplasty for repeated loss, success rates are similar, regardless of the number of previous miscarriages.[106,107] Hysteroscopic resection of the septum should be considered as first-line management.[108,109] Transabdominal approaches should be reserved for difficult resections where complete resection is not possible. Any degree of recurrence or intrauterine adhesion formation after resection should be approached initially with the hysteroscope.[110]

A second area of controversy is the mode of delivery after an abdominal metroplasty. As a general rule, cesarean section is recommended. Earlier data describing management of pregnancy after a metroplasty suggest labor may be permitted.[1,4] Rates of cesarean section in these reports varied from 36 to 70%. Interestingly, in one series, 63% of cesarean sections were performed with an indication of abnormal presentation, one of the precise indications for performance of the metroplasty itself.[4] Although these data suggest that an attempt at vaginal delivery may be permitted in certain patients after appropriate counseling, delivery by cesarean section is generally recommended.

The quality of the evidence and strength of the recommendations for metroplasty in septate uterus deserve explicit emphasis in an evidence-based environment.[88] This literature is composed largely of observational studies rendering these recommendations weak at best (Level II). Two additional points (and the questions they imply) are relevant to the critical analysis of this literature. These include the lack of a standard, quantitative definition and diagnostic criteria for a septate uterus (what is normal?) and the observations that reproductive outcomes tend to improve in this setting without intervention (what happens when nothing is done?). A critical need for standardized definitions of a normal and an abnormal uterine cavity has long been recognized.[111] In 1962, Pendleton Tompkins suggested that these abnormalities be viewed on a spectrum from clearly normal to clearly abnormal.[112] He suggested that the case for or against intervention rested on subtle distinctions. No debate can be mustered, for example, when there is no question that a cavity is at either end of the normal–abnormal spectrum. However, debate exists over the management of those configurations in-between. Subjective standards continue to be used to differentiate normal from abnormal: what may be septate to one examiner may be arcuate to another.

The second issue is the likely improvement in outcomes regardless of intervention. In 1960, M.M. White noted that reproductive outcomes in patients with mullerian abnormalities improved with repeated pregnancies regardless of intervention. Though resection of the uterine septum continues to be the standard of care, these observations suggest that some cases may be amenable to intervention and resection of the septum and others may function perfectly well without any surgery. Surgery may not be the answer to every case of a septate uterus. Both issues should be included in any counseling session to review options and reach an informed understanding of the process.

Summary and Recommendations

The decision to proceed with surgical management of septate, didelphic, or bicornuate uteri should be reached after careful consideration of all potential contributory factors. Not all patients with a history of repeated pregnancy loss require immediate surgical intervention. Consideration of the risks and benefits of the procedure, the age of the patient, and the patient's reproductive history can aid in identifying patients most likely to benefit from a surgical procedure. On the basis of the available literature, the following recommendations are made:

- HSG and diagnostic laparoscopy are two complementary diagnostic tools. Transabdominal and transvaginal ultrasound examination and MRI provide detailed information and, in select cases, may obviate the need for laparoscopy.
- In patients with a septate uterus, an endoscopic approach using either hysteroscopy with microscissors, hysteroscopy with laser fibers, or resectoscope and operating loop provides the most convenient and least invasive approach. These techniques may be performed with either laparoscopic or transabdominal ultrasound guidance.
- If hysteroscopic resection of a septum is impossible or incomplete, consideration may be given to a transabdominal approach using a Jones or Tompkins metroplasty.
- In patients with bicornuate or didelphic uteri, transabdominal metroplasty is necessary. A Strassmann metroplasty should be performed, with consideration of resection of vaginal septum unification of cervices, or both, if present.
- To reduce the likelihood of intrauterine adhesion formation high-dose estrogen (2.5 mg of conjugated estrogen, twice a day for 30 days) followed by a progestin challenge (10 mg of medroxyprogesterone for 10 days) to induce reliable withdrawal may be considered. In select circumstances, a Foley catheter or balloon device may be used. Postoperative use of an IUD has been abandoned. Comparative data of treatment versus no treatment however reveal similar results.
- A follow-up evaluation should be performed, using either HSG or hysteroscopy to assess the adequacy of resection and check for the formation of any intrauterine adhesions.
- Prior to ART, a septum should be removed and normalcy of the endometrial cavity after surgery verified. In this setting, it is appropriate to take a more aggressive approach and recommend excision rather than observation.

- In cases of bicornuate or bicollis uteri, the side into which the embryos are transferred should be guided by the ease of passage through the cervical canal (in bicollis) and the most favorable endometrium (in both bicornuate and bicollis).

References

1.   Granberry HW, Faust FL. Duplicity of the uterus and vagina. Am J Obstet Gynecol 1938;35:1042–1046.

2.   Findley P. Pregnancy in uterus didelphys. Am J Obstet Gynecol 1926;12:318–322.

3.   Van der Velde M. Geburtsstorungen Durch: entwicklungsfehler der gebarmutter, monatcher. F Geburtsch U Gynak Berl 1915;42:307–321.

4.   Miller NF. Clinical aspects of uterus didelphys. Am J Obstet Gynecol 1922;4:398–408.

5.   Ruge P. Fall von Schwangerschaft bei uterus septus. Zascha Geburtsch Gynaekol 1884;10:141–143.

6.   Strassmann P. Die operative vereinigung eines doppeltein uterus. Zentrabl Gynaekol 1907;31:1322–1326.

7.   Tompkins P. Comments on the bicornuate uterus and twinning. Surg Clin North Am 1962;42:1049–1054.

8.   Jones HW, Jones GS. Double uterus as an etiological factor in repeated abortion: indications for surgical repair. Am J Obstet Gynecol 1953;65:375–389.

9.   Jarcho J. Malformations of the uterus. Am J Surg 1946;71:106–166.

10.   American Society for Reproductive Medicine. Classification of adnexal adhesions, distal tubal occlusion, tubal occlusion secondary to tubal ligation, tubal pregnancies, Mullerian anomalies, and intrauterine adhesions. Fertil Steril 1988;49:944–955.

11.   Carson SA, Simpson JL, Elias S, et al. Genetics of Mullerian aplasia. Fertil Steril 1983;40:86–90.

12.   Sarto GE, Simpson JL. Abnormalities of the Mullerian and Wolffian duct systems. Birth Defect 1978;14:37–40.

13.   Mecke S, Passaro E. Encephalocele, polycystic kidneys and polydactyly as an autosomal recessive trait simulating certain other disorders. The Meckel syndrome. Ann Genet 1971;14:97–99.

14.   Fraser GR. Our genetic "load". A review of some aspects of genetic malformations. Ann Hum Genet 1962;25:387–399.

15.   Rudiger RD, Schmidt W, Loose DA, Passarge E. Severe developmental failure with coarse facial features, distal limb hypoplasia, thickened palmar creases, bifid vulva and ureteral stenosis: a previously unidentified familial disorder with lethal outcome. J Pediatr 1971;79:977–979.

16.   Poznanski AK, Kuhns LR, Lapides J, Stern AN. A new family with the hand-foot-genital syndrome – wider spectrum of the hand-foot-uterus syndrome. Birth Defect 1975;11:127–131.

17.   Simpson JL. Genes and chromosomes that cause female infertility. Fertil Steril 1985;44:725–736.

18. Rock JA, Schlaff WD. The obstetric consequences of uterovaginal anomalies. Fertil Steril 1986;43:681–692.

19. Semmens JP. Congenital anomalies of the female genital tract. Obstet Gynecol 1962;19:328–350.

20. Homer HA, Li Tin-Chiu, Cooke ID. The septate uterus: a review of management and reproductive income. Fertil Steril 2000;73:1–14.

21. Fedele L, Zamberletti D, D'Alberton A, et al. Gestational aspects of uterus didelphys. J Reprod Med 1988;33:353–357.

22. Fleming H, Ostor AG, Pickel H, Fortune DW. Arteriovenous malformation of the uterus. Obstet Gynecol 1989;73:209–214.

23. Stege JG, Oosterhof H, Lander M, Aarnoudse JG. Lacking anastomoses between left and right uterine arteries in uterus bicornis during pregnancy as demonstrated by Doppler velocimetry. Br J Obstet Gynecol 1992;99:922–923.

24. Soberon-Arrendondo F, Lorez de Mola R, Shalansky-Goldberg R, Tureck RW. Uterine arteriovenous malformation in a patient with recurrent pregnancy loss and a bicornuate uterus. J Reprod Med 1997;42:239–243.

25. Ghosh TK. Arteriovenous malformations of the uterus and pelvis. Obstet Gynecol 1986;68:405–425.

26. Burchell RC, Creed F, Rasoulpour M, Whitcomb M. Vascular anatomy of the human uterus in pregnancy wastage. Br J Obstet Gynaecol 1978;85:698–706.

27. Miller ME, Dunn PM, Smith DW. Uterine malformation and fetal deformation. Pediatrics 1979;94:387–390.

28. Homsi RI, Sidky IH, Yang A, et al. Uterus didelphys and unilateral lower limb amelia in a discordant monozygotic twin. J Reprod Med 1994;39:481–484.

29. Marabini A, Gubbini G, Stagnozzi R, et al. Hysteroscopic metroplasty. Ann N Y Acad Sci 1994;734:488–492.

30. Buttram VC. Mullerian abnormalities and their management. Fertil Steril 1983;40:159–164.

31. Joki-Erkkila MM, Heinonen PK. Presenting and long-term clinical implications and fecundity in females with obstructing vaginal malformations. J Ped Adolesc Gynecol 2003;16:307–312.

32. Sorenson SS. Fundal contour of the uterine cavity in the new syndrome of minor Mullerian anomalies and oligomenorrhea. Am J Obstet Gynecol 1983;145:659–666.

33. Woolf RB, Allen WN. Concomitant malformations: the frequent occurrence of congential malformations of the reproductive and urinary tracts. Obstet Gynecol 1953;2:236–240.

34. Jones WS. Obstetric significance of female genital anomalies. Obstet Gynecol 1957;10:113–127.

35. Proctor JA, Haney AF. Recurrent first trimester pregnancy loss is associated with uterine septum but not with bicornuate uterus. Fertil Steril 2003;80:1212–1215.

36. Fedele L, Dorta M, Brioschi D, et al. Re-examination of the anatomic indications for hysteroscopic metroplasty. Eur J Obstet Gynecol Reprod Biol 1991;39:127–131.

37. March CM. Uterine surgical approaches to reduce prematurity. Clin Perinatol 1992;19:319–331.

38. Musich JR, Behrman SJ. Obstetric outcome before and after metroplasty in women with uterine anomalies. Obstet Gynecol 1978;52:63–66.

39. Heinnonen PK, Pystynen PP. Primary infertility in uterine abnormalities. Fertil Steril 1983;40:311–315.

40. Beaver MG, Abbott KH. Normal pregnancies and delivery in bicornuate uteri. California Western Med 1937;41:41–42.

41. Jones TB, Fleischer AC, Daniell JF, et al. Sonographic characteristics of congenital uterine abnormalities and associated pregnancy. J Clin Ultrasound 1980;8:435–437.

42. Fedele L, Ferrazzi E, Dorta M, et al. Ultrasonography in the differential diagnosis of double uteri. Fertil Steril 1988;50:361–363.

43. Nicolini U, Bellott M, Bonazzi B, et al. Can ultrasound be used to screen uterine malformations? Fertil Steril 1987;47:89–94.

44. Pellerito JS, McCarthy SM, Doyle MD, et al. Diagnosis of uterine anomalies: relative accuracy of MR imaging. Endovaginal sonography and hysterosalpingography. Radiology 1992;183:795–800.

45. Rauter KL, Daly DC, Cohen SM. Septate versus bicornuate uteri: errors in imaging diagnosis. Radiology 1989;172:749–752.

46. Randolph JR, Ying YK, Maier DB, et al. Comparison of real time ultrasonography, hysterosalpingography, and laparoscopy/hysteroscopy in the evaluation of uterine abnormalities and tubal patency. Fertil Steril 1986;46:828–832.

47. Raga F, Bonilla-Musoels F, Blanes J, Osborne NG. Congenital mullerian anomalies: diagnostic accuracy of three dimensional ultrasound. Fertil Steril 1996;65:523–528.

48. Wu MH, Hsu CC, Huang KE. Detection of congenital mullerian duct anomalies using three-dimensional ultrasound. J Clin Ultrasound 1997;25:487–492.

49. Jurkovic D, Geipel A, Gruboeck K, et al. Three-dimensional ultrasound for the assessment of uterine anatomy and detection of congenital anomalies: a comparison with hysterosalpingography and two-dimensional sonography. Ultrasound Obstet Gynecol 1995;5:233–237.

50. McCarthy S. Magnetic resonance imaging in the evaluation of infertile women. Magn Reson Q 1990;4:339–449.

51. Doyle MD. Magnetic resonance imaging in Mullerian fusion defects. J Reprod Med 1992;37:33–38.

52. Wagner BJ, Woodward PJ. Magnetic resonance evaluation of congenital uterine anomalies. Semin Ultrasound CT MRI 1994;15:4–17.

53. Carrington BM, Hricak H, Nuruddin RN, et al. Mullerian duct anomalies: MR imaging evaluation. Radiology 1990;76:715–720.

54. Letterie GS, Haggerty M, Lindee G. A comparison of pelvic ultrasound and magnetic resonance imaging as diagnostic studies for Mullerian tract abnormalities. Int J Fertil 1995;40:34–38.

55. Fischetti SG, Politi G, Lomeo E, Garozzo G. Magnetic resonance in the evaluation of Mullerian duct anomalies. Radiol Med 1995;89:105–111.

56. Querleu D, Brasme TL, Parmentier D. Ultrasound-guided transcervical metroplasty. Fertil Steril 1990;54:995–998.

57. Heinonen PK, Kuismanen K, Ashorn R. Assisted reproduction in women with uterine anomalies. Eur J Obstet Gynecol Reprod Biol 2000;89:181–184.

58. Jones HW, Wheeless CR. Salvage of the reproductive potential of women with anomalous development of the mullerian ducts: 1868–1968–2068. Am J Obstet Gynecol 1969;104:348–366.

59. Golan A, Langer R, Neuman M, et al. Obstetric outcome in women with congenital uterine malformation. J Reprod Med 1992;37:233–236.

60. Blum M. Prevention of spontaneous abortion by cervical suture of the malformed uterus. Int Surg 1977;62:213–215.

61. Ludmir J, Samuels P, Brooks S, Mennuti M. Pregnancy outcome of patients with uncorrected uterine anomalies managed in a high risk obstetric setting. Obstet Gynecol 1990;75:906–910.

62. Sanfilippo JS, Levine RL. Uterus didelphys with microscopic communication between horns. Am J Obstet Gynecol 1986;55:1055–1056.

63. Toaff ME, Lev-Toaff AJ, Toaff R. Communicating uteri: review and classification with introduction of two previously unreported types. Fertil Steril 1984;41:661–679.

64. Strassmann EO. Fertility in unification of the double uterus. Fertil Steril 1966;17:165–170.

65. Fedele L, Bianchi S. Hysteroscopic metroplasty for septate uterus. Obstet Gynecol Clin North Am 1995;22:473–489.

66. Elchalal U, Schenker JG. Hysteroscopic resection of uterus septus versus abdominal metroplasty. J Am Col Surg 1994;178:637–644.

67. Gaucherand P, Awada A, Rudigoz RC, Dargent D. Obstetrical prognosis of the septate uterus: a plea for treatment of the septum. Eur J Obstet Gynecol Reprod Biol 1994;54:109–112.

68. Fedele L, Bianchi S, Gruft L, et al. Danazol versus a gonadotropin-releasing hormone agonist as preoperative preparation for hysteroscopic metroplasty. Fertil Steril 1996;65:186–188.

69. Valle RF, Sciarra JJ. Hysteroscopic treatment of the septate uterus. Obstet Gynecol 1986;67:253–257.

70. DeCherney AH, Russell JB, Graebe RA, Polan ML. Resectoscopic management of Mullerian fusion defects. Fertil Steril 1986;45:726–728.

71. Rock JA, Murphy AA, Cooper WH. Resectoscopic technique for the lysis of a class 5 complete uterine septum. Fertil Steril 1987;48:495–496.

72. Vercellini P, Vendola N, Colombo A, et al. Hysteroscopic metroplasty with resectoscope or microscissors for the correction of septate uterus. Surg Gynecol Obstet 1993;176:439–442.

73. Cararach M, Penella J, Ubeda A, Labastida R. Hysteroscopic incision of the septate uterus: scissors versus resectoscope. Hum Reprod 1994;9:87–89.

74. Barranger E, Gervaise A, Doumerc S, Fernandez H. Reproductive performance after hysteroscopic metroplasty in the hypoplastic uterus: a study of 29 cases. Br J Obstet Gynaecol 2002;109:1331–1334.

75. Fedele L, Bianchi S, Marchini M, et al. Residual uterine septum of less than 1 cm after hysteroscopic metroplasty does not impair reproductive outcome. Hum Reprod 1996;11:727–729.

76. Vercellini P, Ragni G, Trespidi L, et al. A modified technique for correction of the complete septate uterus. Acta Obstet Gynecol Scand 1994;73:425–428.

77. Valle JA, Lifchez AS, Moise J. A simpler technique for reduction of uterine septum. Fertil Steril 1991;56:1001–1005.

78. Choe JK, Baggish MS. Hysteroscopic treatment of the septate uterus with the Neodymium-YAG laser. Fertil Steril 1992;57:81–84.

79. Candiani GB, Vercellini P, Fedele L, et al. Argon laser versus microscissors for hysteroscopic incision of uterine septa. Am J Obstet Gynecol 1991;164:87–90.

80. Fedele L, Marchini M, Baglioni A, et al. Endometrial reconstruction after hysteroscopic incisional metroplasty. Obstet Gynecol 1989;73:492–495.

81. Candiani GB, Vercellini P, Fedele L, et al. Repair of the uterine cavity after hysteroscopic septal incision. Fertil Steril 1990;54:991–994.

82. Israel R, March CM. Hysteroscopic incision of the septate uterus. Am J Obstet Gynecol 1984;149:66–73.

83. Nawroth F, Schmidt T, Freise C, et al. Is it possible to recommend an "optimal" postoperative management after hysteroscopic metroplasty. A retrospective study with 52 infertile patients showing a septate uterus. Acta Obstet Gynecol Scand 2002;81:55–57.

84. Vercellini P, Fedele L, Arcaini L, et al. Value of intrauterine device insertion and estrogen administration after hysteroscopic metroplasty. J Reprod Med 1989;34:447–450.

85. Heinonen PK. Clinical implications of the didelphic uterus: long-term follow-up of 49 cases. Eur J Obstet Gynecol Reprod Biol 2000;91:183–190.

86. Pabuccu R, Gomel V. Reproductive outcome after hysteroscopic metroplasty in women with septate uterus and unexplained infertility. Fertil Steril 2004;81:1675–1678.

87. Letterie GS. Assessing the quality of evidence in support of resection of a uterine septum. Fertil Steril (abstract) 2000;74:5147.

88. White MM. Uteroplasty in infertility. Proc R Soc Med 1960;53:1006–1009.

89. Kirk EP, Chuong CJ, Coulam CB, Williams TJ. Pregnancy after metroplasty for uterine anomalies. Fertil Steril 1993;59:1164–1168.

90. Maneschi F, Marana R, Muzii L, Mancuso S. Reproductive performance in women with bicornuate uterus. Acta Eur Fertil 1993;24:117–120.

91. Fenton AN, Singh BP. Pregnancy associated with congenital abnormalities of the female reproductive tract. Am J Obstet Gynecol 1952;63:744–755.

92. Khalifa E, Toner JP, Jones HW Jr. The role of abdominal metroplasty in the era of operative hysteroscopy. Surg Gynecol Obstet 1993;176:208–212.

93. Raga F, Bauset C, Remohi J, et al. Reproductive impact of congenital Mullerian anomalies. Hum Reprod 1997,12.2277–2281.

94.   Heinonen PK, Kuismanen K, Ashorn R. Assisted reproduction in women with uterine anomalies. Eur J Obstet Gynecol Reprod Biol 2000;89:181–184.

95.   Heinonen PK. Clinical implications of the didelphic uterus: long-term follow-up of 49 cases. Eur J Obstet Gynecol Reprod Biol 2000;91:183–190.

96.   Stein AL, March CM. Pregnancy outcome in women with mullerian duct anomalies. J Reprod Med 1990;35:411–414.

97.   Candiani GB, Fedele L, Parazzini F, Zamberletti D. Reproductive prognosis after abdominal metroplasty in bicornuate or septate uterus: a life table analysis. Br J Obstet Gynaecol 1990;97:613–617.

98.   Moutos DM, Damewood MD, Schlaff WD, Rock JA. A comparison of the reproductive outcome between women with a unicornuate uterus and women with a didelphic uterus. Fertil Steril 1992;58:88–93.

99.   Ayhan A, Yucel I, Tuncer ZS, Kisnisci HA. Reproductive performance after conventional metroplasty: an evaluation of 102 cases. Fertil Steril 1992;57:1194–1196.

100.   Patton PE, Novy MJ, Lee DM, Hickok LR. Diagnosis and reproductive outcome after surgical treatment of septate uterus, duplicated cervix and vaginal septum. Am J Obstet Gynecol 2004;190:1669–1675.

101.   Fayez JA. Comparison between abdominal and hysteroscopic metroplasty. Obstet Gynecol 1986;68:399–403.

102.   Daly DC, Walters CA, Soto-Albors CE, Riddick DH. Hysteroscopic metroplasty: surgical technique and obstetric outcome. Fertil Steril 1983;39:623–628.

103.   Daly DC, Maier D, Soto-Albors C. Hysteroscopic metroplasty: six years' experience. Obstet Gynecol 1989;73:201–205.

104.   Zhioua F, Mouelhi C, Hamdoun L, et al. Hysteroscopic metroplasty of uterine septa. J Gynecol Obstet Biol Reprod (Paris) 1993;22:600–604.

105.   Goldenberg M, Sivan E, Sharabi Z, et al. Reproductive outcome following hysteroscopic management of intrauterine septum and adhesions. Hum Reprod 1995;10:2663–2665.

106.   Fedele L, Arcaini L, Parazzini F, et al. Reproductive prognosis after hysteroscopic metroplasty in 102 women: life-table analysis. Fertil Steril 1993;59:768–772.

107.   Ayhan A, Yucel I, Tuncer ZS, Kisnisci HA. Reproductive performance after conventional metroplasty: an evaluation of 102 cases. Fertil Steril 1992;57:1194–1196.

108.   Venturoli S, Colombo FM, Vianello F, et al. A study of hysteroscopic metroplasty in 141 women with septate uterus. Arch Gynecol Obstet 2002;266:157–159.

109.   Colacurci N, De Franciscis P, Fornaro F, et al. The significance of hysteroscopic treatment of congenital uterine malformations. Reprod Biomed Online 2002;4:52–54.

110.   Fedele L, Vercellini P, Ricciardiello O, et al. Second-look hysteroscopy after conservative surgery of the uterus. Acta Eur Fertil 1986;17;341–343.

111.   Hay D. Diagnosis and significance of minor defects of uterine abnormality in relation to pregnancy. J Obstet Gynecol Brit Emp 1958;65:557–561.

112.   Tompkins P. Comments on the bicornuate uterus and twinning. Surg Clin North Am 1962;42:1049–1062.

7 Uterine Abnormalities Resulting from DES Exposure

The drug was shown to be beneficial in the treatment of threatened abortion and of . . . abortions that would be anticipated because of previously lost gestations . . .
— O. W. Smith and G. V. S. Smith, 1948

The administration of DES . . . did not reduce the incidence of abortion, prematurity or postmaturity.
— W. J. Dieckmann, 1953

Although the majority of mullerian anomalies are congenital in nature, a unique group of anatomic abnormalities of the male and female reproductive tracts are secondary to in utero exposure to diethylstilbestrol (DES). The history of DES presents an interesting study in the application of basic science to clinical care and what is known in contemporary parlance as "evidence-based medicine". Interest in nonsteroidal estrogens in the 1920s and 1930s focused on developing orally active preparations.[1] In 1933 DES was synthesized by E. C. Dodds in Middlesex, London.[2] There was considerable clinical interest in DES because of its unique effectiveness when administered orally.[3,4] Intensive laboratory and clinical studies investigating its potential role in a variety of clinical settings were carried out shortly thereafter.[5] DES was the most widely researched of the synthetic estrogens and found clinical applications in gynecology, endocrinology, and oncology. Early investigations through the late 1930s and early 1940s demonstrated a marked improvement in the relief of menopausal symptoms in dosages varying from 0.2 to 0.5 mg per day.[6]

In 1948, an article by Smith suggested that DES prevented recurrent pregnancy loss, preterm labor, and preeclampsia.[7] The study was observational, descriptive, without control groups, and based on the extrapolation of laboratory observations to clinical events. Several similar studies followed, and the drug gained an intense following.[8] The efficacy of DES was tested in 1953 by Dieckmann and colleagues in a prospective, double-blind study of 840 women who received the recommended dosage and 806 women to whom placebos were administered.[9] The investigators found no benefits among the patients who took DES. The significance of these conclusions was not recognized at the time.

DES continued to gain popularity. It was used in expanding clinical circumstances, including menopausal hormone replacement therapy. DES had its most profound effect (as revealed by long-term follow-up) when used to prevent first-trimester loss, an effect not related to a reduction in first-trimester abortion but to long-term consequences of the offspring. So widespread was the use of DES that it was included in a variety of preparations, including prenatal vitamins (Figure 7-1). Inclusion of DES in a broad array of medications made tracking patients with in utero exposure to DES

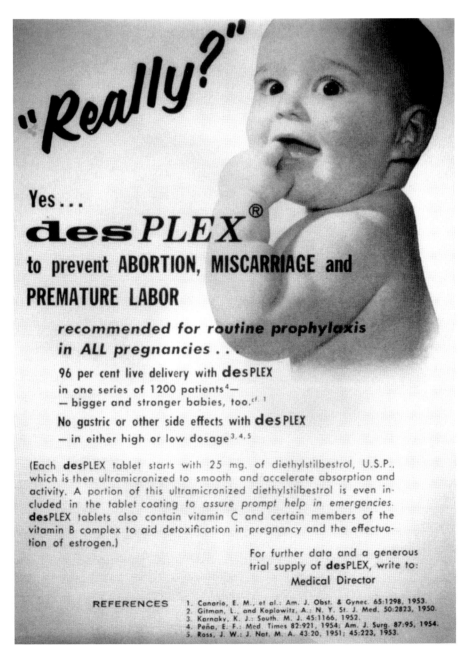

Figure 7-1   Advertisement circa 1955 for desPLEX, a combination of 25 mg DES and vitamins B and C.

particularly difficult. The drug was used throughout the 1950s and 1960s, and its molecular structure varied somewhat to yield a variety of DES-type drugs (Table 7-1). This prescription pattern gained momentum through the

Table 7-1. DES-Type Drugs that May Have Been Prescribed to Pregnant Women		
Nonsteroidal estrogens		
Benzestrol	Gynben	Restrol
Chlorotrianisene	Gyneben	Stilbal
Comestrol	Hexestrol	Stilbestrol
Cyren A and B	Hexoestrol	Stilbetin
Delvinal	Menocrin	Stilbinol
DesPlex	Meprane	Stilboestrol
Dibestil	Mestilbol	Stilestrate
Diestryl	Microest	Stilpalmitate
Dienestrol	Mikarol	Stilphostrol
Dienoestrol	Milestrol	Stilronate
Diethylstilbestrol	Neo-Oestranol I	Stilrone
Digestil	Nulabort	Stils
Domestrol	Oestrogenine	Synestrin
Estilben	Oestromenin	Synestrol
Estrobene	Oestromon	Synthoestrin
Estrosyn	Orestol	Tace
Fonatol	Pabestrol D	Vallestril
	Palestrol	
Nonsteroidal estrogen–progesterone combination		
Progravidium		
Vaginal cream suppositories with nonsteroidal estrogens		
AVC cream with dienestrol	Dienestrol cream	

183

late 1950s and early 1960s despite six controlled clinical trials between 1955 and 1965 that failed to demonstrate the efficacy of such therapy. During this time period, an estimated 500,000 to 2 million women in the United States used DES during their pregnancy.[10]

When the early studies by Smith and Smith in the 1940s were performed, they were state-of-the-art clinical investigations. Later refinement in experimental techniques and evaluation placed these studies in better perspective. They did not control confounding variables such as observation bias or recognize the need for randomization or placebo control. The study by Dieckmann was well executed, but its design and conclusions were exceptions to the established trends. At a time when little recognition was given to study design and quality of clinical data, the significance of the strength of the conclusions was lost. A recent recalculation of these data revealed that DES significantly increased abortions, neonatal deaths, and premature births.[11] A review of early DES literature revealed that all of the DES studies that showed clinical benefit lacked control groups and were not blinded, whereas those reports that failed to show benefit were more carefully designed and had controlled cohorts.[12] Even in the 1950s, a negative study failed to captivate the community as powerfully as a positive study.

DES usage peaked through the 1960s. Physicians continued to prescribe the hormone to many women until 1971 when Herbst reported the association of in utero DES exposure and clear cell adenocarcinoma in young women.[13] The association was described in a series of eight cases in which seven patients used DES and none of the mothers of 32 matched controls used the drug. The studies by Herbst were carefully executed case–control studies and observed a strong association between DES and subsequent vaginal cancer. These studies did not prove cause and effect but clearly implicated DES as the etiologic agent. The association was confirmed in other studies of young patients with clear cell adenocarcinoma of the vagina or cervix whose mothers described prenatal use of nonsteroidal estrogens, including DES, dienestrol, and hexestrol.[14] The influence of DES on the endometrial cavity in particular and the reproductive tract in general was subsequently described.[15] These descriptions led to the establishment of an international registry for the study of vaginal adenocarcinoma in patients with a history of in utero exposure to nonsteroidal estrogens. The unusual nature of the tumor in young patients contributed to general public alarm and the drug was shortly abandoned for prenatal use. An FDA bulletin in 1971 contraindicated its use in pregnancy.

The scope of the risk and size of the exposed population remained unknown for some time. Studies from the National Cooperative Diethylstilbestrol Adenosis Project (DESAD) soon showed that the risk of adenocarcinoma of the vagina among daughters exposed to DES in utero was lower than some investigators had initially feared.[16,17] However, concerns began to grow about the risks for other disease, not only among these daughters, but also among the mothers who had taken DES during pregnancy and sons who had been exposed in utero to DES. Concern for anyone exposed to the drug led to the formulation of a unique nomenclature for these groups – DES daughters, DES mothers, and DES sons. Distribution of DES was prohibited in the United States in 1971, and in 1973, the Committee on Safety of Medicines in the United Kingdom advised against use of DES during pregnancy.[18] Additional registries were formed to track outcomes and calculate risks (Table 7-2).

The demographics of this population make DES a relevant topic today. Many of those exposed in utero are now 30 to 50 years of age. They have reached and in some cases passed through the reproductive phase of their lives. Assisted reproductive technologies and oocyte donation may extend the reproductive potential well beyond age 50. Patients who were exposed to DES will be reaching age 45 in the years ranging from 2000 (for those exposed during 1955, a peak year for prescribing the drug) to 2019 (for those exposed during 1973, the final year for use.[18,19] Whether in utero exposure to stilbestrol has any consequences for women entering menopause and

Table 7-2. DES Cohort Studies	
Project Name	**Project Description**
• Diethylstilbestrol Adenosis Project (DESAD)	• Initiated in 1974 • 4014 DES daughters and 1033 unexposed women • Determine any increased risk of DES daughters to a variety of health-related problems
• DES Mothers Study	• Initiated in 1980 • 3000 women exposed to DES while pregnant (the mothers) and 3000 unexposed women • Determine the degree of risk of women exposed to DES while pregnant for any increased cancer risk
• Connecticut Mothers Study	• 1706 DES-exposed mothers and 1405 unexposed mothers
• Dieckmann Cohort	• Initiated in 1974 to study DES-related health risks • Cohort included 800 women exposed to DES while pregnant and 800 unexposed mothers; 400 DES daughters and 400 control group women, and 400 men exposed to DES before birth and 400 unexposed men
• British Medical Council (BRMC) Study	• Included DES daughters and DES sons identified through follow-up study to include 79 DES-exposed and 72 unexposed people
• British Randomized Trial	• Designed to study DES-related health effects and includes 379 mothers, 144 DES daughters and 177 DES sons and a control group of 371 unexposed mothers, 170 unexposed daughters and 163 unexposed sons
• Registry for Research on Hormonal Transplacental Carcinogenesis	• Initiated in 1971 to track the incidence of clear cell adenocarcinoma of the cervix and vagina • Now includes 750 cases of these malignancies

showed a 25% rate of spontaneous first-trimester abortion and term delivery at a mean of 37 weeks' gestation. Patients without upper or lower tract changes and colposcopic abnormalities only had a spontaneous first-trimester abortion rate of 12% and delivery at a mean of 39.8 weeks' gestation.[71] These findings lead to two important suggestions: (1) upper tract changes may not result in an increase in preterm delivery or shortening of gestation (based on similar durations of 37 weeks and 39 weeks) and (2) cervical incompetence is probably rare in patients with lower tract changes (comparing first-trimester spontaneous abortion rates of 25 and 12%) and thus questions the need for cerclage placement. These findings suggest that conservative management may result in a favorable outcome.

In patients who have upper and lower tract changes and who have consistently unfavorable outcomes of either repeated mid-trimester loss or prematurity, consideration should be given to the placement of a cerclage or gestational surrogacy. In utero DES exposure resulting in both upper and lower tract changes may be managed with the placement of a cerclage early in pregnancy. In one series without a control group, a higher rate of term pregnancy was described.[49] In patients with a history of recurrent pregnancy loss and a constricted, T-shaped uterine cavity, resectoscopic and abdominal metroplasty resulted in a decrease in the incidence of first-trimester loss and prematurity but did not result in any enhancement of fertility in patients with a history of infertility.[72–75] Extreme care is required in recommending either resectoscopic or abdominal metroplasty in this setting. Cerclage or resectoscopic metroplasty is based on extremely limited series without adequate controls. Before any recommendation for either modality can be made, especially given favorable outcomes with conservative management, larger prospective and comparative studies are necessary. Gestational surrogacy may offer a less invasive option for reproductive potential.

In patients with a history of infertility, IVF is an effective means of achieving pregnancy, with pregnancy rates comparable with those in a normal, unexposed population.[56,57] In patients with a markedly contracted uterine cavity and a history of repeated first-trimester loss or prematurity, gestational host surrogacy may be offered. IVF outcomes demonstrated pregnancy rates for DES-exposed patients similar to rates for controls, a 23% pregnancy rate per patient and 19% per embryo transfer (data from 1988, 1990 and 1992).[76–78]

Outcomes Analysis

The influence of DES exposure on reproductive outcomes is controversial. Viewed most favorably, DES exposure has no adverse influence on any aspect of reproduction, whether infertility or repeated first-trimester loss. A number of case-control studies describe no differences in reproductive outcomes between exposed and unexposed daughters.[79] Two studies, however, found that DES daughters have a higher incidence of infertility than controls.

These studies are in the exceptions. Overall, there is no increase in infertility. Viewed most cautiously, reproductive outcomes for DES daughters are adversely influenced, with increases in first-trimester loss, prematurity, and ectopic pregnancy. In some series, the first-trimester spontaneous abortion rate is doubled, the incidence of preterm deliveries tripled, and term delivery rate reduced to 55%. The survival rate of infants is 67%, owing to preterm labor and preterm delivery. Among patients with cervical and vaginal changes, a preterm delivery rate of 74% may be expected.[56] Nevertheless, 80% of DES daughters have delivered at least one live-born infant.[56]

The possibility exists that DES exposure may result in increases in the incidence of all neoplastic processes.[18,19,80] A 25-year follow-up on the subjects of the Dieckmann study showed an increase in breast cancer among DES mothers, but this increase was not statistically significant.[81,82] A follow-up study of women seen at the Mayo Clinic who had received smaller doses than did the women in the Dieckmann study did not show an increase in breast cancer among the DES mothers. The association between DES exposure and testicular cancers in DES sons remains controversial. Exposure to DES has also been linked to immune system disorders and psychosexual effects in DES sons and daughters. No evidence for transgenerational effects exists. The risk for many cancers of the reproductive tract does not begin until after the age of 50. Hence, the long-term impact of DES on daughters' well-being is unclear. Continued monitoring of this group for any neoplastic changes in mullerian-derived structures is warranted. All men and women born between the years 1938 and 1971 should attempt to ascertain their DES exposure status for both purposes of reproductive potential and for the possibility of long-term adverse outcomes of both male and female reproductive tract cancers. Further research is needed to define long-term health effects related to DES exposure. Such research would provide a basis for counseling persons exposed to DES and would further understanding of environmental and pharmacologic compounds similar to DES.[83]

Summary and Recommendations

The short-term effects of in utero exposure to DES are well defined. Reproductive issues, still a concern as DES daughters continue to explore their reproductive potential, become more complicated as these patients pass age 40. Not only must the possible influence of DES exposure on their reproductive outcomes be addressed, but in addition, they must contend with the issue of age-related infertility. The long-term effects of in utero exposure to DES are unknown. There is a suggestion that the mothers of DES daughters are at an increased risk of breast cancer. The risk to the daughters is unknown. The literature describing the influence of in utero exposure to DES on reproductive outcome mainly presents case-control studies. There appears to be no increase in infertility but an increased incidence of adverse outcomes. Several recommendations and conclusions can be drawn:

expression such as menstrual timing, race, and uniformity in microarray platforms.[22] Microarray analysis should provide insight regarding the differential expression of genes in myomatous tissue and hopefully targeted therapy that will be patient specific, non-surgical, and durable.[23]

These data suggest that specific chromosomal and genetic abnormalities could characterize the same tumor type, regardless of histologic appearance. The possibilities of genetic variability of myomas within the same patient or across different patients could explain their differential growth patterns and response to a similar hormonal milieu.[24,25] Variable growth patterns of myomas may be observed within the same uterus, that is, differential growth of various myomas within one specimen, or between different patients. The variable growth suggests a unique interaction between the individual myoma and either the hormonal milieu of the individual or the underlying myometrium secondary to the specific genetics of each myoma. This genetic heterogeneity of the tumors may be present within different myomas in the same uterus and thus account for the varied growth. Somatic mutations may also confer a selective growth advantage of one tumor to another on the basis of modifying responsiveness to identical hormonal environments.

Ovarian Steroids

Differences in biologic behavior may also be caused by a variable endocrine milieu rather than a distinctive property of the myomas. Ovarian steroids are clearly contributory factors to the growth of myomas in complex ways not fully understood. Estradiol stimulation and activation of estrogen-sensitive uterine genes may be one primary reason why these tumors proliferate.[26] A dependency on cyclic secretion of estradiol, progesterone, or both for growth and development may underlie the occurrence and increase in size and number of myomas during the reproductive years and their regression at menopause. In addition, continuous estradiol secretion, uninterrupted by pregnancy and lactation, is another risk factor in the development of these tumors. Any process that interrupts the cyclic process of rising and falling gonadal steroids decreases the risk of these tumors. Pregnancy confers protection and the relative risk of myomas decreases with each additional term pregnancy. An association of myomas and nulliparity further suggests the increased risk of continuous, uninterrupted menstrual cycling. Oral contraceptives reduce the risk of myomas by approximately 17% with each 5 years of usage. Cigarette smoking also reduces the risk of myomas, possibly related to changes in estradiol secretion. Women who smoke more than 10 cigarettes per day have an 18% lower risk than do nonsmokers.[10,27]

Reduction in estradiol and progesterone secretion reduces size. Gonadotropin-releasing hormone (GnRH) agonists have provided an insightful method to investigate the dependence of these tumors on ovarian steroids. The induction of a reversible medical menopause with GnRH agonists results in a reduction of myoma size. These observations have further substantiated their estrogen and/or progesterone dependence.[28] Both the shrinkage and the consistent finding of increased size with discontinuation of the GnRH agonists and return of cyclical ovarian function support this.

The clinical observation of the dependency of these tumors on estrogen secretion is also supported by studies of their steroid receptor content. Analysis of steroid receptor content of myomas demonstrates a significant increase in cytoplasmic receptors for 17-β estradiol and progesterone within uterine myomas that exceeds that of the surrounding myometrium and endometrium.[29] Though estradiol receptors are consistently present, progesterone receptors are variably expressed. These observations suggest a differential receptivity of myomas to the same hormonal milieu. In culture studies, growth pattern depends on the amount of estrogen, with variable responses to both progesterone and insulin.[30] The demonstration of mitoses and identical S-phase fraction in response to estradiol suggests that myomas are sensitive to this steroid. Tissue cultures of normal myometrium and myomas, however, do not consistently demonstrate that estradiol is differentially mitogenic. These results suggest a clear-cut dependency on but differential response to ovarian steroids in support of the marked clinical diversity of these tumors.

The role of progesterone in myoma growth may be more critical than originally thought. Two lines of evidence make a compelling case for this concept. Mifepristone is a powerful antiglucocorticoid and antiprogesterone. The drug has found application in a variety of clinical circumstances in which steroid metabolism is critical. This agent mediates its effect largely through interaction with progesterone receptors. It blocks receptor function at multiple steps including the binding of progesterone to the receptor, altering conformational changes associated with this binding, blocking both dissociation of associated proteins and receptor dimerization. Mifepristone reduces myoma size, suggesting that progesterone in some fashion, perhaps in synergism with estradiol, exerts a proliferative effect on myoma growth.

These responses of myomas to an antiprogesterone raise several questions regarding the estrogen dependence hypothesis. These findings with the observation that the medroxyprogesterone acetate may increase myoma size in GnRH agonist-suppressed patients (when these agents are started concomitantly) suggests that the paradigm that estradiol stimulates and progesterone inhibits myoma growth should be reevaluated. Mifepristone may act as a noncompetitive antiestrogen by its ability to antagonize the mitogenic effects of estrogen. The action of mifepristone may also be mediated through its action on a variety of growth factors. The finding that epidermal growth factor mRNA in myomas is elevated during the luteal phase of the menstrual cycle suggests that progesterone may provide a stimulation to myoma growth mediated through increasing concentrations of epidermal growth factor.

Mifepristone provides yet another medical management for uterine myomas. This reduction in myoma size appears to occur in spite of serum estradiol concentrations consistent with luteal phase levels. This provides an obvious advantage in avoiding the hypoestrogenism and bone loss attendant to long-term use of GnRH agonists. Further use of these agents in investigating myoma response may also provide insight regarding the exact mechanisms of growth of these unique uterine tumors.

Growth Factors

Growth factors provide a third explanation for the unique growth patterns of myomas. Several factors have a role in cell proliferation and differentiation of epithelial and stromal cell lines and, as such, may play a critical role in the initiation and growth of myomas. These factors include epidermal growth factor, platelet-derived growth factor (PDGF), insulin-like growth factor (IGF), insulin, keratinocyte growth factor, and transforming growth factor.

EGF is a single chain polypeptide that stimulates cellular growth and affects smooth muscle proliferation via both autocrine and paracrine mechanisms mediated in part by estrogen. Receptors for EGF are present in myometrium and myomas. The messenger RNA (mRNA) encoding for EGF has been detected in both normal myometrium and myoma cells. Production of EGF in myomas appears to be cycle dependent and increases during the secretory phase suggesting that an initial priming by estradiol and subsequent stimulation by progesterone may be necessary to fully express EGF. This finding also calls into play an increased role for progesterone. The exact role of EGF in the growth of myomas, however, may be considerably more complex. Conflicting reports describe EGF content in myomas throughout the menstrual cycle as both a steady state and increased concentration in the follicular and luteal phases noted. In addition, EGF receptors, although present in both normal myometrium and myomas, is similar to and in some studies less than that found in the myometrium. The exact role of EGF in the growth of myomas is speculative and may be mediated through a complex interaction with estrogen and progesterone in conjunction with other growth factors.

PDGF is a second growth factor implicated in the growth of myomas. PDGF binds to both normal human myometrium and myomas. The receptor for PDGF has been demonstrated by in situ hybridization probes and immunofluorescence in human endometrium and cultured myometrial cells. They contribute to the growth of fibroids through a mitogenic effect in conjunction with IGF-1. Transforming growth factor beta-1 (TGFβ-1) and TGFβ-3 have also been demonstrated to be highly expressed in myomas. The concentration of TGFβ and TGFβ receptor mRNA were suppressed during treatment with GnRH analogs suggesting that TGFβ and receptor expression may have a role in both myoma growth and during myoma regression.

Insulin-like growth factors I and II have emerged as prominent factors in myoma growth. Both IGF-I and IGF-II genes are expressed in the myometrium, myomas, and leiomyosarcomas. They have a differential, tissue-specific sensitivity to estrogen. The IGF-I gene within a myoma is estrogen dependent while the IGF-II gene is neither cycle nor estrogen dependent. Both are concentrated within uterine myomas. Increased contents of mRNAs for IGF-I and IGF-II have been described in both myomas and leiomyosarcomas. Similarly, mRNA for IGF binding proteins (IGFBP) in uterine myomas and their underlying myometrium is also present. Transcripts for the five major binding proteins have been found in normal myometrium and myomas. They may provide a vehicle for the expression of the ovarian steroids at a cellular level. The effect of GnRH agonist treatment for a period of 4 to 6 months decreases the secretion of IGF-I and IGF-II in cultures of tissue from women treated with GnRH agonists compared with controls. This suggests that another mechanism by which GnRH agonist therapy may exert a decrease in fibroid size is by decreasing IGFs in both myometrium and myoma.

IGF-I and IGF-II and their binding proteins (IGFBP) exhibit a sensitivity to ovarian steroids that parallels clinical observations of growth of myomas. This sensitivity may result in their growth-promoting effect on myomas through both an autocrine and paracrine interaction involving estrogen and progesterone. IGF binding proteins may be further modulated by either an autocrine or paracrine mechanism of IGF-I action in this tissue. To exert their mitogenic and growth-promoting activity, these growth factors interact through their receptors in the normal myometrium and myoma. Myomas have an increased concentration of IGF-I but not IGF-II receptors when compared with normal myometrium. IGF-I but not IGF-II was identified as a mediator of estradiol action in the growth of myomas. Increased concentrations of type 1 IGF-I receptors in myoma compared with the normal myometrium may provide myomas with a differential growth advantage compared with the surrounding myometrium and may in part be responsible for the differential growth of these tumors.

Cyclins are major cell cycle regulators responsible for the progression of cells through various phases of the cycle. Cyclins are associated with a family of cyclin-dependent protein kinases with a link to oncogenesis. Cyclin G1 may be responsible in part for the growth of uterine leiomyomas. It has been demonstrated that cyclin G1 is overexpressed in these tumors and may be responsible for the cellular proliferation noted within these tumors.

Unanswered questions regarding myoma growth and their natural history include the varying growth patterns of myomas within the same uterus and exposed to the same hormonal milieu; variable recurrence rates that may be related to myoma size, numbers, and age of initial occurrence; differential and variable responses of a myoma and myometrium, possibly secondary to the heterogeneity of receptor content, variable cytogenetics, and differential responses to systemic and local hormonal milieu; and the consistent response to GnRH analogs secondary to a decrease in estrogen and progesterone.[31]

Clinical Correlates

Myomas may be single, multiple, and of varying size. The macroscopic appearance is that of a firm, round tumor with a surrounding pseudo-capsule. They may be located on the serosal surfaces (subserosal), within the myometrium (intramural) or just beneath the endometrium (submucous). Those that are subserosal may occasionally develop on a stalk and are labeled as pedunculated. Occasionally, these may obtain preferential blood supply from adjacent organs such as the omentum or bowel and become "parasitic". In other cases, subserosal myomas may protrude into the broad ligament to form an intraligamentous myoma. Submucosal myomas are located immediately beneath the endometrium. They may also become pedunculated within the endometrial cavity and at times they protrude through the cervical os or may grow to substantial sizes and occupy the entire endometrial cavity.

The microscopic appearance of the tumors differs considerably depending on the degree of interlacing smooth muscle fibers and fibrous tissue and the degree of calcification and degeneration. Three specific types of degeneration – hyalin, cystic, and calcific – that further modify the histologic appearance have been described.[32] Histologically, myomas are composed of whirling bundles of smooth muscle cells that resemble the architecture of the uninvolved myometrium. The individual muscle cells are usually uniform in size and shape, with a characteristic oval nucleus and bipolar slender cytoplasmic processes. When degenerative changes occur, these foci appear as ischemic areas of necrosis with hemorrhage and in extreme cases, collapsed cells in various stages of degradation. Mitotic figures are scarce, creating a compelling histologic picture of a benign process. The histologic appearance of myomas may be modified after GnRH agonist therapy. GnRH agonist therapy may increase cellularity and hyalinization when compared with controls. There are no changes in mitotic activity, fibrosis, pleomorphism, and necrosis after GnRH agonist therapy.[33–35]

Myomas are usually benign. However, malignant degeneration (leiomyosarcoma) is a clear concern in any patient with a fibroid that rapidly increases. The incidence of sarcoma in such patients is extremely low accounting for only 0.23% of all uterine sarcomas.[36,37] (Rapid uterine growth may be defined as an increase by 6 weeks' gestational size on clinical examination during 1 year.) Rare forms of manifestations as leiomyomatosis include intravenous extension of leiomyomas of the uterus and leiomyomatosis peritonealis disseminata.[38,39] Intravenous leiomyomatosis is the extension into the venous channels of histologically benign smooth muscle tumors arising from a uterine myoma or from smooth muscle cells of neighboring vessels. These tumors may extend for considerable distances within vessel lumens. Intracardiac spread has been described. Leiomyomatosis peritonealis disseminata is a rare clinical entity consisting of subperitoneal nodules seemingly composed of smooth muscle disseminated throughout the abdominal cavity.[40,41]

The cases reported to date suggest the possibility of hormonal influence leading to these changes. Myomas have been rarely described within the ovarian substance itself.[38,39]

Myomas are present in 20 to 50% of women older than 30 years, and 20 to 50% of women with myomas have symptoms that can be attributed to these tumors.[12,18,42] The symptoms associated with myomas are usually related to either the size or the location of the tumor. Occasionally degeneration, torsion, infarction, or infection may cause acute symptoms. The overwhelming majority of patients will present secondary to complications of size or location. The most common myoma-related symptoms are caused by the mass effect of an enlarged uterus on adjacent pelvic organs and to excessive menstrual bleeding. Most myomas are asymptomatic, are noted incidentally on clinical examination or on ultrasound examination performed for other indications, and do not require treatment.

Several symptoms require evaluation and decisions regarding whether management, if any, is required and of what specific type.[43] Specific clinical scenarios that require evaluation and possible therapy can be categorized into four groups: gynecologic indications for abnormal uterine bleeding, pelvic pain, or lower urinary tract symptoms; reproductive disorders, such as infertility and repeated pregnancy loss; pregnancy-related indications both prior to conception and during pregnancy; and prior to IVF depending on myoma size and location. Recommendations for management may vary depending on which type of indication is present.

Gynecologic Indications

Indications for intervention commonly are irregular bleeding and symptoms secondary to mass effect of the myomas, such as pelvic pain, pressure, and urinary frequency. Menstrual irregularities are noted in 30% of women who have myomas.[44,45] Various theories have been proposed to explain the etiology of the irregular bleeding. The likelihood that a specific myoma will result in any menstrual abnormality depends on its size and location. Increased blood loss is secondary to an increase in the surface area of the uterine cavity when the myoma is submucous. An increase in the amount of prostaglandins in menstrual effluent in patients who have myomas may also contribute[10] and probably leads to further increases in dysmenorrhea and blood loss. Marked congestion and dilatation of the endometrial venus plexuses surrounding the myomas, also occurs which further impede the normal coagulation process.

Myomas may result in acute pain that is sometimes associated with febrile morbidity and peritoneal signs. Such symptoms may be associated with degeneration of a myoma or, occasionally, torsion of a pedunculated tumor. In these circumstances, a conservative approach is warranted until the acute episode resolves. In other circumstances, dull lower abdominal pelvic pain or pressure may result from a mass effect as the myoma grows within the pelvis. Urinary frequency or constipation may be noted when these tumors increase in size, either anteriorly or posteriorly, and exert pressure either on the bladder or rectum, respectively. Hydronephrosis may result when myomas increase substantially in size and compress the ureter against the pelvic side wall. These tumors are typically not associated with stress-related urinary incontinence. Hence, any patient presenting with this symptom should undergo a complete urogynecologic evaluation.

Reproductive Indications

The influence of myomas on infertility and reproduction is expressed in several ways.[46] Uterine myomas, whether submucosal or intramural, are significant if large enough or if they distort the endometrial cavity.[47–49] In these circumstances, myomas are associated with increased risks of first-trimester loss, preterm delivery, abnormal presentation in labor, and both postpartum hemorrhage and sepsis. Up to 15% of patients presenting with infertility have asymptomatic uterine myomas, including submucous myomas.[50] A meta-analysis of patients undergoing in vitro fertilization suggested that the relative risk of pregnancy for women with submucous myomas was 0.32 (95% confidence interval: 0.13–0.70). After resection, the relative risk of pregnancy rose to 1.72 (CI 1.13–2.58). Several observations suggest that uterine myomas are significant factors in reproduction. In uncontrolled studies, pregnancy rates after abdominal myomectomy in one of the earliest studies in 1991 revealed a marked increase in fertility after the surgery. In subsequent studies, fertility increased with myomectomy regardless of whether the procedure is done transabdominally, laparoscopically, or hysteroscopically.

Uterine myomas may also impact outcomes after assisted reproductive technologies.[51] Regardless of the impact of the myomas on the endometrial cavity, if large enough, the presence of myomas reduce the efficacy of any ART treatment. Pregnancy rates and implantation rates appear to be lowest when the myomas exceed 5 cm in size or are located in an intramural or submucosal position. The issue is not without controversy.[52] Myoma size and location continue to be a debated issue. In patients with normal uterine cavities and myomas less than 7 cm, some studies have suggested that myomectomy is not necessary. Outcomes after in vitro fertilization in some studies are identical when the endometrial cavity is normal and the uterine myoma is less than 7 cm. In other studies any intramural myomas appear to adversely impact outcome after assisted reproductive technologies. In one study analyzing only patients with intramural myomas $\leq$ 5 cm in size, implantation and pregnancy rates were one-half that of matched control patients.[53,54] In this study, logistic regression analysis demonstrated that the presence of intramural fibroids was one of the most significant variables impacting the likelihood of a live birth (odds ratio 0.46; CI 0.24–0.88; $P = 0.019$). Hence, even small intramural myomas not impacting the shape of the endometrial cavity can negatively affect outcomes after assisted reproductive technologies.

One possible explanation for this impact of myomas on implantation may be related to changes in the endometrial micro-environment and several important proteins.[55] Glycodelin is a glycoprotein present in both serum and uterine flushings. It has been implicated in the process of implantation and angiogenesis. During the luteal phase of the menstrual cycle, progesterone secretion is related to glycodelin production by the endometrium. Endometrial glycodelin levels are significantly increased in patients with endometrial polyps and myomas. Both myomas and polyps are associated with significantly greater plasma glycodelin levels and endometrial/uterine glycodelin. These elevations are noted both in the follicular and periovulatory period in addition to the luteal phase of the menstrual cycle. Myomas may impact cycle-dependent glycodelin secretion and ultimately endometrial function. Alterations in glycodelin secretion may adversely impact both fertilization and implantation.

Several other hypotheses regarding impact of myomas on reproduction have been suggested. Classic theories include altered uterine contractility, impaired sperm transport, and impaired implantation.[49–59] Another potential mechanism for infertility secondary to submucosal myomas may involve changes in the endometrial structure overlying the myoma. In these regions, histologic study of the endometrium revealed either no endometrial glands or marked reduction in the number of glands. When present, glands were significantly fewer in number (97 per 2-mm section versus 82.6 per 2-mm section for the control group).[60] A significant difference was noted in the analysis of the thickness of the myometrium between the myomas and overlying endometrium in these groups.

Obstetric Indications

Obstetric complications occur in one-third of patients with myomas.[61] These reports are primarily descriptive and suggest a correlation between myomas and specific adverse obstetric outcomes. Cause and effect has not been proven. These complications include premature rupture of the membranes and preterm labor and delivery. Preterm labor occurs in 20 to 30% of patients with myomas, influenced by the size and location of the myomas.[62] Patients with myomas smaller than 3 cm appear at minimal risk, while those with sizes ranging from 3 to 5 cm and larger than 5 cm are at 20 and 28% risk of preterm labor, respectively.[63]

The most common antenatal complication associated with myomas is abnormal fetal presentation. The most frequent presentation is breech in 91%, with the second most common being transverse. In one study of 113 women, a significant increase in malpresentation with multiple myomas (24%) when compared with patients with single myomas (11%) was described.[63] Dysfunctional labor, placental abruption, postpartum hemorrhage, and postpartum sepsis have all been associated with myomas. Presence of myomas carries with it a relative risk of 2.4 for cesarean section due to labor abnormalities.[64–66] Both myoma size and location are independent predictors of cesarean section, with a relative risk of 2.6 with myomas of diameter larger than 5 cm and a relative risk of 2.4 if they are located in the lower uterine segment.[67] The incidence of cesarean section, however, is influenced by the number of myomas. Placental abruption is increased in patients with myoma volumes greater than 200 cc and in a retroplacental location.[64] Placental abruption has been described in 11% of patients with sonographically demonstrated myomas, compared with approximately 1% in the normal population. Postpartum sepsis in a population of women with myomas in one study was tenfold greater than matched controls. In this series, 75% of women were noted to have cystic degeneration of the myoma. No clear-cut association of hemorrhage has been noted.

Congenital fetal abnormalities and deformities have also been described in association with myomas.[68] The prevalence of localized malformations in pregnancy with myomas is twice that of controls and is consistent across all age groups in one study.[69] Intrauterine growth restriction has also been described.[63,65] Myomas larger than 10 cm appear to have a negative influence on fetal growth.[63] Possible contributing factors may relate a compromise of blood flow and placental function.

Women with myomas depending on size, number and location should be counseled preconceptionally regarding the possibilities of spontaneous abortion, painful degeneration of the myomas, preterm labor, intrauterine growth restriction and fetal malformations.[47,69] Care should be taken in counseling and the quality of evidence included in discussion. Observational data suggest benefit but there are no randomized trials that conclude myomectomy will improve outcome. The final decision should take into account past reproductive history, immediate fertility plans, and the overall interests of the patient.

Diagnosis

Conventional Radiography

The majority of myomas are diagnosed on physical examination or on ultrasound examination. The suspicion of a myoma is usually based on the finding of an enlarged, firm, nontender, and irregularly shaped uterus. Hysterosalpingography (HSG) and conventional radiography of the abdomen may suggest the presence of a myoma. The finding of "egg shell" calcifications on abdominal or pelvic x-rays was frequently the first indication of the presence of myomas. On HSG, the cavity may demonstrate filling defects and an enlarged volume. A characteristic filling pattern may be recognized on fluoroscopy during HSG because the contrast medium flows around the myoma (Figures 8-1 and 8-2). Complete filling of the cavity may result in a

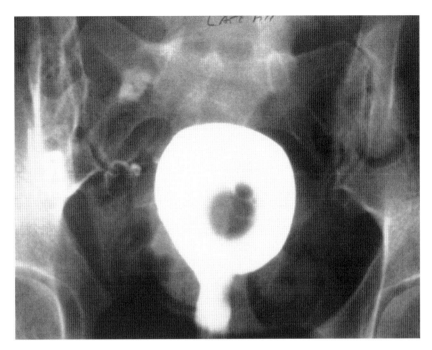

Figure 8-1   Hysterosalpingogram demonstrating marked enlargement and distortion of the uterine cavity with a central filling defect in a patient with a large fundal myoma.

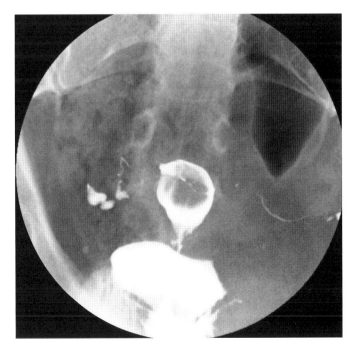

Figure 8-2   Hysterosalpingogram demonstrating a large central filling defect in a patient with an anterior myoma.

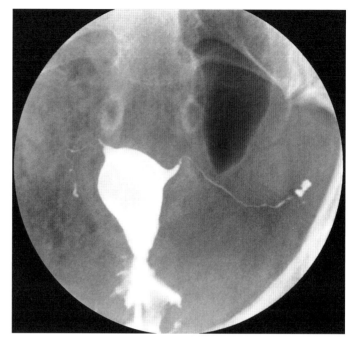

Figure 8-3   Hysterosalpingogram demonstrating anterior distortion of the endometrial cavity in a patient with a large posterior uterine myoma.

distorted, irregular pattern (Figure 8-3). These findings require confirmation by abdominal and pelvic ultrasound examination.

Ultrasound

Myomas are most frequently detected by pelvic ultrasound imaging. Confirmation of findings of clinical examination or HSG by transvaginal or transabdominal ultrasound is essential to define the number and size, evaluate for adenomyosis, and rule out the possibility that the palpated mass is ovarian in nature. Two- and three-dimensional ultrasound examination are the most efficient and cost-effective imaging techniques for diagnosing uterine myomas.[70] Their importance lies in its ability to assess size and location and to completely evaluate the adnexae.[71]

Ultrasound findings of myomas can present a wide spectrum of sonographic features, including deformity of the uterus, displacement of the endometrium when in submucosal location, poor acoustic transmission, and altered echogenicity of the myometrium (Figures 8-4 and 8-5).[70,71] Ultrasound appearance of the myomas may be as a discrete intramural, subserosal, or submucosal collection of tissue with well-defined borders. The myoma is distinct from the surrounding myometrium and may have variable echogenicity ranging from hypoechoic, echogenic, or isoechogenic changes when contrasted to the adjacent myometrium, depending on the composition of the

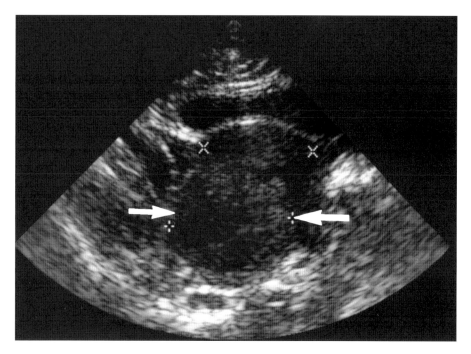

Figure 8-4   Transabdominal transverse ultrasound image of the uterus demonstrating a posterior myoma with posterior wall distortion (arrows).

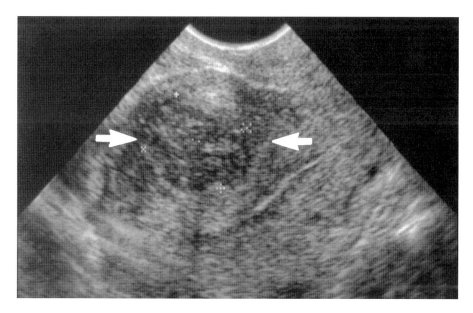

Figure 8-5   Transvaginal ultrasound image of a posterior wall myoma (arrows).

myoma (i.e., the degree of connective tissue and calcification). The echogenicity of the myoma depends in part on the ratio of fibrous tissue to smooth muscle and the degree of degeneration, if any. Cystic areas suggesting degeneration may be noted.

The low penetrance but high acuity of transvaginal scanning makes it ideal for locating intramural or submucosal fibroids. Transvaginal ultrasound scanning is most useful for small myoma. For very large myomas, transabdominal ultrasound scanning may better detect changes particularly if the myoma extends beyond the pelvis. Transabdominal scanning has a high false-negative rate for small myomas less than 2 mm. Transabdominal ultrasound is useful to evaluate larger myomas, especially those in which clinical examination demonstrates enlargement exceeding 6-week size.

Conventional transvaginal sonography for the diagnosis of submucous myomas has a sensitivity of 90% and a specificity of 98% (Figure 8-6 A and B).[70] Tumor size is more accurately assessed through sonography than hysteroscopy. Transvaginal sonography will fail to identify myomas less than 5% of the time. These failures may be due to location and size of the myomas.

Of all sonographic techniques, sonohysterographic evaluation of submucous myoma growth is the most precise.[41,70] Sonohysterography better defines the character of the endometrial cavity suggested on routine pelvic ultrasound examination.[72-74] The depiction of the endometrial surface is highlighted using contrast and particularly helpful in identifying myometrial masses because of the displacement of the characteristic trilaminar appearance of the myometrium. Sonohysterography is a less invasive and more cost-effective diagnostic study to assess these abnormalities before proceeding to more aggressive and costly hysteroscopy. Sonohysterography is particularly useful in demonstrating the exact relationship of the myoma to the endometrium and any degree of cavity distortion (Figures 8-7 A and B and 8-8).[75]

Transabdominal and transvaginal ultrasound evaluation of myomas during pregnancy is of invaluable assistance.[76,77] In addition to myoma size, the ultrasound evaluation of myomas during pregnancy should include definition of position, location, relationship to the placenta, and echogenic character. The ultrasound findings make it possible to identify women at risk for myoma-related complications. Calculation of the volume of the myoma may be of importance in determining patients most likely to experience complications. When myoma volume was related to complications during pregnancy or at delivery, size and volume were significant variables. Myomas with volumes of more than 200 cm^3 showed a higher complication rate than myomas with volumes of 100 cm^3 or less. Ultrasound monitoring of myomas during pregnancy is also useful in monitoring growth. Traditional teaching has been that myomas grow rapidly during pregnancy under the influence of estrogen.[78] In a study of 32 myomas in 29 pregnant women with serial ultrasound examinations, growth curves showed a maximum overall increase in

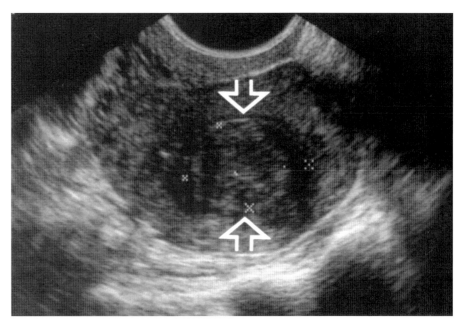

(A)

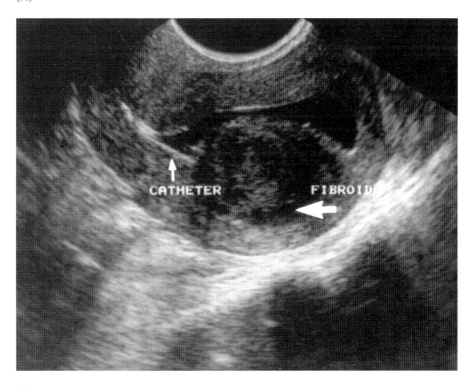

(B)

Figure 8-6   Sonohysterogram (preinjection) of a fundal uterine myoma (A). Post-injection image demonstrates anterior displacement of the cavity (B). Catheter and myoma are labeled with arrows.

(A)

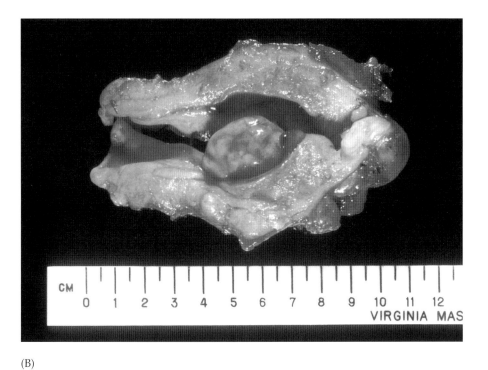

(B)

Figure 8-7   Sonohysterogram of a pedunculated intracavitary myoma (A). Surgical specimen of uterus imaged on SHG (B).

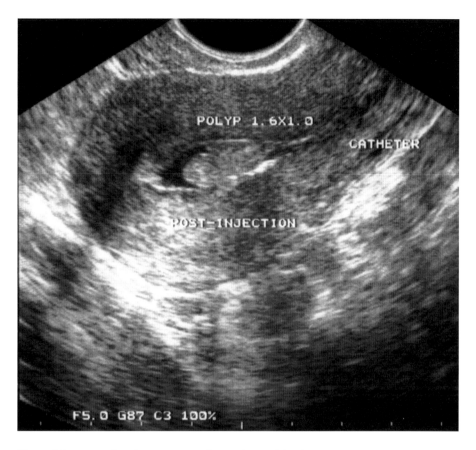

Figure 8-8   Sonohysterogram of an endometrial polyp.

volume of 25%, with most myomas showing a 10% increase of initial mea-surements.[79] During pregnancy, the only statistically significant change occurs in the first trimester, with a 32% increase in size.[80] In contrast to earlier perceptions, myoma growth later in pregnancy does occur, but generally the changes are minimal.

Magnetic Resonance Imaging

Magnetic resonance imaging (MRI) is a sensitive though more complex study for myomas.[81,82] It may be useful especially to confirm findings unclear on ultrasound scanning. MRI may be used to assess the size, location, and volume of myomas and is complimentary to ultrasound imaging (Figure 8-9). It provides more accurate measurement and more precise localization of the myoma than HSG. In addition, MRI provides insight into any extent of degeneration and vascularity of the myoma. Degenerative changes will influ-ence images depending on the type and degree of myomatous degenera-tion.[83] A mixed signal pattern of both low and high signal intensities is characteristic of a myxomatous or cystic degeneration (Figure 8-10). This

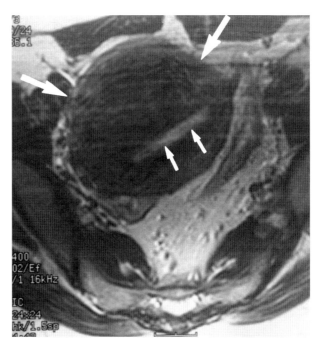

Figure 8-9   Axial magnetic resonance image of a subserosal uterine fibroid (large arrows). The endometrial stripe is recognized by characteristic hyperintense signals immediately beneath the myoma (arrows).

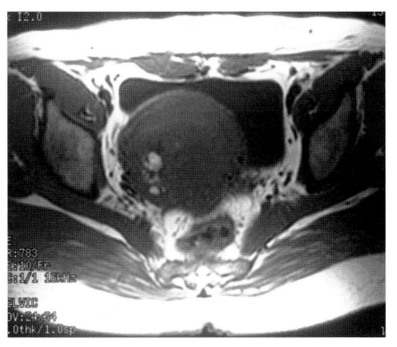

Figure 8-10   Degenerating intramural myoma. Sagittal T2 image demonstrating signal intensities consistent with partial calcification and degeneration of a myoma.

may be of value in monitoring response to GnRH analog therapy, or symptomatology suspected to be secondary to degeneration. In one series, MRI proved more sensitive than ultrasound imaging in assessing the response to therapy.[84] Whether MRI can improve outcome or clinical care, however, has not been conclusively proven.

Identification of the ovaries in cases of large myomas may be compromised during ultrasound examination. MRI provides an additional modality to evaluate the ovaries in this setting.[84] In one study, MRI visualized 44 of 46 ovaries; ultrasound scanning imaged only 21 of 46 in patients with a large myomatous uterus.[81] MRI provides a means to monitor size and progression of myomas when a conservative, expectant approach is elected and provides a means of calculating uterine volume. The quantitative assessment of the myomas in response to GnRH therapy, for example, may be more accurately assessed using MRI. Assessment of volumes using ultrasound may be problematic when the volume of the myoma exceeds 140 mL but does not appear to be problematic when MRI is used.[82]

The clinical role of MRI as superior to ultrasound has not been definitely proven. Decisions regarding therapy can frequently be made with an ultrasound examination and SHG and do not require the more expensive, though more detailed, MRI. At present, the impact of MRI for clinical decision making has not been shown to exceed that of ultrasound. Because of the added expense of MRI, it is not routinely advocated as a first-line diagnostic study; MRI should be used as a backup to both transabdominal and transvaginal ultrasound.

Hysteroscopy

Hysteroscopy is helpful in assessing the size and location of myomas suspected to be submucous, and allows a direct assessment of the uterine cavity for any distortion secondary to myomas in other locations. In conjunction with SHG (particularly if SHG findings are equivocal) it is part of preoperative planning if resectoscopic surgery is being considered. With the advent of SHG, the hysteroscopy is a second-line study for evaluating myomas assuming a more important role prior to ART.

Evaluation Prior to ART

Ultrasound examination and sonohysterography are required to evaluate both the myometrium and endometrial cavity (Table 8-1). Any myoma that is impacting the endometrial cavity may require removal. As noted above, any myoma, regardless of size and location, should be carefully evaluated. For myomas of less than 3 to 5 cm, discussion with the patient regarding their potential impact on outcome should be held. This becomes increasingly important for patients aged 38 years or more. A reevaluation of the endometrial cavity after surgery is essential to make certain that the endometrial cavity walls are smooth and even.

Table 8-1.
Evaluation Prior to ART: Leiomyomas

o Excision of all myomas that impact the endometrial cavity regardless of size

o Excision of all myomas greater than 5 cm regardless of location

o Evaluation of the endometrial cavity prior to surgery/myomectomy to rule out occult polyps

o Careful patient selection regarding resectoscopic myomectomy; when performed, precise use of resectoscope to limit damage to normal endometrium

o Assessment of the cavity postoperatively regardless of type of myomectomy; i.e., transabdominal laparoscopic or resectoscopic

o Questionable role of GnRH analog suppression for myoma shrinkage in patients who are > 35 years

The impact of uterine myomas regardless of size or location on outcomes with in vitro fertilization continues to be a debated point. Conflicting data exist regarding the influence of uterine myomas on implantation and pregnancy rates. This applies equally to intramural and submucosal myomas even when no distortion of the endometrial cavity is noted. In several studies when age, number of eggs, clinical response, and number of embryos are controlled for, the presence of both intramural and submucosal fibroids is associated with diminished implantation and live birth rates. Careful patient selection is essential, taking into consideration the patient's age, previous experiences (i.e., previous losses), size and growth of the myomas and location.

Management

Options for the management of uterine myoma are either nonsurgical or surgical. Nonsurgical methods include observation or expectant management, both agonist and antagonist GnRH analogs, and the antiprogesterone mifepristone. Surgical techniques include transabdominal, resectoscopic or laparoscopic myomectomy, uterine artery embolization and myolysis, and hysterectomy. The focus of surgical management of symptomatic uterine myomas in this chapter will be on techniques of myomectomy and will not include any discussion of hysterectomy. The decision regarding which therapy is most appropriate depends largely on the symptoms a patient experiences, the growth patterns of the myoma, and reproductive plans. The likelihood that myomas will cause symptoms is related to their number, size, and location. Therapy should be initiated in patients experiencing progressive symptoms or in asymptomatic patients with significant myomas prior to ART.

Few data support uterine size as the sole indication for surgical intervention. Conventional guidelines for intervention advocate surgery when uterine size equals or exceeds 12 weeks' gestation on clinical exam, regardless of the presence or absence of significant symptoms. Multiple clinical reasons have been cited in support of this traditional indication: the inability to examine the ovaries, the possibility of malignancy of the enlarged pelvic mass, the potential for compromise of adjacent organ function if uterine leiomyomatous growth continues, the greater risks of future surgical treatment, the potential for greater fertility after surgery on a smaller uterus, and the possibility of continued uterine or myomatous growth resulting from hormone replacement therapy after menopause.[85] None are relevant in contemporary management. These standards, however, were developed in an era in which ultrasonographic assessment of myoma size and growth and ovarian size and structure was not routinely available; clinicians relied primarily on clinical examination to assess the adnexae and the growth patterns of the fibroid. In the absence of symptoms with reliable follow-up, including clinical examination and ultrasound to assess myoma size, surgical intervention is not recommended for patients based solely on size. Patients with increased uterine size secondary to myomatous enlargement are no more likely to experience perioperative complications than those with smaller uteri.[85] The traditional indications for surgery based on uterine size have no clinical foundation when examined critically.[86] The presence and severity of myoma-related symptoms and reproductive plans are the most important considerations in deciding what type and timing of treatment. In patients with asymptomatic myomas and no reproductive plans, expectant management is an option. When symptoms develop, a decision regarding either medical or surgical intervention should be made and a therapy plan formulated, based on severity of symptoms and age of the patient.

Expectant Management

Expectant management is an option for women with mild or no myoma-related symptoms. This approach entails clinical and ultrasonographic examination at 6- to 12-month intervals to assess uterine size, myoma growth patterns, myoma number, and ovarian size and morphology as well as to review symptoms. The decision to pursue expectant management should be tempered in part by the patient's age, with a lower threshold for patients in the perimenopausal age range or in any patient with clinical or laboratory findings suggestive of the perimenopause. For those patients who elect expectant management and who exhibit mild symptoms of abnormal uterine bleeding, management may be initiated using nonsteroidal anti-inflammatory agents, which reduce menstrual blood loss (by up to 50%) and the associated dysmenorrhea.[87] A second option is cyclic or continuous low-dose combination oral contraceptives. They provide a convenient means of controlling bleeding and reliable contraception.[88] In patients who develop symptoms secondary to uterine myomas, medical management may be considered.

Medical Management

With long-acting GnRH analogs, medical management of myomas is an option.[28] GnRH agonists are a group of compounds that are a variation on the decapeptide GnRH. By substitution of a single amino acid in a critical position (position 6), the duration of action of these agents was markedly increased, resulting in a blockage of pituitary secretion of follicle-stimulating hormone (FSH) and luteinizing hormone (LH) and leading to a pseudomenopausal state. The action of these drugs as agonists results in an initial rise in serum concentrations of FSH and LH reflected by a transient rise in estradiol followed by complete blockade of both gonadotropins and estradiol to less than the limits of detectability on assay.

GnRH analogs are important adjuncts in the medical management of myomas.[89–91] As sole medical management, however, they have a limited role. When the medications are discontinued, a gradual but eventual recurrence of the myomas is noted. The maximal benefit for the use of these agents is 8 to 12 weeks after the first injection.[92] No appreciable reduction in growth is noted after 12 weeks in studies that addressed long-term (6 month) analog use in the management of myomas (Figure 8-11). These medications may be safely used for longer than 6 months in select circumstances, for example, for patients in the perimenopause. In this circumstance, consideration should be given to estrogen add-back therapy to maintain bone integrity. Initial injection of GnRH analogs may be given either in the follicular or luteal phase administration, and there is no clear-cut difference in myoma response with either protocol.

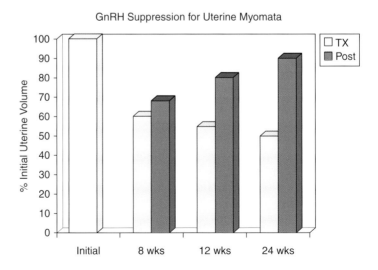

Figure 8-11   Percentage of reduction in uterine volume after 8, 12, and 24 weeks of treatment with a GnRH agonist at 4, 12, and 24 weeks post-treatment.

The largest body of information regarding medical management of myomas has been with GnRH agonist therapy. Powerful and effective GnRH antagonists have brought into the clinical practice a second option for medical management. Early studies using GnRH antagonists were frustrated because of the extremely low potency of the compound and a marked histamine reaction. These side effects have been overcome, creating a variety of compounds that provide immediate and powerful pituitary down-regulation with no side effects and without the attendant flare effect of the agonist. These agents are effective when administered for 3 months leading to reduction in myoma size of approximately 53% after 1 month of therapy. As expected, size reduction was associated with a concomitant reduction in serum estrogen and progesterone levels. The response after discontinuation of the antagonists, however, was similar to that with the agonists and characterized by a gradual return of myoma size after discontinuing the medication. Continuous treatment with these compounds induces an immediate and sustained pituitary and gonadal suppression by circumventing the GnRH agonist-related flare of pituitary gonadotropin secretion and ovarian response. With modifications in duration of action GnRH antagonists may provide an alternative method of the medical management of leiomyomas. No depot forms are available, limiting any wide-spaced clinical use at present.

A second category of drugs possibly effective in the medical management of myomas are the antiprogesterones.[93–95] Mifepristone was the first clinically available antiprogestin. Because of the dependency of uterine myomas on ovarian steroid secretion, mifepristone was investigated as a potential medical management for these tumors. In one study using 50 mg of mifepristone per day for 3 months, myoma size was reduced by 22% at 4 weeks, 39% at 8 weeks, and 49% at 12 weeks.[93] The exact mechanism of action by which these changes occur is unknown. One possible influence is through interaction of mifepristone with the progesterone receptors within the myoma, leading to a reduction in receptor content.[94] The second mechanism may be a reduction in uterine blood flow similar to that observed with GnRH agonists. Uterine blood flow is decreased with mifepristone by 40%.[96] Mifepristone may provide an alternate medical management for myoma when GnRH analog therapy is contraindicated or unsuccessful.

Surgical Management

Surgical management of uterine myomas is indicated in any patient with persistent and progressive symptoms not responsive to conservative management or for sizes greater than 5 cm regardless of location and for submucous myomas regardless of size for patients planning IVF. Symptoms include abnormal uterine bleeding, anemia secondary to chronic blood loss, pelvic pain including bladder pressure, urinary frequency or constipation, and a progressive enlargement in uterine size that results in distortion of abdominal contour and is of general concern to the patient.[97] These indications are relatively straightforward and surgical management in these conditions results in a high rate of subjective improvement of symptoms.

Myomectomy as a sole treatment for infertility continues to be controversial. Since 1900 myomectomy has been reported as therapy for infertility, with a wide range of success rates from 40% to 60% in nonrandomized and uncontrolled studies.[98–101] Many women with myomas readily conceive and carry to term. If and how myomas influence fertility in some women but not others is open to speculation. Early studies that investigated myomectomy were performed in patients who were interested in preserving the potential for childbearing at a time when the prevalent option was hysterectomy. The concern was whether or not a uterus that had been operated on could maintain a pregnancy and function during labor. In early studies by Bonney[7] results were extremely encouraging in this regard. At this time, monitoring outcomes after myomectomy looked less to its efficacy as a fertility-enhancing procedure, but more as a means to assess its safety in patients interested in preserving childbearing potential. Subsequent to this, a series of studies were published that investigated myomectomy as a fertility-enhancing procedure. The success rates have ranged from 30 to 60%. These broad rates were reported regardless of whether the study included adequate evaluation for other factors contributory to infertility and of the duration of follow-up.

The way in which myomas impair fertility is not fully understood (see above). Structure and function may both be adversely effected. Theories include distortion in the cavity and, particularly, the endometrium in submucous myoma; thinned and unresponsive endometrium overlying intramural myoma; and increased prostaglandin secretion.[102] Myomas may interfere with sperm transport, impinge on the tubal lumen, distort the course of the fallopian tube, compress the cervical canal, or alter the position of the cervix.[49] Changes in the micro-environment as noted above may reduce the likelihood of implantation. Further study of endometrial function may provide additional insights. No conclusive proof has been offered to substantiate any theory. Clinical outcomes suggest that myomectomy enhances fertility in certain patients in whom no other factors are present,[58,59] but caution must be exercised. Myomectomy may result in adhesion formation and a reduction in fertility.[103,104]

Several paradigms have been suggested to guide decisions for reproductive enhancement. Pregnancy rates after myomectomy are influenced by the age of the patient, duration of infertility, and the size, location, and number of the myomas and role of ART in the treatment plan.[49] Surgery should be avoided on a solitary myoma less than 3 cm. Surgery should be considered for multiple myomas less than 5 cm or any solitary myoma larger than 5 cm. When ART is considered or with a history of infertility, care is required in patient selection. Blanket recommendations regarding infertility and myomectomy should be avoided and plans individualized. A pregnancy rate of 61.5% in 17 previously infertile patients after removal of a submucosal leiomyoma of at least 5 cm has been reported.[58] The data for patients with subserosal or intramural myomas only are less clear. In one series 15 of 23 patients with subserosal or intramural myomas conceived, and 56%

delivered term infants.[59] In any patient considering IVF, any fibroid greater than 3 to 5 cm regardless of location or in a submucous location regardless of size should be removed. After myomectomy, regardless of technique, evaluation of the endometrial cavity is essential, particularly after any resectoscope procedure.

The studies concerning the effects of myomas on pregnancy outcome present conflicting results, possibly because of the methods used to detect the myomas and populations studied. Early studies describe uterine myomas in approximately 2% of pregnant women.[32,105] These reports suggest that 60 to 70% of women with myomas had obstetric complications related to the myomas. With more sensitive diagnostic techniques, the prevalence of myomas is greater in pregnant women but the complication rate is lower.[65,68,106] Less significant myomas have been detected with increasing frequency. Single myomas have been reported in 88% of patients and multiple myomas in 12% using ultrasound to make the diagnosis. Approximately 10 to 40% of women with myomas have related pregnancy complications.[62,106] The discrepancy between older and contemporary data reflects a bias towards inclusion of larger, more symptomatic tumors in the older literature.

The complications of myomas during pregnancy are divided into those occurring during pregnancy, at delivery, and in the puerperium. Threatened abortion, increased first-trimester loss, preterm labor, abruptio placenta, and pelvic pain are the most common complications during pregnancy.[67] Of patients with myomas larger than 200 cm^3, 82% described painful episodes during pregnancy.[63] Treatment for this syndrome has been medical management with analgesics ranging from nonsteroidal anti-inflammatory drugs (NSAIDs) to narcotics, if necessary.[107] At delivery and in the puerperium, a higher incidence of preterm delivery and premature rupture of the membranes, retained placenta, malpresentation, and postpartum sepsis has been described.[62,106]

Surgery during pregnancy should be considered only under the most extreme and dire circumstances. Though well-described in the literature rarely should it be considered. Two circumstances for myomectomy during pregnancy may be encountered: (1) prior to maturity and at maturity and (2) at the time of cesarean section. Myomectomies have been performed for symptomatic patients with imaging characteristics (either from ultrasound or MRI) consistent with degeneration and failure of aggressive pain management.[108] In one series, 50 antepartum myomectomies were performed for indications primarily of pain uncontrolled with medical management. The complications include hemorrhage, preterm labor and delivery, hysterectomy, and disseminated intravascular coagulation.[106,109,110] The decision to perform myomectomy during cesarean delivery must be made with caution because of the risk of hemorrhage and only when the option to reevaluate in the postpartum period is limited.[63]

The disadvantage of these systems is the absence of a specimen for histologic evaluation and the presence of gas bubbles within the distending media that may enter the vascular system. The monopolar loop electrode is the most commonly used instrument for removal of submucous myomas.

The procedure may be performed under laparoscopic or ultrasound guidance.[133,134] Intraoperative transabdominal ultrasound to guide the procedure provides a means of assessing both the location of the scope and the intramural portion of the myomas (Figure 8-14). By ultrasound guidance, the exact depth of dissection and relationship of the instrumentation to the uterine serosa may be accurately gauged. This method also provides a means of avoiding a concomitant laparoscopy. Resectoscopic myomectomy for the treatment of abnormal uterine bleeding associated with uterine myomas may be combined with endometrial ablation. This dual approach provides a means of achieving amenorrhea in a single procedure.

The day before resectoscopic myomectomy, a laminaria tent should be placed in the cervix, or pretreatment with misoprostol the evening prior to or the morning of surgery. Uterine distension may be achieved using any variety of distending media including low-viscosity nonelectrolyte-containing

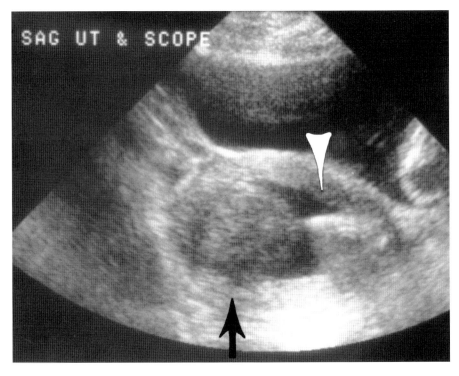

Figure 8-14   An intraoperative sonohysterogram demonstrating the resectoscope (arrowhead), and the submucous myoma filling the fundal region of the cavity (arrow).

solutions, sorbitol (Travinol/Bakstra, Deerfield, IL), and 1% glycine. The ease of use of low-viscosity solutions has made these media the preferred choice. Distending media should be infused with a pump. Intrauterine pressure should not exceed mean arterial pressure. Precise measurement of input and output is essential during the entire procedure. To facilitate this critical aspect, a double flow resectoscope is used. Suction is attached to the outflow for more accurate recording of input and output, and to reduce intrauterine pressures because absorption of fluids may be related to increased intrauterine pressure.

Vasopressin, 5 mL on either side of the cervix, may be used to reduce blood flow and cause myometrial contractility.[135] An undamped cutting current of 45 to 110 W may be used with occasional blending of damped current (coagulating current) to control intraoperative bleeding. Settings should be determined by visual inspection of the tissue effect, with the lowest undamped current used consistent with easy passage of the loop through the myoma. The myoma is progressively shaved from apex to base, extending the dissection to 1 to 2 mm beneath the surrounding endometrium. A 9-mm suction cannula or myoma forceps may be used to extract the fragments of the myoma during the procedure (Figures 8-15 and 8-16). Extreme care is

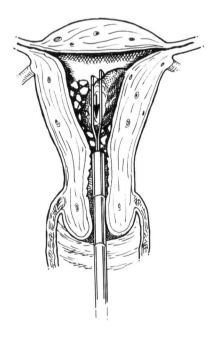

Figure 8-15   Resectoscopic myomectomy. Submucous myoma is serially dissected with sufficient power to permit an effortless passage of the loop through the substance of the myoma. Myoma fragments may collect within the uterine cavity and necessitate evacuation using either polyp forceps or a small-caliber, soft-tipped suction cannula.

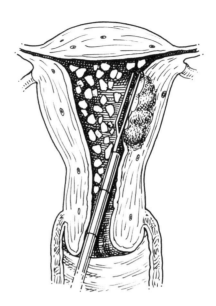

Figure 8-16   Resectoscopic myomectomy. The myoma dissection is carried to the level of the surrounding endometrium. The dissection should be extended to sufficient depth to dissect as much of the intramural portion of the myoma as possible.

required if the procedure is done prior to IVF. Minimal damage to adjacent normal endometrium is important.

Complications have been described with media of both low and high viscosity.[136,137] Severe volume overload and the related complications of electrolyte imbalance may result from the absorption of these fluids during operative hysteroscopy. Meticulous attention to intraoperative fluid balance is imperative. Fluid balance should be checked intraoperatively at 15-minute intervals. To maintain as accurate a balance as possible, all outflow channels are connected to suction canisters for quantitation of fluid retrieval. A multi-channel hysteroscope may be used for the dual purpose of maintaining low intrauterine pressure and for connecting the outflow track to a suction canister. A large plastic drape with a retrieval trap should be attached to a separate suction apparatus to scavenge any fluid that may inadvertently reflux into the vagina. Extensive surgical procedures requiring prolonged operative time (more than 60 min) may need to be performed in stages. Factors contributing to fluid overload are related to elevated intrauterine pressure, extensive myometrial dissection, and prolonged operating room time.[138,139]

Absorption of large volumes of electrolyte-free, low-viscosity fluid may result in volume overload and water intoxication. Volume overload may cause pulmonary edema and lead to hyponatremia, hypo-osmolarity, and cerebral edema (Table 8-2). Postoperative hyponatremia may result after excessive fluid administration or absorption, and occurs in approximately

| Table 8-2. |
| Postoperative Hyponatremia |

Etiology
o Alterations in antidiuretic hormone, renal function, and excessive fluid administration intraoperatively
o Severe symptomatic hyponatremia (< 120 mIU/L) associated with encephalopathies and death
o Premenopausal women are 25 times more likely to suffer sequelae
o Men and women >40 are at less risk

Diagnosis
o May develop within 48 hours of surgery
o Symptoms include nausea and vomiting, headache, visual disturbances, agitation, irritability, weakness, lethargy, disorientation, seizures, or respiratory arrest
o Check serum electrolytes on any patient at risk
o Routine postoperative serum electrolytes in healthy, uncomplicated patients are not necessary

Prevention
o Quantitative monitoring of intraoperative fluids
o Regular, periodic assessments of intake and outputs
o Restriction of intrauterine pressure below mean arterial pressure

Treatment
o Conservative: 3% hypertonic saline with a loop diuretic
o Monitoring of serum sodium concentrations and urinary input and output
o Consultation with nephrologist or intensivist is essential
o Anticonvulsants for seizures

4.4% of all surgical patients.[140] Prevention of postoperative hyponatremia is related to careful selection and administration of intravenous fluids. The treatment is similarly directed towards fluid resuscitation, with gentle administration of 3% hypertonic saline in conjunction with loop diuretics. Careful monitoring of serum sodium concentrations, fluid input, and urinary output is absolutely essential.[141-144] High-viscosity media such as dextran-70 may cause volume overload secondary to the oncotic effect of intravascular dextran. Dextran-70 has also been associated with anaphylaxis and coagulation disorders. Most complications related to the use of these media can be avoided by meticulous fluid assessment.

A vasopressin pack may be used to manage refractory bleeding after myoma resection. Twenty units of vasopressin may be diluted with 30 mL of normal saline and a 2.5 cm gauze pack soaked in the dilute solution and packed into the uterus in the region of the bleeding beds. The pack can be used for 1 hour.

Complete resection improves long-term results of transcervical resection of submucosal myomas for control of abnormal uterine bleeding and polyps.[145] Transcervical resection of submucous myomas with more than 50% intramural extension should be performed in separate procedures; complete resection usually necessitates repeat procedures.[146] The alternative is to perform myolysis of the remaining intramural component. Nd:YAG laser hysteroscopy may be used for large submucous myomas.[147] Different techniques may be employed, depending on the degree of myoma within the endometrial cavity compared with the degree within the intramural portion. In patients in whom a portion of the myoma is within the uterine wall, a partial myomectomy may be performed by resecting the protruding portion of the myoma. Thereafter, a laser fiber may be directed as perpendicularly as possible to the remaining or intramural portion of the myoma and introduced in the myoma to a length of 5 to 10 mm. Application of laser energy causes myoma coagulation.

Uterine Artery Embolization

The embolization of pelvic vessels in the management of a variety of gynecologic problems is not new. Dating back to 1979, transcatheter arterial embolization was used in the management of postpartum hemorrhage and postoperative bleeding. Embolization also found application to manage hemorrhagic ectopic pregnancies. Uterine artery embolization has emerged as a nonsurgical conservative option for symptomatic uterine myomas. This procedure has proven to be clinically effective and cost-effective. The main indication for uterine artery embolization is to reduce the size of the myomata and to treat any excessive uterine bleeding. In general, the smaller the embolization particles, the more likely they are to occlude the smaller vessels inside the myometrium, thus causing a large area of ischemia and infarction. The procedure is most appropriate when the fibroid is < 9 cm. Each additional centimeter increase in the diameter of the myoma contributes a 10% increase in failure. The procedure is well tolerated and effective with the follow-up available thus far. Uterine artery embolization provides an excellent option for patients who are interested in conservative management of uterine fibroids and provides excellent relief from abnormal uterine bleeding, pelvic pain, and pelvic pressure secondary to uterine size. Early studies suggest that uterine artery embolization is associated with normal reproductive function and obstetric outcomes.

Procedure

Prior to embolization, detailed transvaginal and transabdominal ultrasound examination of the uterus and myomas is necessary. In some circumstances, when bleeding is the primary clinical concern then endometrial biopsy is appropriate to rule out endometrial carcinoma. Though used primarily in patients in whom reproductive issues are not of concern, a limited but growing number of patients become pregnant and carry to term after uterine artery embolization. As an interesting sidelight, the patients who were managed in the late 1970s and early 1980s with embolization in the management of postpartum hemorrhage do not appear to have any compromise of their reproductive potential, drawing into question whether or not this is an option for patients whose reproductive plans have not yet been completed. The procedure may be performed under intravenous sedation (Figure 8-17 A and B). The catheters are inserted through a single inguinal puncture, usually on the right. A 5 Fr catheter may be used to cannulate through the aortic bifurcation utilizing anteroposterior and oblique digital arteriograms. After

(A)

(B)

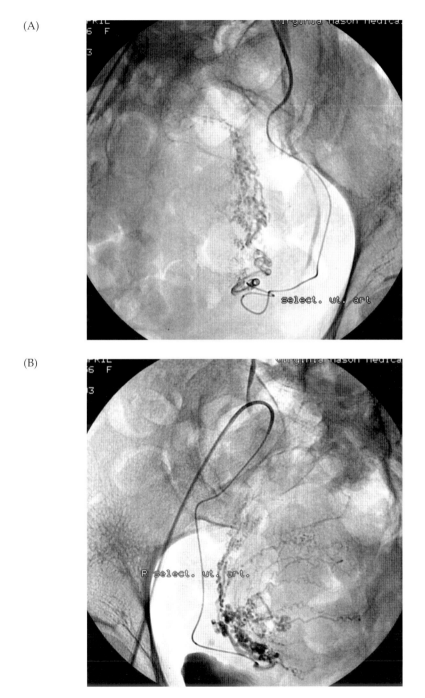

Figure 8-17   Uterine artery embolization. Catheter is threaded into region of myoma (A). Note blush in region of myoma (B).

the uterine artery has been identified and catheterized, the microcatheter is advanced deep within the uterine artery and embolized with polyvinyl alcohol (PVA). Myomas undergo size reduction secondary to necrosis. Histologic evaluations of myomas after uterine artery embolization suggest a hyaline-type necrosis and acute suppurative necrosis.

Reduction in volume of the myomas and uterus occurs in 75–80% of the patients with resolution of abnormal uterine bleeding in approximately 80% of the patients. Considerable cost savings have been noted with uterine artery embolizations. The estimated cost for hospitalization for uterine artery embolization and abdominal hysterectomy is $3193 and $5598, respectively. The primary cause for the discrepancy is related to the hospital care and operating room costs associated with the myomectomy.

Uterine artery embolization is associated with risks, however. The most serious involve ischemia and necrosis of the fibroids leading to uterine abscess and sepsis.[152] One death has been reported due to septicemia after a uterine artery embolization. Bowel obstruction associated with necrosis of a subserous myoma has been described. Additional complications of the procedure include pain associated with ischemic infarction of the myomas. This usually occurs anywhere from 24–48 hours after the procedure and may last for approximately 2 weeks. Sepsis, bowel obstruction, post-embolization fever, uterine infection and chronic salpingitis have been described after uterine artery embolization. Treatment failures occur in 5–10% of patients. In these circumstances, hysterectomy or myomectomy may be recommended. Factors that influence success include: age of the patient, with younger patients at higher risk for failure; and size of the uterus and myomas with the increased likelihood of failure as myoma sizes exceed 8 cm and mean uterine volume exceeds 1400 ml.

From the standpoint of reproductive potential, decreased ovarian function, infertility, and premature menopause have been described after uterine artery embolization.[153] Because of the potential adverse impact on ovarian function and because of the persistence, possibly, of at least part of the myoma, this procedure is not recommended in patients who are planning future fertility. Assessment of its ultimate impact on reproductive potential in the future, including ovarian function, may modify this approach. Overall, treatment failure, defined as a lack of or minimal shrinkage of a myoma or leading to hysterectomy, will occur in approximately 5 to 10% of patients. These failures occur between 2 and 24 weeks after uterine embolization and are primarily manifested by recurrence of symptoms.[154–156]

Laparoscopic Myolysis

Laparoscopic myolysis has a small role for managing subserosal and intramural myomas.[157] Laparoscopic myolysis using a Nd:YAG was introduced in 1990.[158] Dense adhesion formation noted after this procedure resulted in the design of a bipolar instrument that appeared to be as effective as the laser without the attendant excessive adhesion formation. The bipolar instrument consists of two 5-cm steel needles connected to a standard bipolar generator. A second approach is cryomyolysis that uses a dedicated cryoablation system to eliminate vascular supply to the myoma. The concept behind myolysis is to coagulate the myometrial and myomatous tissue and vasculature.[159] The end result of this is an initial shrinkage of the myomas and eventual stabilization in their growth.

In this technique, the laser fiber or needle is passed serially into the depth of the myomas depending on size. A 10% vasopressin solution (Parke-Davis, Morris Plains, NJ) is injected into the serosa and body of the myomas. As mentioned above, the laser with a 600- to 1000-μm fiber at 50 W of power or bipolar needle at 50 to 200 W of continuous power may be used to drill the myoma. Repeated concentric passes of the fiber into the myoma should be continued to coagulate the entire myoma. A total of 70 to 100 punctures generally suffice for a 5-cm myoma. A 5-mm corkscrew may be used to stabilize the uterus and myoma and, in conjunction with an intrauterine manipulator, control uterine position. The laser or bipolar needle tip should be passed in two planes, an anteroposterior (i.e., front-to-back) and lateral (i.e., side-to-side) motion. The former may be achieved by passing the laser fiber or bipolar needle through suprapubic punctures. The latter may be achieved by passing the instruments through either the laparoscopic channel or a second midline puncture. Coagulation of the myoma regardless of technique results in tissue damage approximately 3 to 5 mm in diameter and creates multiple areas of desiccated vasculature, thus effectively destroying the entire myoma. The technique is applicable for both subserosal and serosal myomas.

The results for either the coagulation with the Nd:YAG laser or the bipolar needle are similar. Myomas decrease in size with a resolution in symptoms in most patients. For patients interested in fulfilling reproductive potential, however, two negative aspects of the procedure are the possibility of adhesion formation and the possibility of uterine rupture secondary to the uterine wall damage that may result from the coagulation process.[160,161] Ideal candidates have myomas less than 10 cm in diameter and less than 4 in number. Those patients whose myomas are larger than 10 cm or are greater than 4 in number are not candidates. The procedure is not first line management for symptomatic myomas.

Outcomes Analysis

Myomectomy for the treatment of pelvic pain and irregular bleeding is appropriate therapy for patients whose symptoms do not respond to medical management. For patients with submucous myomas, a resectoscopic myomectomy is an effective surgical approach. For intramural or subserosal myomas, laparoscopic or abdominal myomectomy is appropriate therapy. Conversion rates for laparoscopic procedures are 5%.

Laparoscopically assisted myomectomy combining operative laparoscopy and mini-laparotomy may be an alternative, in rare cases where laparoscopic myomectomy is difficult or removal of the bulk of the myoma is impossible. In a series of 57 patients, laparoscopically assisted myomectomy was performed on myomatous uteri ranging in size from 8 to 26 weeks.[123] In this series, the weight of the myomas ranged from 28 to 998 g, with operative times from 40 to 285 minutes. In a follow-up of 284 patients over a 10-year period, resectoscopic myomectomy resulted in clinical and functional improvement in 95% of cases with a 1-year postoperative follow-up. Continued improvement occurred in 87% and 76% at 3 and 5 years respectively.[162]

Myomectomy as a sole treatment for infertility is a complex issue. Several retrospective and observational studies suggest an enhancement of fertility after these procedures.[163–171] In one of the largest series, 477 of 1193 (40%) patients from 18 studies who underwent myomectomy became pregnant postoperatively.[163] However, many of these patients had multiple factors contributing to their infertility, making the importance of myomectomy as a sole fertility-enhancing procedure difficult to evaluate. In a review of the cumulative data of seven investigators over a 10-year interval, 60% conceived with follow-up that ranged from 10 to 112 months.[59] The cumulative pregnancy rates in patients undergoing myomectomy solely for infertility ranged from 40 to 70%. Of these, 53% occurred within the first 6 months and 74% within the first year.[166] Patients with infertility longer than 2 years duration prior to surgery appeared to benefit the most. These studies fall short of the randomized, controlled study necessary to adequately evaluate the impact of myomectomy on fertility. A significant shift in this paradigm has been in myoma management prior to IVF. Any myoma that distorts the endometrial cavity regardless of size or is greater than 3 to 5 cm regardless of location appears to adversely impact pregnancy rates. Excision in these circumstances is recommended.[167–169]

Pelvic adhesions after the myomectomy have been shown to significantly reduce the chance of conception.[170,172] Adhesion formation ranges from 2–3% to 40%.[113,142] In one study, adhesions of varying stages were documented in 68% of patients who underwent abdominal surgery at a later date. Myomectomy incisions on the posterior uterine wall are associated with more and a higher degree of adnexal adhesions than are incisions on the fundus and anterior wall. Blood transfusions with abdominal myomectomy are rarely needed – 4% of patients had an estimated blood loss of more than 1000 mL, and 70% of transfused patients receive autologous blood. The total transfusion rate has been reported as 20%.[172]

Based on several large studies with adequate follow-up, the likelihood of recurrence is low. In one study of more than 3000 patients, recurrent myomas were discovered in 15% of patients.[173,174] Of these, 10% required subsequent surgical therapy for a variety of indications. The reported range is 5 to 30%. The cumulative 10-year recurrence rate by life table analysis was

27%.[175] When operation is required, it is usually at an interval exceeding 3 years from the original myomectomy. Factors such as the initial surgery, age at which the surgery was performed, and the number, size, and location of the myomas may all influence the likelihood of recurrence.

In the event of pregnancy after myomectomy, the need for cesarean section for delivery is controversial. Formerly, it was held that entrance into the endometrial cavity during myomectomy was an absolute indication for delivery by cesarean section. With contemporary surgical techniques, this concept may no longer be valid and vaginal delivery may be attempted. Invasion of the myometrial cavity and extent of the myomectomy should be considered and obstetric plans individualized.

Summary and Recommendations

Uterine myomas are responsible for a variety of symptoms, such as pressure, pain, bleeding, and (though controversial) infertility. Their management depends on symptoms and fertility plans. The medical management of uterine myomas includes the long-acting GnRH analogs and mifepristone to induce shrinkage of the myomas. This management may be instituted prior to an operative procedure to reduce operative time and complications or as an alternative to surgery, timed according to the patient's age and pending menopause. Surgical management has changed dramatically from being dependent solely on transabdominal myomectomies to employing endoscopic techniques. Hysteroscopic management of submucous myomas is effective in controlling abnormal uterine bleeding and enhancing fertility in selected patients. One of the most controversial topics in the management of myomas focuses on their management when no other factors are found in an infertility evaluation and during pregnancy. On the basis of current literature, the following recommendations may be made:

- Both medical and surgical management provide viable options for the management of symptoms of uterine myomas, especially pain and pressure.
- Medical management with current GnRH agonists, GnRH antagonists, and mifepristone are important tools in the management of myomas. These agents increase the likelihood of converting a potential transabdominal procedure to an endoscopic one.
- No large-scale, prospective, controlled studies clearly support myomectomies when no other contributing factors to infertility can be found. The literature does suggest that myomectomies may enhance fertility in certain settings, based on size and location. Excision is a prerequisite prior to IVF.
- Adhesion formation after abdominal myomectomies is well-described and could potentially compromise a patient's fertility. This aspect must be included in any counseling session prior to a myomectomy.
- Ultrasound monitoring, regardless of the size and location of the myomas,

is all that is required for pregnant patients. Previous literature describing the complications of myomas during pregnancy overstated the incidence of complications. A conservative and watchful-waiting approach to myomas during pregnancy is warranted.

- Myolysis and cryomyolysis using either a bipolar needle or a laser fiber has a limited role for both laparoscopic and hysteroscopic treatment of myomas. It is not first-line management and is done only in select cases.
- Uterine artery embolization is an effective option. Plans for pregnancy after the procedure do not appear to be a contraindication, pending long-term follow-up.

References

1. Kelly HA. Operative gynecology. New York: Appleton & Co., 1898.

2. Alexander W. Denucleation of uterine fibroids. Br Gynecol Soc 1898;1:47–74.

3. Finn WF, Muller PF. Abdominal myomectomy: special reference to subsequent pregnancy and the reappearance of fibromyomas of the uterus. Am J Obstet Gynecol 1959;60:109–115.

4. Kelly HA, Noble CP. Gynecology and abdominal surgery. Philadelphia: WB Saunders, 1908.

5. Davids AM. Myomectomy; surgical technique and results in a series of 1,150 cases. Am J Obstet Gynecol 1952;63:592–604.

6. Rubin JE. Progress in myomectomy. Am J Obstet Gynecol 1952;44:196–212.

7. Bonney V. Myomectomy or hysterectomy. Br Med J 1918;i:276–280.

8. Franks RT. The hormonal causes of premenstrual tension. Arch Neurol Psychol 1931;126:1051–1060.

9. Graham H. Gynecology made safe. In: Eternal Eve. Altrincham, William Heinemann Medical Books, 1950:524–552.

10. Buttram VC Jr, Reiter RC. Uterine leiomyomata: etiology, symptomatology, and management. Fertil Steril 1981;36:433–445.

11. Nisolle M, Gillerot S, Casanas-Roux F, et al. Immunohistochemical study of the proliferation index, oestrogen receptors and progesterone receptors A and B in leiomyomata and normal myometrium during the menstrual cycle and under gonadotrophin-releasing hormone agonist therapy. Hum Reprod 1999;14:2844–2850.

12. Cramer SF, Patel A. The frequency of uterine leiomyomas. Am J Clin Pathol 1990;94:435–438.

13. Nilbert M, Helm S. Uterine leiomyoma cytogenetics. Genes Chromosome Cancer 1990;2:3–12.

14. Townsend DE, Sparkes RS, Baluda MC, McClelland G. Unicellular histogenesis of uterine leiomyomas as determined by electrophoresis by glucose-6-phosphate dehydrogenase. Am J Obstet Gynecol 1970;107:1168–1173.

15. Sargent MS, Weremowicz S, Rein MS, Morton CC. Translocations in 7q22 define a critical region in uterine leiomyomata. Cancer Genet Cytogenet 1994;77:65–68.

16. Vanni R, Lecca U, Faa G. Uterine leiomyoma cytogenetics. II. Report of forty cases. Cancer Genet Cytogenet 1991;53:247–256.

17. Hug K, Doney MK, Tyler MJ, et al. Physical mapping of the uterine leiomyoma t(12;14)(q13–15;q24.1) breakpoint on chromosome 14 between SPTB and D14S77. Genes Chromosome Cancer 1994;11:263–266.

18. Wanschura S, Hennig Y, Deichert U, et al. Molecular-cytogenetic refinement of the 12q14-->q15 breakpoint region affected in uterine leiomyomas. Cytogenet Cell Genet 1995;71:131–135.

19. Quade BJ, Weremowicz S, Neskey DM, et al. Fusion transcripts involving HMGA2 are not a common molecular mechanism in uterine leiomyomata with rearrangements in 12q15. Cancer Res 2003;63:1351–1358.

20. Tsibris JC, Segars J, Coppola D, et al. Insights from gene arrays on the development and growth regulation of uterine leiomyomata. Fertil Steril 2002;78:114–121.

21. Wang H, Mahadevappa M, Yamamoto K, et al. Distinctive proliferative phase differences in gene expression in human myometrium and leiomyomata. Fertil Steril 2003;80:266–276.

22. Catherino WH, Segars JH. Microarray analysis in fibroids: which gene list is the correct list? Fertil Steril 2003;80:293–294.

23. Tsibris JC, Porter KB, Jazayeri A, et al. Human uterine leiomyomata express higher levels of peroxisome proliferator-activated receptor gamma, retinoid X receptor alpha, and all-trans retinoic acid than myometrium. Cancer Res 1999;59:5737–5744.

24. Freije WA. Genome biology and gynecology: the application of oligonucleotide microarrays to leiomyomata. Fertil Steril 2003;80:277–278.

25. Tsibris JC, Segars J, Enkemann S, et al. New and old regulators of uterine leiomyoma growth from screening with DNA arrays. Fertil Steril 2003;80:279–281.

26. Li S, McLachlan JA. Estrogen-associated genes in uterine leiomyoma. Ann N Y Acad Sci 2001;948:112–120.

27. Vollenhoven BJ, Lawrence AS, Healy DL. Uterine fibroids: a clinical review. Br J Obstet Gynaecol 1990;97:285–298.

28. Filicori M, Hall DA, Loughlin JS, et al. A conservative approach to the management of uterine leiomyoma: pituitary desensitization by a luteinizing hormone-releasing hormone analogue. Am J Obstet Gynecol 1983;147:726–727.

29. Soules MR, McCarty KS Jr. Leiomyomas: steroid receptor content. Variation within normal menstrual cycles. Am J Obstet Gynecol 1982;143:6–11.

30. van der Ven LT, Gloudemans T, Roholl PJ, et al. Growth advantage of human leiomyoma cells compared to normal smooth-muscle cells due to enhanced sensitivity toward insulin-like growth factor I. Int J Cancer 1994;59:427–434.

31. Healy DL, Vollenhoven BJ. The role of GnRH agonists in the treatment of uterine fibroids. Br J Obstet Gynaecol 1992;99:23–26.

32. Pritts EA. Fibroids and infertility: a systematic review of the evidence. Obstet Gynecol Surv 2001;56:483–491.

33. Cohen D, Mazur MT, Jozefczyk MA, Badawy SZ. Hyalinization and cellular changes in uterine leiomyomata after gonadotropin releasing hormone agonist therapy. J Reprod Med 1994;39:377–380.

34. Upadhyaya NB, Doody MC, Googe PB. Histopathological changes in leiomyomata treated with leuprolide acetate. Fertil Steril 1990;54:811–814.

35. Deligdisch L, Hirschmann S, Altchek A. Pathologic changes in gonadotropin releasing hormone agonist analogue treated uterine leiomyomata. Fertil Steril 1997;67:837–841.

36. Romero R, Chervenak FA, DeVore G, et al. Fetal head deformation and congenital torticollis associated with a uterine tumor. Am J Obstet Gynecol 1981;141:839–840.

37. Meyer WR, Mayer AR, Diamond MP, et al. Unsuspected leiomyosarcoma: treatment with a gonadotropin-releasing hormone analogue. Obstet Gynecol 1990;75:529–532.

38. Pearce PH. Leiomyomatosis peritonealis disseminata. Am J Obstet Gynecol 1982;144:133–134.

39. Leibsohn S, d'Ablaing G, Mishell DR Jr, Schlaerth JB. Leiomyosarcoma in a series of hysterectomies performed for presumed uterine leiomyomas. Am J Obstet Gynecol 1990;162:968–76.

40. Cicinelli E, Romano F, Anastasio PS, et al. Transabdominal sonohysterography, transvaginal sonography, and hysteroscopy in the evaluation of submucous myomas. Obstet Gynecol 1995;85:42–47.

41. Timmis AD, Smallpeice C, Davies AC, et al. Intracardiac spread of intravenous leiomyomatosis with successful surgical excision. N Engl J Med 1980;303:1043–1044.

42. National Center for Health Statistics. Health, United States, 1990. Hyattsville, MD: Public Health Service, 1991. DHHS publication [PHS] 91–1232.

43. Broder MS, Bovone S. Improving treatment outcomes with a clinical pathway for hysterectomy and myomectomy. J Reprod Med 2002;47:999–1003.

44. Carlson KJ, Miller BA, Fowler FJ Jr. The Maine Women's Health Study: II. Outcomes of nonsurgical management of leiomyomas, abnormal bleeding, and chronic pelvic pain. Obstet Gynecol 1994;83:566–572.

45. Parazzini F, La Vecchia C, Negri E, Cecchetti G, Fedele L. Epidemiologic characteristics of women with uterine fibroids: a case-control study. Obstet Gynecol 1988;72:853–857.

46. Hart R. Unexplained infertility, endometriosis, and fibroids. BMJ 2003;327:721–724.

47. Itzkowic D. Submucous fibroids: clinical profile and hysteroscopic management. Aust N Z J Obstet Gynaecol 1993;33:63–67.

48. Stevenson CS. Myomectomy for improvement of fertility. Fertil Steril 1964;15:367–384.

49. Verkauf BS. Myomectomy for fertility enhancement and preservation. Fertil Steril 1992;58:1–15.

50.   Jun SH, Ginsburg ES, Racowsky C, et al. Uterine leiomyomas and their effect on in vitro fertilization outcome: a retrospective study. J Assist Reprod Genet 2001;18:139–143.

51.   Donnez J, Jadoul P. What are the implications of myomas on fertility? A need for a debate? Hum Reprod 2002;17:1424–1430.

52.   Nawroth F, Foth D. IVF outcome and intramural fibroids not compressing the uterine cavity. Hum Reprod 2002;17:2485–2486.

53.   Stovall DW, Parrish SB, Van Voorhis BJ, et al. Uterine leiomyomas reduce the efficacy of assisted reproduction cycles: results of a matched follow-up study. Hum Reprod 1998;13:192–197.

54.   Seracchioli R, Rossi S, Govoni F, et al. Fertility and obstetric outcome after laparoscopic myomectomy of large myomata: a randomized comparison with abdominal myomectomy. Hum Reprod 2000;15:2663–2668.

55.   Richlin SS, Ramachandran S, Shanti A, Murphy AA, Parthasarathy S. Glycodelin levels in uterine flushings and in plasma of patients with leiomyomas and polyps: implications for implantation. Hum Reprod 2002;17:2742–2747.

56.   Hart R, Khalaf Y, Yeong CT, et al. A prospective controlled study of the effect of intramural uterine fibroids on the outcome of assisted conception. Hum Reprod 2001;16:2411–2417.

57.   Check JH, Choe JK, Lee G, Dietterich C. The effect on IVF outcome of small intramural fibroids not compressing the uterine cavity as determined by a prospective matched control study. Hum Reprod 2002;17:1244–1248.

58.   Rosenfeld DL. Abdominal myomectomy for otherwise unexplained infertility. Fertil Steril 1986;46:328–330.

59.   Pritts EA. Fibroids and infertility: a systematic review of the evidence. Obstet Gynecol Surv 2001;56:483–491.

60.   Patterson-Keels LM, Selvaggi SM, Haefner HK, Randolph JF Jr. Morphologic assessment of endometrium overlying submucosal leiomyomas. J Reprod Med 1994;39:579–584.

61.   Gehlbach DL, Sousa RC, Carpenter SE, Rock JA. Abdominal myomectomy in the treatment of infertility. Int J Gynaecol Obstet 1993;40:45–50.

62.   Celik C, Acar A, Cicek N, et al. Can myomectomy be performed during pregnancy? Gynecol Obstet 2002;53:79–83.

63.   Glavind K, Palvio DH, Lauritsen JG. Uterine myoma in pregnancy. Acta Obstet Gynecol Scand 1990;69:617–619.

64.   Rice JP, Kay HH, Mahony BS. The clinical significance of uterine leiomyomas in pregnancy. Am J Obstet Gynecol 1989;160:1212–1216.

65.   Vergani P, Ghidini A, Strobelt N, et al. Do uterine leiomyomas influence pregnancy outcome? Am J Perinatol 1994;11:356–358.

66.   Exacoustos C, Rosati P. Ultrasound diagnosis of uterine myomas and complications in pregnancy. Obstet Gynecol 1993;82:97–101.

67.   Gainey H, Keeler JE. Submucous myoma in term pregnancy. Am J Obstet Gynecol 1949;58:727–731.

68.   Winer-Muram HT, Muram D, Gillieson MS. Uterine myomas in pregnancy. J Can Assoc Radiol 1984;35:168–170.

69.   Matsunaga E, Shiota K. Ectopic pregnancy and myoma uteri: teratogenic effects and maternal characteristics. Teratology 1980;21:61–69.

70.   Fedele L, Bianchi S, Dorta M, et al. Transvaginal ultrasonography versus hysteroscopy in the diagnosis of uterine submucous myomas. Obstet Gynecol 1991;77:745–748.

71.   Fleischer AC, Gordon AN, Entman SS. Transabdominal and transvaginal sonography of pelvic masses. Ultrasound Med Biol 1989;15:529–533.

72.   Dubinsky TJ, Parvey HR, Gormaz G, Makland N. Transvaginal hysterosonography in the evaluation of small endoluminal masses. J Ultrasound Med 1995;14:1–6.

73.   Lev-Toaff AS, Toaff ME, Liu JB, et al. Value of sonohysterography in the diagnosis and management of abnormal uterine bleeding. Radiology 1996;201:179–184.

74.   Cicinelli E, Romano F, Anastasio PS, et al. Transabdominal sonohysterography, transvaginal sonography, and hysteroscopy in the evaluation of submucous myomas. Obstet Gynecol 1995;85:42–47.

75.   Leone FP, Lanzani C, Ferrazzi E. Use of strict sonohysterographic methods for preoperative assessment of submucous myomas. Fertil Steril 2003;79:998–1002.

76.   Strobelt N, Ghidini A, Cavallone M, et al. Natural history of uterine leiomyomas in pregnancy. J Ultrasound Med 1994;13:399–401.

77.   Muram D, Gillieson M, Walters JH. Myomas of the uterus in pregnancy: ultrasonographic follow-up. Am J Obstet Gynecol 1980;138:16–19.

78.   Brown AB, Chamberlain R, Te Linde RW. Myomectomy. Am J Obstet Gynecol 1956;71:759–763.

79.   Rosati P, Exacoustos C, Mancuso S. Longitudinal evaluation of uterine myoma growth during pregnancy. A sonographic study. J Ultrasound Med 1992;11:511–515.

80.   Aharoni A, Reiter A, Golan D, et al. Patterns of growth of uterine leiomyomas during pregnancy. A prospective longitudinal study. Br J Obstet Gynaecol 1988;95:510–513.

81.   Yamashita Y, Torashima M, Takahashi M, et al. Hyperintense uterine leiomyoma at T2–weighted MR imaging: differentiation with dynamic enhanced MR imaging and clinical implications. Radiology 1993;189:721–725.

82.   Hricak H, Tscholakoff D, Heinrichs L, et al. Uterine leiomyomas: correlation of MR, histopathologic findings, and symptoms. Radiology 1986;158:385–391.

83.   Kawakami S, Togashi K, Konishi I, et al. Red degeneration of uterine leiomyoma: MR appearance. J Comput Assist Tomogr 1994;18:925–928.

84.   Dudiak CM, Turner DA, Patel SK, et al. Uterine leiomyomas in the infertile patient: preoperative localization with MR imaging versus US and hysterosalpingography. Radiology 1988;167:627–630.

85.   Friedman AJ, Haas ST. Should uterine size be an indication for surgical intervention in women with myomas? Am J Obstet Gynecol 1993;168:751–755.

86.   Reiter RC, Wagner PL, Gambone JC. Routine hysterectomy for large asymptomatic uterine leiomyomata: a reappraisal. Obstet Gynecol 1992;79:481–484.

87.   Makarainen L, Ylikorkala O. Primary and myoma-associated menorrhagia: role of prostaglandins and effects of ibuprofen. Br J Obstet Gynaecol 1986;93:974–978.

88.   Parazzini F, Negri E, La Vecchia C, et al. Oral contraceptive use and risk of uterine fibroids. Obstet Gynecol 1992;79:430–433.

89.   Healy DL. The role of GnRH agonists in the treatment of uterine fibroids. Br J Obstet Gynecol 1992;9:23–26.

90.   Lethaby A, Vollenhoven B, Sowter M. Efficacy of preoperative gonadotropin hormone releasing analogues for women with uterine fibroids undergoing hysterectomy or myomectomy: a systematic review. Br J Obstet Gynecol 2002;109:1097–1108.

91.   Lethaby A, Vollenhoven B, Sowter M. Pre-operative GnRH analogue therapy before hysterectomy or myomectomy for uterine fibroids. Cochrane Database of Systematic Reviews 2003.

92.   Letterie GS, Coddington CC, Winkel CA, et al. Efficacy of a gonadotropin-releasing hormone agonist in the treatment of uterine leiomyomata: long-term follow-up. Fertil Steril 1989;51:951–956.

93.   Murphy AA, Kettel LM, Morales AJ, et al. Regression of uterine leiomyomata in response to the antiprogesterone RU 486. J Clin Endocrinol Metab 1993;76:513–517.

94.   Murphy AA, Morales AJ, Kettel LM, Yen SS. Regression of uterine leiomyomata to the antiprogesterone RU486: dose-response effect. Fertil Steril 1995;64:187–190.

95.   Eisinger SH, Meldrum S, Fiscella K, et al. Low-dose mifepristone for uterine leiomyomata. Obstet Gynecol 2003;101:243–250.

96.   Reinsch RC, Murphy AA, Morales AJ, Yen SS. The effects of RU 486 and leuprolide acetate on uterine artery blood flow in the fibroid uterus: a prospective, randomized study. Am J Obstet Gynecol 1994;170:1623–1628.

97.   Vessey MP, Villard-Mackintosh L, McPherson K, et al. The epidemiology of hysterectomy: findings in a large cohort study. Br J Obstet Gynaecol 1992;99:402–407.

98.   Marchionni M, Fambrini M, Zambelli V, et al. Reproductive performance before and after abdominal myomectomy. Fertil Steril 2004;82:154–159.

99.   Munnell EW, Martin FW Jr. Abdominal myomectomy, advantages and disadvantages. Am J Obstet Gynecol 1951;62:109–120.

100.   Miller H, Tyrone CH. A survey of myomectomies with a follow-up. Am J Obstet Gynecol 1946;51:804–815.

101.   McCormick TA. Myomectomy with subsequent pregnancy. Am J Obstet Gynecol 1958;75:1128–1130.

102.   Deligdish L, Loewenthal M. Endometrial changes associated with myomata of the uterus. J Clin Pathol 1970;23:676–680.

103.   Berkeley AS, DeCherney AH, Polan ML. Abdominal myomectomy and subsequent fertility. Surg Gynecol Obstet 1983;156:319–322.

104. Takeuchi H, Kinoshita K. Evaluation of adhesion formation after laparoscopic myomectomy by systematic second-look microlaparoscopy. J Am Assoc Gynecol Laparosc 2002;9:442–446.

105. Barter RH, Parks J. Myoma uteri associated with pregnancy. Clin Obstet Gynecol 1958;1:519–533.

106. Davis JL, Ray-Mazumder S, Hobel CJ, et al. Uterine leiomyomas in pregnancy: a prospective study. Obstet Gynecol 1990;75:41–44.

107. Dildy GA 3rd, Moise KJ Jr, Smith LG Jr, et al. Indomethacin for the treatment of symptomatic leiomyoma uteri during pregnancy. Am J Perinatol 1992;9:185–189.

108. Angtuaco TL, Shah HR, Mattison DR, Quirk JG Jr. MR imaging in high-risk obstetric patients: a valuable complement to US. Radiographics 1992;12:91–110.

109. Lois D, Zikopoulos K, Paraskevaidis E. Surgical management of leiomyomata during pregnancy. Int J Gynaecol Obstet 1994;44:71–72.

110. Lolis DE, Kalantaridou SN, Makrydinas G, et al. Successful myomectomy during pregnancy. Human Reprod 2003;18:1699–1702.

111. Friedman AJ, Daly M, Juneau-Norcross M, Rein MS. Predictors of uterine volume reduction in women with myomas treated with a gonadotropin-releasing hormone agonist. Fertil Steril 1992;58:413–415.

112. Mencaglia L, Tantini C. GnRH agonist analogs and hysteroscopic resection of myomas. Int J Gynaecol Obstet 1993;43:285–288.

113. Carr BR, Marshburn PB, Weatherall PT, et al. An evaluation of the effect of gonadotropin-releasing hormone analogs and medroxyprogesterone acetate on uterine leiomyomata volume by magnetic resonance imaging: a prospective, randomized, double blind, placebo-controlled, crossover trial. J Clin Endocrinol Metab 1993;76:1217–1223.

114. Di Gregorio A, Maccario S, Raspollini M. The role of laparoscopic myomectomy in women of reproductive age. Reprod Biomed Online 2002;4 Suppl 3:55–58.

115. Dubuisson JB, Fauconnier A, Chapron C, et al. Reproductive outcome after laparoscopic myomectomy in infertile women. J Reprod Med 2000;45:23–30.

116. Malzoni M, Rotond M, Perone C, et al. Fertility after laparoscopic myomectomy of large uterine myomas: operative technique and preliminary results. Eur J Gynaecol Oncol 2003;24:79–82.

117. Di Gregorio A, Maccario S, Raspollini M. The role of laparoscopic myomectomy in women of reproductive age. Reprod Biomed Online 2002;4 Suppl 3:55–58.

118. Marret N, Chevillot M, Giraudeau B, et al. A retrospective study comparing myomectomy by laparoscopy and laparotomy in current surgical practice. Eur J Obstet Gynecol Reprod 2004;117:82–86.

119. Seinera P, Farina C, Todros T. Laparoscopic myomectomy and subsequent pregnancy: results in 54 patients. Hum Reprod 2000;15:1993–1996.

120. Parker WH, Rodi IA. Patient selection for laparoscopic myomectomy. J Am Assoc Gynecol Laparosc 1994;2:23–26.

121. Frederick J, Fletcher H, Simeon D, et al. Intramyometrial vasopressin as a haemostatic agent during myomectomy. Br J Obstet Gynaecol 1994;101:435–437.

122. Pelosi MA 3rd, Pelosi MA. Laparoscopic-assisted transvaginal myomectomy. J Am Assoc Gynecol Laparosc 1997;4:241–246.

123. Nezhat C, Nezhat F, Bess O, et al. Laparoscopically assisted myomectomy: a report of a new technique in 57 cases. Int J Fertil Menopausal Stud 1994;39:39–44.

124. Tulandi T, Murray C, Guralnick M. Adhesion formation and reproductive outcome after myomectomy and second-look laparoscopy. Obstet Gynecol 1993;82:213–215.

125. Neuwirth RS. Hysteroscopic management of symptomatic submucous fibroids. Obstet Gynecol 1983;62:509–511.

126. Corson SL, Brooks PG. Resectoscopic myomectomy. Fertil Steril 1991;55:1041–1044.

127. Loffer FD. Removal of large symptomatic intrauterine growths by the hysteroscopic resectoscope. Obstet Gynecol 1990;76:836–840.

128. Indman PD. Hysteroscopic treatment of menorrhagia associated with uterine leiomyomas. Obstet Gynecol 1993;81:716–720.

129. Valle RF. Hysteroscopic removal of submucous leiomyomas. J Gynecol Surg 1990;6:89–96.

130. Derman SG, Rehnstrom J, Neuwirth RS. The long-term effectiveness of hysteroscopic treatment of menorrhagia and leiomyomas. Obstet Gynecol 1991;77:591–594.

131. Hallez JP. Single-stage total hysteroscopic myomectomies: indications, techniques, and results. Fertil Steril 1995;63:703–708.

132. Goldenberg M, Sivan E, Sharabi Z, et al. Outcome of hysteroscopic resection of submucous myomas for infertility. Fertil Steril 1995;64:714–716.

133. Letterie GS, Kramer DJ. Intraoperative ultrasound guidance for intrauterine endoscopic surgery. Fertil Steril 1994;62:654–656.

134. Tempany CM, Stewart EA, McDannold N, et al. MR imaging-guided focused ultrasound surgery of uterine leiomyomas: a feasibility study. Radiology 2003;226:897–905.

135. Corson SL, Brooks PG, Serden SP, et al. Effects of vasopressin administration during hysteroscopic surgery. J Reprod Med 1994;39:419–423.

136. Baggish MS, Brill AI, Rosenzweig BA, et al. Fatal acute glycine and sorbitol toxicity during operative hysteroscopy. J Gynecol Surg 1993;9:137–143.

137. Shirk GJ, Kaigh J. The use of low-viscosity fluids for hysteroscopy. J Am Assoc Gynecol Laparosc 1994;2:11–21.

138. Vulgaropulos SP, Haley LC, Hulka JF. Intrauterine pressure and fluid absorption during continuous flow hysteroscopy. Am J Obstet Gynecol 1992;167:386–391.

139. Baumann R, Magos AL, Kay JD, Turnbull AC. Absorption of glycine irrigating solution during transcervical resection of endometrium. BMJ 1990;300:304–305.

140. Arieff AI. Hyponatremia, convulsions, respiratory arrest, and permanent brain damage after elective surgery in healthy women. N Engl J Med 1986;314:1529–1535.

141.   Kayan N, Karsli B, Zorlung B, Dosemic L, Erman M. Hysteroscope syndrome. Eur J Anaesthesiol 2002;19:770–772.

142.   Ayus JC, Krothapalli RK, Arieff AI. Treatment of symptomatic hyponatremia and its relation to brain damage. A prospective study. N Engl J Med 1987;317:1190–1195.

143.   Arieff AI, Ayus JC. Endometrial ablation complicated by fatal hyponatremic encephalopathy. JAMA 1993;270:1230–1232.

144.   Ayus JC, Arieff AI. Symptomatic hyponatremia: correcting sodium deficits safely. J Crit Illness 1990;5:905–918.

145.   Varasteh NN, Neuwirth RS, Levin B, Keltz MD. Pregnancy rates after hysteroscopic polypectomy and myomectomy in infertile women. Obstet Gynecol 1999;94:168–171.

146.   Wamsteker K, Emanuel MH, de Kruif JH. Transcervical hysteroscopic resection of submucous fibroids for abnormal uterine bleeding: results regarding the degree of intramural extension. Obstet Gynecol 1993;82:736–740.

147.   Donnez J, Gillerot S, Bourgonjon D, et al. Neodymium:YAG laser hysteroscopy in large submucous fibroids. Fertil Steril 1990;54:999–1003.

148.   Pinto I, Chimeno P, Romo A, et al. Uterine fibroids: uterine artery embolization versus abdominal hysterectomy for treatment – a prospective, randomized, and controlled clinical trial. Radiology 2003;226:425–431.

149.   Pelage JP, Le Dref O, Soyer P, et al. Fibroid-related menorrhagia: treatment with superselective embolization of the uterine arteries and midterm follow-up. Radiology 2000;215:428–431.

150.   Hutchins FL Jr, Worthington-Kirsch R, Berkowitz RP. Selective uterine artery embolization as primary treatment for symptomatic leiomyomata uteri. J Am Assoc Gynecol Laparosc 1999;6:279–284.

151.   Braude P, Reidy J, Nott V, et al. Embolization of uterine leiomyomata: current concepts in management. Hum Reprod Update 2000;6:603–608.

152.   Robson S, Wilson K, Munday D, Sebben R. Pelvic sepsis complicating embolization of a uterine fibroid. Aust N Z J Obstet Gynaecol 1999;39:516–517.

153.   Tulandi T, Sammour A, Valenti D, et al. Ovarian reserve after uterine artery embolization for leiomyomata. Fertil Steril 2002;78:197–198.

154.   Felemban A, Stein L, Tulandi T. Uterine restoration after repeated expulsion of myomas after uterine artery embolization. J Am Assoc Gynecol Laparosc 2001;8:442–444.

155.   Liu WM, Ng HT, Wu YC, et al. Laparoscopic bipolar coagulation of uterine vessels: a new method for treating symptomatic myomas. Fertil Steril 2001;75:417–422.

156.   Klein A, Schwartz ML. Uterine artery embolization for the treatment of uterine fibroids: an outpatient procedure. Am J Obstet Gynecol 2001;184:1556–1563.

157.   Chapman R. Treatment of uterine myomas by interstitial hyperthermia. Gynecol Endoscopy 1993;2:227–230.

158.   Nisolle M, Smets M, Malvaux V, et al. Laparoscopic myolysis with the Nd:YAG laser. J Gynecol Surg 1993;9:95–99.

159.   Dubuisson JB, Chapron C, Fauconnier A, Kreiker G. Laparoscopic myomectomy and myolysis. Curr Opin Obstet Gynecol 1997;9:233–238.

160.   Donnez J. Laparoscopic myolysis with Nd-YAG laser. J Gynecol Surg 1993;9:95–97.

161.   Phillips DR. Laparoscopic leiomyoma coagulation (myolysis). Gynaecol Endosc 1995;4:5–7.

162.   Hallez JP. Single stage total hysteroscopic myomectomies: indications, techniques, and results. Fertil Steril 1995;63:703–708.

163.   Ingersoll FM. Fertility following myomectomy. Fertil Steril 1963;14:596–602.

164.   Brown JM, Malkasian GD Jr, Symmonds RE. Abdominal myomectomy. Am J Obstet Gynecol 1967;99:126–129.

165.   Loeffler FE, Noble AD. Myomectomy at the Chelsea Hospital for Women. J Obstet Gynaecol Br Commonw 1970;77:167–170.

166.   Acien P, Quereda F. Abdominal myomectomy: results of a simple operative technique. Fertil Steril 1996;65:41–51.

167.   Fauconnier A, Dubuisson JB, Ancel PY, Chapron C. Prognostic factors of reproductive outcome after myomectomy in infertile patients. Hum Reprod 2000;15:1751–1757.

168.   Eldar-Geva T, Meagher S, Healy DL, et al. Effect of intramural, subserosal, and submucosal uterine fibroids on the outcome of assisted reproductive technology treatment. Fertil Steril 1998;70:687–691.

169.   Surrey ES, Lietz AK, Schoolcraft WB. Impact of intramural leiomyomata in patients with a normal endometrial cavity on in vitro fertilization-embryo transfer cycle outcome. Fertil Steril 2001;75:405–410.

170.   Mais V, Ajossa S, Piras B, et al. Prevention of de-novo adhesion formation after laparoscopic myomectomy: a randomized trial to evaluate the effectiveness of an oxidized regenerated cellulose absorbable barrier. Hum Reprod 1995;10:3133–3135.

171.   Campo S, Campo V, Gambadauro P. Reproductive outcome before and after laparoscopic or abdominal myomectomy for subserous or intramural myomas. Eur J Obstet Gynecol Reprod Biol 2003;110:215–219.

172.   LaMorte AI, Lalwani S, Diamond MP. Morbidity associated with abdominal myomectomy. Obstet Gynecol 1993;82:897–900.

173.   Fedele L, Parazzini F, Luchini L, et al. Recurrence of fibroids after myomectomy: a transvaginal ultrasonographic study. Hum Reprod 1995;10:1795–1796.

174.   Fedele L, Vercellini P, Bianchi S, et al. Treatment with GnRH agonists before myomectomy and the risk of short-term myoma recurrence. Br J Obstet Gynaecol 1990;97:393–396.

175.   Candiani GB, Fedele L, Parazzini F, Villa L. Risk of recurrence after myomectomy. Br J Obstet Gynaecol 1991;98:385–389.

9 Intrauterine Adhesions

A stenosis or blocking of the internal cervical os may occur under certain conditions producing amenorrhea . . .
— *Joseph G. Asherman, 1948*

Though frequently credited to Asherman, intrauterine adhesions and amenorrhea were initially described in Germany by Fritsch in 1894.[1] His case report described a 24-year-old woman with a 2-year history of amenorrhea who underwent a curettage 3 weeks after delivery. Asherman in 1948 described adhesions in the cervical canal and cervical stenosis in 29 patients as a cause of amenorrhea.[2] These cases followed curettage for postpartum hemorrhage, incomplete abortion, or missed abortion. Subsequently, Asherman expanded the series to include both intracervical and intrauterine adhesions resulting in cervical stenosis, obliteration of the cervical canal, and partial or complete obliteration of the uterine cavity. Asherman observed that adhesion formation occurred frequently after curettage of missed rather than incomplete first-trimester loss, suggesting a time sensitivity to the formation of adhesions. In Asherman's original manuscript, a note at the conclusion of the paper described a Scandinavian series published in 1937 by Stamer of 37 cases, between 1894 and 1933, of "uterine atresia" after curettage.[3] The cases were very similar to those described by Asherman and further contributed to establishing the clinical significance of intrauterine adhesions.

Since these original descriptions, the frequency and clinical significance of intrauterine adhesions have become more thoroughly documented and appreciated.[4,5] Adhesions between the anterior and posterior uterine walls resulting in menstrual irregularities, repeated pregnancy loss, and infertility have evolved into a distinct clinical entity known as *Asherman's syndrome* or intrauterine adhesions. This chapter describes contributory factors to the development of intrauterine adhesions, their clinical consequences, and their surgical management.

Etiology

Any intrauterine manipulation can cause the formation of adhesions within the uterine cavity. The typical scenario is the development of intrauterine adhesions shortly after a terminated event of pregnancy.[6,7] The incidence varies from 3 to 40% depending on the population studied and the sensitivity of the diagnostic tests used.[8] In fertile patients with regular menstrual cycles investigated by hysteroscopy at the time of tubal ligation, 3% have intrauterine adhesions.[9] The incidence increases considerably in patients evaluated for secondary amenorrhea or hypomenorrhea and whether diagnostic studies include hysterosalpingography (HSG) or hysteroscopy, in which case, 30 to 40% of patients have evidence of intrauterine adhesions.[10]

Factors that predispose to Asherman's syndrome include any form of intrauterine manipulation, whether as a diagnostic dilatation and curettage, or after any event of pregnancy, whether term delivery or spontaneous abortion, that requires dilatation and curettage (D&C). In approximately 90% of patients, the etiology of intrauterine adhesions may be traced to events surrounding an event of pregnancy, such as a D&C for a missed abortion or for retained products of conception.[11–13] As yet undefined aspects surrounding pregnancy predispose to formation of intrauterine adhesions when the intrauterine cavity is manipulated. A postoperative or postpartum infection, previously thought to be a threshold event in the development of the adhesions, is not a prerequisite. The critical period, during which time the endometrium is most susceptible to trauma and the development of adhesions (i.e., formation of scar tissue between the anterior and posterior walls), appears to be the first 2 to 4 weeks after delivery. This interval is associated with low serum concentrations of estrogen and lack of endometrial stimulation, which may contribute to a prolonged exposure of the basalis on the contiguous uterine walls.

Insight into the process of adhesion formation may be gained through study of the normal process of menstruation. The repair of the endometrium is estrogen-dependent and may be impeded in circumstances where estrogen levels are low, such as after an event of pregnancy. Regeneration of normal endometrium after menstruation is initiated by the basalis within 24 hours after normal menstrual shedding.[14] This process begins on cycle day 1 and continues in response to increasing serum concentrations of estrogen. Endometrial repair continues as the menstrual cycle progresses and estrogen levels rise with the formation of a thickened endometrium progressing throughout the follicular phase. The formation of intrauterine adhesions may represent a perturbation of this process. Any delay in the reformation of the endometrium secondary to hypoestrogenism may provide an opportunity for adhesion formation between contiguous denuded endometrial walls. Evidence suggesting that lack of hormonal stimulation may contribute is the observation of higher incidence of intrauterine adhesions in breastfeeding women when resumption of ovarian function may be delayed.

Repeated D&C for first-trimester loss may contribute to the formation and severity of adhesions. The incidence of intrauterine adhesions following sharp curettage after one and two spontaneous first-trimester losses is 8 and 15%, respectively. In this setting, adhesions are mild and filmy and occupy less than one-quarter of the uterine cavity. The incidence after three or more spontaneous abortions, however, increases significantly to 32%. In addition, 58% of intrauterine adhesions diagnosed in this setting are more severe, both in character and extent.[15] The occurrence of intrauterine adhesions in one study did not appear to be related to serum estradiol concentration on the day of the curettage, nor to any estrogen treatment used after the procedure.[16] The high incidence and severity of intrauterine adhesions in patients with three or more spontaneous abortions justifies a diagnostic hysteroscopy as part of any evaluation for repeated pregnancy loss managed by D&C prior to any ART.[17] A D&C performed for a first-trimester missed abortion may be an independent risk factor beyond that posed after incomplete or complete spontaneous abortion. Patients who undergo D&C for a missed or spontaneous abortion, develop adhesions in 30% versus 6% respectively.[18] The difference suggests a potential time factor between the loss of viability and curettage. The technique of evacuation may play a role. It is unclear whether the soft or rigid suction cannula or sharp curette for elective first-trimester abortion contributes more extensively to the formation of intrauterine adhesions.

Another factor that contributes to the development of intrauterine adhesions are mullerian abnormalities. In a study of adhesion formation and uterine abnormalities, intrauterine adhesions were described in 8% of patients with mullerian abnormalities and 4% of patients with infertility and an otherwise unremarkable evaluation and normally shaped uterine cavity – a significant difference.[19] This finding was strongly correlated for patients with a septate uterus. This association suggests the possibility that an intrinsic defect may be present in the endometrium of these patients to prevent normal endometrial regeneration.

Intrauterine adhesions may be a long-term complication of any complex operative hysteroscopy with the frequency dependent on the pathology initially treated in the case of resectoscopic myomectomy. The degree of dissection, wattage, and manipulation of the cavity may influence the occurrence of intrauterine adhesions. In addition, hypoestrogenism secondary to GnRH analog therapy, a frequent preoperative treatment for resection of myomas, endometrial polyps, or uterine septum, may persist after the procedure and discontinuation of the analog. This setting may increase the possibility of intrauterine adhesions. Hence, any patient undergoing these procedures should be considered at risk for intrauterine adhesions and consideration given to second-look in-office hysteroscopy or HSG to assess the normalcy of the endometrial cavity.

Other variables, such as an intrauterine device (IUD), do not contribute to intrauterine adhesions. In the past, infectious processes such as tuberculosis contributed significantly to formation of intrauterine adhesions. Except in endemic areas, it is rare to discover this process as a cause in contemporary practice.[20]

Clinical Correlates

The most frequent complaints of patients with intrauterine adhesions are changes in menstrual frequency and character of menstrual flow (i.e., either amenorrhea or hypomenorrhea), infertility, and repeated pregnancy loss.[8,10] The extent of the change in menstrual flow offers no insight into the extent of intrauterine adhesions. A suggestion of the diagnosis is made by the patient's history, for example, hypomenorrhea or amenorrhea after intrauterine manipulation regardless of type. A typical history elicited in a patient with intrauterine adhesions is curettage after an event of pregnancy, then a series of spontaneous menstrual cycles that decrease in intensity followed by amenorrhea. Amenorrhea and cyclic abdominal and pelvic pain may be initial complaints when isolated adhesions in the lower uterine segment block menstrual flow. The most dramatic clinical presentations are secondary to obstruction of menstrual flow and result in the development of hematometra requiring immediate evaluation and drainage. The history in this circumstance is typically one of a cessation of menses with gradual cyclic abdominal and pelvic pain suggestive of severe dysmenorrhea. The pain initially is restricted only to the time of expected menses but becomes progressively more severe and occupies more and more of the month. In this circumstance, emergency evaluation may be required. Only a small amount of critically placed adhesions is necessary to result in this clinical picture.

Menstrual changes are not prerequisites to the diagnosis. Sugimoto found that 39% of patients with Asherman's syndrome clearly defined by hysteroscopy had no change in their menstrual histories.[21] The extent of the intrauterine adhesions correlates poorly with the extent of changes in the menstrual pattern. Patients with severe intrauterine adhesions may continue with regular monthly menses, depending on the degree of function of the remaining endometrium. Conversely, patients with mild adhesions may complain of marked changes in their menstrual pattern and considerable diminution in the amount of flow. Approximately 13% of patients have cyclic menses, and 72% are completely asymptomatic.[10] The causes of this differential response are unknown. Limited information from MRI suggests that change in the function and responsiveness of endometrium surrounding but not part of the intrauterine adhesions may be involved.[22] In a series of cases of amenorrhea associated with intrauterine adhesions, MRI revealed endometrial and junctional signals of low intensity throughout the cavity, suggesting a dysfunctional endometrium. This pattern persisted in spite of prolonged high-dose estrogen stimulation. These findings suggest that in areas free of adhesion, endometrial damage of sufficient intensity and depth may exist and prevent regeneration of endometrium in response to hormonal stimulation. These findings support the concept that events contributory to intrauterine adhesion formation may occur on a continuum. Extreme damage to regions of the endometrium and basalis may result in coalescence of the opposing uterine walls and eventual organization into intrauterine adhesions. In other areas, damage to the basalis may be of sufficient intensity to prevent regeneration of functioning endometrium but not so severe as to contribute to adhesion formation or obliteration of the cavity. These areas may appear free of adhesions on HSG or hysteroscopy but may be without the ability to respond to hormonal stimulation. Other surrounding areas may be mildly damaged, with regeneration of normally functioning endometrium contributing to monthly menses.

Patients may also present with a history of infertility. The incidence of adhesions in an infertile population is 21% and in a normal fertile population 3.2%. Of patients with intrauterine adhesions and infertility, 80% have been infertile for at least 1 year, and menstrual changes are an accompanying complaint in 30 to 40% of the patients. The etiology of the infertility associated with intrauterine adhesions is unclear. Two possible contributing factors may be the location of the intrauterine adhesions and endometrial function and receptivity. Adhesions partially blocking the endocervical canal or the tubal ostia may result in infertility by an obstructive phenomenon. There may also be changes in endometrial responsiveness and receptivity in damaged regions surrounding but not directly affected by the adhesions, as noted above.

In addition to the clinical changes in menstrual patterns and infertility, patients may also present with complaints of recurrent pregnancy loss, a history of placental implantation abnormalities, both previa and accreta, as well as premature rupture of the membranes and abnormal fetal presentation.[23–27] Hence, factors contributing to infertility, repeated loss, and abnormal obstetric events may be related to a decrease in actual cavity space and capacity, to poor distension of the uterine walls, and possibly to changes in functional aspects of the endometrium itself.

Diagnosis

Clinical Examination

There are no findings evident on clinical examination suggestive of intrauterine adhesions. At times, difficulty passing a uterine sound, an endometrial biopsy curette, or a Pipelle curette may provide a hint that intrauterine adhesions are present. Otherwise, the presence of intrauterine adhesions is detected only by an imaging technique or direct visualization.

Hysterosalpingography

HSG is the mainstay for diagnosis of intrauterine adhesions. Characteristic appearance on HSG shows multiple intrauterine filling defects, which may range from small isolated areas of intrauterine shadowing scattered within an otherwise normal cavity (Figure 9-1) to loss of 50% or more of the cavity (Figure 9-2) to nearly complete obliteration of the cavity. At times, outright failure to fill the cavity occurs or there is filling of only the very lower-most portion of the intrauterine cavity (Figure 9-3). Careful inspection of the endometrial cavity in any patient with septate or bicornuate uterus is essential given the predisposition of this group of patients to form adhesions (Figure 9-4).

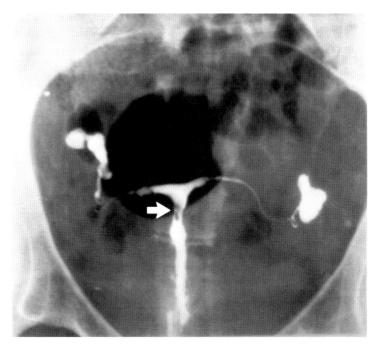

Figure 9-1   Hysterosalpingogram showing mild intrauterine adhesions in the lower uterine segment (arrow).

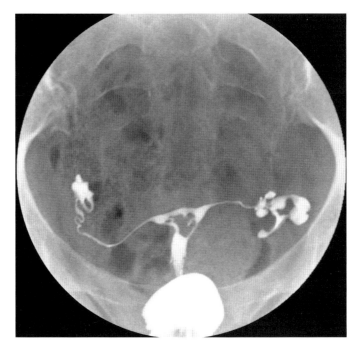

Figure 9-2   Hysterosalpingogram showing moderate intrauterine adhesions occupying the central portion of the endometrial cavity.

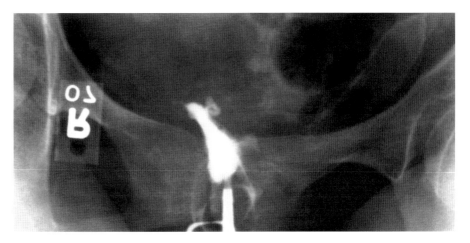

Figure 9-3   Hysterosalpingogram showing filling of only the endocervical canal in a patient with complete obliteration of the endometrial cavity (severe adhesions). Such an image may be consistent with either obstructive adhesions at the internal cervical os or severe adhesions. Final diagnosis required additional imaging with ultrasound and MRI.

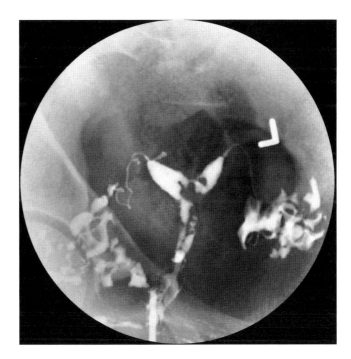

Figure 9-4   Hysterosalpingogram in a patient with a septate uterus. Multiple intrauterine filling defects throughout all segments of the uterine cavity are demonstrated.

Intrauterine adhesions are classified according to the extent of uterine cavity occlusion seen on HSG and the type of intrauterine adhesions observed at hysteroscopy. Accurate classification is important because prognosis is related to the degree of cavity obliteration and character of adhesions. Two classification systems have been described. In the first,[11,28,29] the extent of cavity occlusion is divided into three categories: (1) severe – more than 75% of the uterine cavity involved, ostial areas and upper cavity occluded, and agglutination or thick adhesive bands present in the uterine walls; (2) moderate – 25 to 75% of the uterine cavity involved, ostial areas and upper fundus partially occluded, and adhesions only (no agglutination of the uterine walls); and (3) minimal – less than 25% of the uterine cavity involved, ostial areas and upper fundus minimally involved or clear, and thin or filmy adhesions. This straightforward system is convenient and is based solely on visualization on HSG.

The second system is a numerical scoring system.[30] This classification consists of an objective scoring system that incorporates both HSG and hysteroscopic assessment of the intrauterine adhesions. The scheme takes into consideration the extent of the cavity involved, the character of the adhesions (i.e., whether dense or filmy), and the clinical history of the patient's menstrual pattern. The exact location of adhesions may be incorporated into a drawing for documentation and explanation. Both classification systems provide information regarding the extent of intrauterine adhesions and are convenient ways of communicating findings on HSG or hysteroscopy. No classification scheme provides an accurate predictor of likelihood of recurrence, resumption of menses, or pregnancy. These systems are useful, however, in counseling patients and offer a descriptive tool.

Ultrasonography

Although the data are limited, ultrasound assessment of the endometrial cavity may be useful for the diagnosis of intrauterine adhesions.[31] Adhesions appear as dense, highly echogenic structures in the region of the endometrial stripe and, with severe intrauterine adhesions, completely replace the endometrial stripe (Figures 9-5, 9-6, and 9-7). Transvaginal ultrasound may also be used as a means of diagnosing and assessing the degree of intrauterine adhesions. In one study of 77 women, adhesions were diagnosed with a sensitivity of 91% and a specificity of 100%. In this study, transvaginal sonography was useful in diagnosing and classifying intrauterine adhesions.[32] Preoperative assessment of endometrial pattern by transvaginal sonography may also provide some insight regarding outcome after surgical repair in patients with severe intrauterine adhesions.[33] Patients with minimal endometrium seen on transvaginal sonography during the last luteal phase are at risk of having severe adhesions or cavity obliteration. However, those patients with a clearly defined, well-developed endometrium on ultrasound may have mild adhesions or adhesions restricted to the lower uterine segment. These patients are in the most favorable category and usually

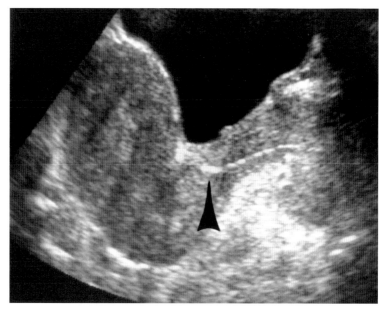

Figure 9-5   Transabdominal ultrasound demonstrating hyperechoic densities in the lower uterine segment (arrowhead) in a patient with intrauterine adhesions. Hysteroscope demonstrated complete obstruction of the lower uterine segment in the region of these densities and moderate intrauterine adhesions throughout the endometrial cavity.

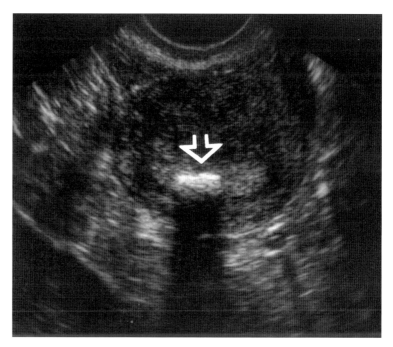

Figure 9-6   Transvaginal ultrasound demonstrating hyperechoic densities (arrow) in the mid and upper endometrial cavity.

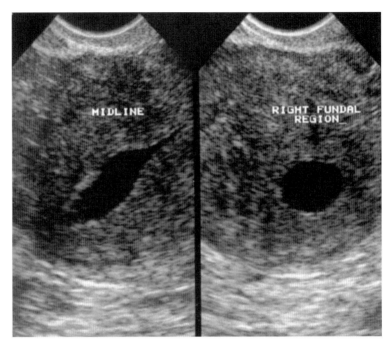

Figure 9-7   Transvaginal ultrasound demonstrating multiple sonolucencies throughout the endometrial cavity in the midline and right fundal region. This patient had complete obliteration of the lower one-third of the uterine cavity and obstruction of the outflow tract.

resume normal menstruation after hysteroscopy. Transvaginal ultrasound assessment of the endometrial pattern also permits identification of patients who may require preoperative suppression to facilitate hysteroscopic lysis of adhesions. If the endometrium is thickened in some areas adjacent to the adhesions, endometrial debris may occlude the operative field and suppression may be beneficial. Ultrasound can also demonstrate hematometra in patients in whom adhesions block the egress of menstrual flow or may be useful in identifying areas of loculation (Figure 9-8). Ultrasound evaluation is an essential preoperative evaluation to assess the endometrial stripe and rule-out any areas of hematometra.

Both two-dimensional and three-dimensional sonohysterography may be used as an adjunct to transvaginal ultrasonography.[34,35] In circumstances where transvaginal sonography is normal but a high index of suspicion regarding the possibility of intrauterine adhesions is present, sonohysterography has been shown to provide an enhanced image of the endometrial cavity and increased the diagnostic sensitivity and specificity for diagnosing intrauterine adhesions. Though essential in preoperative planning, transabdominal and transvaginal ultrasound assessment and sonohysterography are second-line diagnostic studies and complementary to HSG. HSG and hysteroscopy continue to provide the most sensitive techniques for diagnosis and classification.

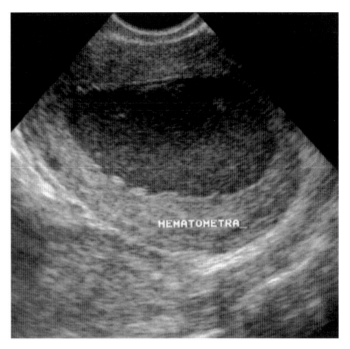

Figure 9-8   Transvaginal ultrasound demonstrating a hematometra in a patient with complete obliteration of the lower uterine segment and internal cervical os.

Magnetic Resonance Imaging

MRI provides a noninvasive technique to detect a variety of intrauterine abnormalities, through its ability to detect subtle variations in signal intensities. MRI has been reported for the detection of intrauterine synechia.[22,36] As a technique to define intrauterine anatomy and the functional status of the endometrium, MRI provides information on the presence or absence of intrauterine adhesions and the functional status of the endometrium.[37,38] Findings suggestive of intrauterine adhesions are low-density signals on T2-weighted scans within the endometrial cavity and loss of zonal definition (distinct junctional and endometrial zones may be poorly defined). The changes in signal intensity may be in a region of otherwise normal endometrial architecture.[36,37] In milder cases, MRI has also demonstrated hypointense signals of the endometrium and junctional zones in areas surrounding the intrauterine adhesions (Figure 9-9). Findings of hypointense endometrial, junctional, and normal myometrial signals suggest that the residual endometrium surrounding the adhesions may have an altered function, a possible explanation for the varying menstrual histories (as noted above). MRI may help in assessing endometrial function, before and after stimulation with high-dose estrogens, in order to identify possible contributory factors to changes in menstrual history and infertility. Though capable of providing insightful clinical information, MRI is not an integral study in the evaluation

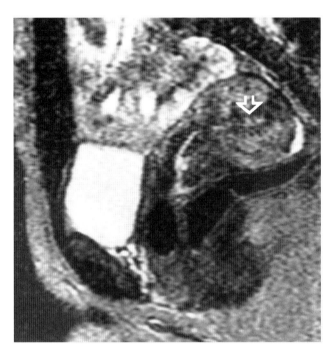

Figure 9-9   Sagittal magnetic resonance image demonstrating hypointense endometrial and junctional signals (arrow) throughout the endometrial cavity in a patient with moderate intrauterine adhesions.

of intrauterine adhesions. Cost considerations and a lack of data demonstrating clear-cut benefit and improvement in outcomes preclude its routine use.

Hysteroscopy

Diagnostic hysteroscopy provides direct visualization of the cavity and, in some series, a more sensitive diagnostic technique than HSG. The procedure may be carried out using conventional or flexible micro-hysteroscopic equipment.[28,39] For diagnosis, Sugimoto's criteria are useful: namely that the adhesions be attached at the uterine wall at two points, either central or marginal.[21] Histologic confirmation is not necessary. On direct visualization with hysteroscopy, intrauterine adhesions may assume one of two appearances. The simplest (and easiest to lyse) are adhesions that are fibrous and avascular and found scattered throughout the endometrial cavity. The second type are vascular, dense, and rigidly bind the anterior to the posterior wall. The latter circumstance may present difficulty in achieving adequate uterine distension and visualization. In extreme cases, the adhesions may be sufficiently dense to result in complete obliteration of the intrauterine cavity and preclude any visualization. As many as 45% of patients undergoing diagnostic hysteroscopy may have some degree of intracavitary adhesions depending on history.[19,21]

Management

Management of intrauterine adhesions consists of lysis of adhesions under direct visualization using hysteroscopy.[40,41] Hysteroscopy has made direct diagnosis of intrauterine adhesions possible and offers a visually controlled approach to therapy.[42–45] Preoperative HSG and ultrasound are essential. Reference to the HSG not only provides guidance intraoperatively but enables a more informed counseling session to present all possible outcomes prior to surgery, especially for patients who have severe adhesions or complete cavity obliteration and who may require either a second hysteroscopic procedure or hysterotomy. Reference to the ultrasound scan may assist in deciding whether endometrial suppression is needed and may predict both surgical difficulty and ultimate outcome.[33] If there are thickened areas of the endometrium on ultrasound in a patient with continued menses, suppression with gonadotropin-releasing hormone (GnRH) analogs is advised. Suppression provides an enhanced visualization of the intrauterine cavity regardless of the extent of adhesions. GnRH suppression is not necessary in all patients.[45]

Operative Technique: Hysteroscopic Lysis of Intrauterine Adhesions

In performing hysteroscopic lysis of adhesions, extreme care must be used in inserting the hysteroscope. Perforation is a distinct possibility because of the limited distensibility of the uterine cavity, especially in severe cases. Insertion of a laminaria 12 to 24 hours before the procedure may facilitate insertion of the hysteroscope. Misoprostol may also be used to soften the cervix 12–18 hours before surgery. The drug may be taken orally the night before or vaginally 4 hours before surgery. The scope should be advanced to the level of the internal os and full visualization of the entire endometrial cavity made. The degree of adhesions and adherence of the anterior and posterior walls may initially limit distension of the cavity and restrict the field of view. Adequate distension of the cavity is essential for complete identification and lysis of adhesions. The HSG should be available for review in the operating room to assist in the dissection. Dilute methylene blue as a vital stain may help differentiate normal endometrial tissue from dense fibrous adhesions in some circumstances.

Different hysteroscopic operative procedures have been used to divide intrauterine adhesions. Microscissors are most commonly used for mild or moderate disease. A loop resectoscope may also be used, but the possibility of thermal injury to surrounding normal endometrium limits its application. Laser fibers with both carbon dioxide and Nd:YAG and KTP 532 laser are an alternative.[39,46,47] The adhesions are lysed using hysteroscopic microscissors under direct visualization. The scissors are advanced into the cavity and the adhesions cut serially at their midpoint. With this dissection, the adhesions usually retract to the anterior and posterior uterine walls. The bands may be filmy, dense, avascular, or vascular and require sharp incision. Equipment for coagulation by laser or cautery should be available. The dissection should be initiated at the lowermost portion of the cavity and carried superiorly as the cavity broadens. The bands are under some tension; as the dissection is performed, the adhesive bands usually retract to the anterior and posterior walls. Seldom is actual excision and removal required.[48,49] In cases where distension is restricted by the adhesions, lysis of the lowermost adhesions may improve visualization. The process requires patient, gradual progress.

Difficult or impossible visualization of the endometrial cavity and endometrium may be encountered in cases of severe intrauterine adhesions. Visualization may be compromised due to a reduction in cavity volume and inadequate cavity distension. For extensive lysis of adhesions, it may also be impossible after dissection to distinguish denuded myometrium from scar tissue. One option in these circumstances is to discontinue the procedure and cycle the patient postoperatively on high-dose estrogens in the hope of establishing some degree of endometrial regeneration.[50] Endometrial thickness may be assessed postoperatively by transvaginal ultrasound. After maximal regeneration has been achieved, consideration may be given to a second procedure to identify and lyse the remaining adhesions. Partial lysis from the first procedure may permit easier and more complete uterine distension and visualization.

In difficult cases, intraoperative transabdominal or laparoscopic ultrasound guidance or diagnostic laparoscopy may be required to guide the dissection.[51,52] In cases in which the extent of dissection is questionable, an intraoperative HSG may be advisable. Intrauterine adhesiolysis should be continued until normal uterine architecture is restored. One criterion to determine if the cavity is restored is identification of the tubal ostia. The ostia of both cornua should be visualized easily by moving the scope from side to side. In addition, the overall appearance of the cavity should be fuller and broader on panorama and have a normal or nearly normal appearance at the conclusion of the adhesiolysis. Most procedures can be performed under direct visualization with an operative hysteroscope. In some cases, a resectoscope and operative loop may be used, especially if the adhesions appear vascular and the need to use cautery or laser frequently is anticipated. In approximately 5% of patients, the adhesions are so extensive they preclude insertion of the scope into the cavity, and prevent access to the upper part of the cavity. In these circumstances, a hysterotomy may be required. There is no advantage of resectoscopic lysis with an operative loop over hysteroscopic resection using microscissors to reduce recurrence. A balloon may also be inserted into the endometrial cavity for lysis of intrauterine adhesions.

A transabdominal approach may be necessary after failed hysteroscopic lysis of adhesions or as an initial approach in select cases, such as with complete obliteration of the cavity. It may also be required in those patients who have recurrent severe intrauterine adhesions after a successful hysteroscopic procedure.[53] The procedure is performed as a variation of a Tompkins metroplasty. The uterus itself is divided in the midline, the intrauterine cavity identified, and the walls sharply separated using scissors, taking care to differentiate endometrial and myometrial tissues from adhesions. This technique should be applied only in extremely difficult circumstances that preclude a hysteroscopic approach.

Alternative Techniques for Lysis of Adhesions

There is no place for blind D&C as this technique may result in an aggravation of the condition rather than a solution to the problem. As a blind approach if hysteroscopy is not possible, a Pratt dilator may be used. In the most simple approach to the reconstruction of the endometrial cavity, a single Pratt cervical dilator is passed through the cervix with the curved tip pointing lateral toward the uterine cornua. The procedure is performed under laparoscopic guidance. After alignment of the dilator in the plane of the endometrial cavity, the Pratt dilator is swept from side to side under laparoscopic guidance. This has resulted in recreation of a normal endometrial cavity. Pressure lavage under ultrasound has been proposed as one therapy alternative to hysteroscopic resection of adhesions. This technique may be performed as an in-office procedure. This may be applicable to mild adhesions but its role in thick adhesions remains to be seen.

Postoperative Care

A major focus of care after lysis is the prevention of recurrence. An intrauterine stent and hormonal therapy have been used for variable periods of time after surgery. The choice of which therapy to use and for how long may be guided in part by the appearance and extent of the adhesions noted on the hysteroscopy. No prospective data support one modality over another. However, postoperative hormonal therapy is frequently used. High-dose estrogen therapy (i.e., 5 mg of conjugated estrogens daily for 30 days), followed by 10 mg of medroxyprogesterone for 10 days is one option. In a limited, comparative study, hormonal therapy, an IUD, or balloon showed no advantage when compared with a control group.[54] In one comparative study, estrogen had no apparent improvement in the likelihood of recurrence of the intrauterine adhesions.[55] Application of adhesion-preventing gel (Seprafilm) may have a role in prevention of recurrent adhesions.

Postoperative HSG is absolutely essential for final evaluation of the cavity. In one series, persistent intrauterine abnormalities suggestive of intrauterine adhesions were associated with poor outcome, that is, no pregnancies or repeated first-trimester loss. Placenta previa, placenta accreta, malpresentation, and obstetric hemorrhage have also been described secondary to persistent intrauterine adhesions.[23–27] Adhesions noted on the postoperative HSG, if significant, should be managed with a second procedure.

Hysteroscopy is necessary to evaluate any suggestion of intrauterine adhesions detected on HSG or sonohysterography. If cavity distortion or significant adhesions are detected, lysis is required prior to ART. After lysis of intrauterine adhesions, evaluation of the cavity postoperatively is necessary. In cases of severe intrauterine adhesions requiring extensive resection, observation of endometrial thickness by transvaginal ultrasound during the late luteal phase over 2 to 3 cycles postoperatively is suggested. These observations will provide insight regarding the responsiveness of the endometrium to gonadal steroids. In some cases, the endometrium may be persistently thin and irregular. Structure may be restored but function may be absent or reduced. In extreme cases, a normal endometrial cavity may result after lysis of adhesions. But the endometrium may be functionally deficient and unresponsive. In these circumstances, a trial of estrogen may be required to assess responsiveness. Failure to respond to high-dose estrogen and/or progestin further supports this impression of a denuded, unresponsive endometrium. These findings suggest persistent endometrial damage and compromised function in spite of an anatomically normal cavity. In this setting, observation over additional cycles may reveal resolution. However, persistence of a thin and irregular endometrium and a history of a failed IVF cycle (i.e. no pregnancy with quality embryos), should prompt a discussion of surrogacy.

Outcomes Analysis

Clinical observations in cases of untreated intrauterine adhesions are unfavorable enough to weigh against any conservative approach and mandate treatment. In one study of 792 patients who attempted pregnancy without treatment, 15% conceived, 53% delivered a viable infant, and 13% had placenta accreta.[11] The literature describing outcomes after treatment of intrauterine adhesions is primarily observational and uncontrolled. Outcomes after surgery have frequently been compared with outcomes in the same patients before surgery. With this database, favorable outcomes have been described in a variety of settings after lysis of adhesions. Final outcome depends on the exact indications for surgery, the extent of the intrauterine adhesions, and the restoration of normal structure and function.[56,57] In patients with repeated loss, 82% of patients with mild adhesions and 32% with severe adhesions achieved pregnancy. Of patients with this history who do achieve pregnancy, 80% deliver at term, 18% end in spontaneous first-trimester loss, and 3% have ectopic pregnancy.[58] In one series, a pregnancy rate of 93% and term-delivery rate of 87% was noted for patients with mild adhesions and a pregnancy rate of 57% and term delivery rate of 55% for severe adhesions.[59] Normal menstruation was restored after hysteroscopic resection in 90% of patients with menstrual changes such as amenorrhea or hypomenorrhea as the primary complaint. Six percent had recurrent hypomenorrhea or amenorrhea.[44,59]

Of patients whose only apparent cause of infertility was intrauterine adhesions, a pregnancy rate of 60 to 75% has been described.[44] Variable outcomes may be influenced by patients who had multiple factors contributing to their infertility in addition to the intrauterine adhesions. In any patient, a complete evaluation of all factors possibly contributing to their infertility and recurrent pregnancy loss is essential. The initial severity of the adhesions correlate with recurrence. The impact of intrauterine adhesions on infertility rates may be related in part to endometrial atrophy and loss of endometrial function in the area of the adhesions, even after adequate restoration of the cavity. Although contemporary treatment via hysteroscope has dramatically improved the prognosis, the term-pregnancy rate following treatment of severe disease is only 32%.[28] In the treatment of recurrent pregnancy loss, 70% will carry to term after lysis of mild adhesions. Pregnancy and term delivery rates are reduced to 43 and 10%, respectively, in the case of moderate and severe adhesions. Adverse obstetric outcomes after lysis of adhesions have also been described.[26] Patients must be counseled regarding the possibility of attendant obstetrical complications. Recurrence of adhesions is influenced by several factors in patients with minimal to mild adhesions, but the likelihood of recurrence is extremely low. Adhesion reformation in patients who have several adhesions is as high as 50–60%.

Summary and Recommendations

A high index of suspicion for intrauterine adhesions should exist for any patient with a history of curettage regardless of menstrual pattern. Changes in menstrual patterns, presence of infertility, or history of recurrent pregnancy loss should heighten suspicion. The diagnosis, treatment, and outlook for patients with intrauterine adhesions has improved considerably with the introduction of sensitive diagnostic studies and endoscopic techniques for lysis. On the basis of available literature describing outcomes measures, the following recommendations are made:

- The mainstay for diagnosis of intrauterine adhesions continues to be HSG. This technique provides a means not only of localizing the adhesions, but also a way to classify the adhesions according to current classification techniques.
- Ultrasound and MRI are attractive but as yet unproven modalities for diagnosis of intrauterine adhesions. Transvaginal ultrasound should be performed preoperatively to assess endometrial thickness. This measurement may be used to decide the need for endometrial suppression and to provide some insight into outcome.
- Hysteroscopy is the most sensitive technique for diagnosing intrauterine adhesions and assessing their character. It represents a more invasive and costly diagnostic study than HSG.
- In patients with either infertility or repeated pregnancy loss, surgical management is indicated. Hysteroscopic lysis of adhesions is the method of

choice. Patients should be counseled preoperatively about the possible need for a second procedure, the recurrence of the adhesions, or the need for a hysterotomy if severe intrauterine adhesions exist and hysteroscopic lysis is incomplete. Possible adverse obstetric events should be discussed.

- Postoperative HSG or hysteroscopy is essential. Outcomes have been unfavorable for patients with persistent intrauterine adhesions. If persistent or recurrent adhesions are present, a repeat lysis should be performed.
- Postoperative high-dose estrogen and progestins are indicated. However, comparative data of postoperative treatment versus no treatment describe similar outcomes.
- Other options such as an intrauterine balloon or Seprafilm may be considered to reduce recurrence.
- Adverse obstetric outcomes after lysis have been described. Communication of extent of adhesions and procedure for lysis to their attending obstetrician is essential.
- Prior to ART and after lysis of adhesions, the cavity should be re-evaluated with HSG or hysteroscopy and the endometrium should be measured at mid-cycle and late luteal phase to verify a normally responsive endometrium.
- Verification of normal structure and a restored endometrial cavity is essential prior to any ART cycle. In cases of a thin endometrium in spite of maximum doses of estrogen, consideration should be given to surrogacy.

References

1. Fritsch H. Ein fall von volligen Schwund der Gebarmutterhohle nach Auskratzung. Zentralbl Gynakol 1894:18:1337–1339.

2. Asherman JG. Traumatic intrauterine adhesions. J Obstet Gynaecol Br Commonw 1948;55:23–27.

3. Stamer S. Partial and total atresia of the uterus after excochleation. Acta Obstet Gynecol Scand 1946;26:263–268.

4. Hald H. On uterine atresia consequent to curettage. Acta Obstet Gynecol Scand 1949;28:169–172.

5. Asherman JG. Traumatic intrauterine adhesions. J Obstet Gynecol Br Commonw 1950;57:892–896.

6. Eriksen J, Kaestel C. The incidence of uterine atresia after post-partum curettage. A follow-up examination of 141 patients. Dan Med Bull 1960;7:50–51.

7. Adoni A, Palti Z, Milwidsky A, Dolberg M. The incidence of intrauterine adhesions following spontaneous abortion. Int J Fertil 1982;27:117–118.

8. Bergman P. Traumatic intra-uterine lesions. Acta Obstet Gynecol Scand 1961;40:1–39.

9. Taylor PJ, Cumming DC, Hill PJ. Significance of intrauterine adhesions detected hysteroscopically in eumenorrheic infertile women and role of antecedent curettage in their formation. Am J Obstet Gynecol 1981;139:239–242.

10. Lancet M, Kessler I. A review of Asherman's syndrome, and results of modern treatment. Int J Fertil 1988;33:14–24.

11. March CM. Intrauterine adhesions. Obstet Gynecol Clin North Am 1995;22:491–505.

12. Schenker JG. Etiology of and therapeutic approach to synechia uteri. Eur J Obstet Gynecol Reprod Biol 1996;65:109–113.

13. Westendorp IC, Ankum WM, Mol BW, Vonk J. Prevalence of Asherman's syndrome after secondary removal of placental remnants or a repeat curettage for incomplete abortion. Hum Reprod 1998;13:3347–3350.

14. Ferenczy A, Bertrand G, Gelfand MM. Proliferation kinetics of human endometrium during the normal menstrual cycle. Am J Obstet Gynecol 1979;133:859–867.

15. March CM, Israel R. Intrauterine adhesions secondary to elective abortion. Hysteroscopic diagnosis and management. Obstet Gynecol 1976;48:422–424.

16. Friedler S, Margalioth EJ, Kafka I, Yaffe H. Incidence of post-abortion intra-uterine adhesions evaluated by hysteroscopy – a prospective study. Hum Reprod 1993;8:442–444.

17. Shaffer W. Role of uterine adhesions in the cause of multiple pregnancy losses. Clin Obstet Gynecol 1986;29:912–924.

18. Rabau E, David A. Intrauterine adhesions: Etiology, prevention, and treatment. Obstet Gynecol 1963;22:626–629.

19. Stillman RJ, Asarkof N. Association between mullerian duct malformations and Asherman syndrome in infertile women. Obstet Gynecol 1985;65:673–677.

20. Klein SM, Garcia CR. Asherman's syndrome: a critique and current review. Fertil Steril 1973;24:722–735.

21. Sugimoto O. Diagnostic and therapeutic hysteroscopy for traumatic intrauterine adhesions. Am J Obstet Gynecol 1978;131:539–547.

22. Letterie GS, Haggerty MF. Magnetic resonance imaging of intrauterine synechiae. Gynecol Obstet Invest 1994;37:66–68.

23. Friedman A, DeFazio J, DeCherney A. Severe obstetric complications after aggressive treatment of Asherman syndrome. Obstet Gynecol 1986;67:864–867.

24. Deaton JL, Maier D, Andreoli J Jr. Spontaneous uterine rupture during pregnancy after treatment of Asherman's syndrome. Am J Obstet Gynecol 1989;160:1053–1054.

25. Dmowski WP, Greenblatt RB. Asherman's syndrome and risk of placenta accreta. Obstet Gynecol 1969;34:288–299.

26. Jewelewicz R, Khalaf S, Neuwirth RS, Vande Wiele RL. Obstetric complications after treatment of intrauterine synechiae (Asherman's syndrome). Obstet Gynecol 1976;47:701–705.

27. Georgakopoulos P. Placenta accreta following lysis of uterine synechiae (Asherman's Syndrome). J Obstet Gynaecol Br Commonw 1974;81:730–733.

28.   Valle RF, Sciarra JJ. Intrauterine adhesions: hysteroscopic diagnosis, classification, treatment, and reproductive outcome. Am J Obstet Gynecol 1988;158:1459–1470.

29.   Nasr AL, Al-Inany HG, Thabet SM, Aboulghar M. A clinicohysteroscopic scoring system of intrauterine adhesions. Gynecol Obstet Invest 2000;50:178–181.

30.   The American Fertility Society. The American Fertility Society classifications of adnexal adhesions, distal tubal occlusion, tubal occlusion secondary to tubal ligation, tubal pregnancies, mullerian anomalies and intrauterine adhesions. Fertil Steril 1988;49:944–955.

31.   Confino E, Friberg J, Giglia RV, Gleicher N. Sonographic imaging of intrauterine adhesions. Obstet Gynecol 1985;66:596–598.

32.   Fedele L, Bianchi S, Dorta M, Vignali M. Intrauterine adhesions: detection with transvaginal US. Radiology 1996;199:757–759.

33.   Schlaff WD, Hurst BS. Preoperative sonographic measurement of endometrial pattern predicts outcome of surgical repair in patients with severe Asherman's syndrome. Fertil Steril 1995;63:410–413.

34.   van Roessel J, Wamsteker K, Exalto N. Sonographic investigation of the uterus during artificial uterine cavity distention. J Clin Ultrasound 1987;15:439–450.

35.   Sylvestre C, Child TJ, Tulandi T, Tan SL. A prospective study to evaluate the efficacy of two- and three-dimensional sonohysterography in women with intrauterine lesions. Fertil Steril 2003;79:1222–1225.

36.   Bacelar AC, Wilcock D, Powell M, Worthington BS. The value of MRI in the assessment of traumatic intra-uterine adhesions (Asherman's syndrome). Clin Radiol 1995;50:80–83.

37.   Dykes TA, Isler RJ, McLean AC. MR imaging of Asherman syndrome: total endometrial obliteration. J Comput Assist Tomogr 1991;15:858–860.

38.   Demas BE, Hricak H, Jaffe RB. Uterine MR imaging: effects of hormonal stimulation. Radiology 1986;159:123–126.

39.   Hamou J, Salat-Baroux J, Siegler AM. Diagnosis and treatment of intrauterine adhesions by microhysteroscopy. Fertil Steril 1983;39:321–326.

40.   March CM, Israel R, March AD. Hysteroscopic management of intrauterine adhesions. Am J Obstet Gynecol 1978;130:653–657.

41.   Levine RU, Neuwirth RS. Simultaneous laparoscopy and hysteroscopy for intrauterine adhesions. Obstet Gynecol 1973;42:441–445.

42.   McComb PF, Wagner BL. Simplified therapy for Asherman's syndrome. Fertil Steril 1997;68:1047–1050.

43.   Magos A. Hysteroscopic treatment of Asherman's syndrome. Reprod Biomed Online 2002;4 Suppl 3:46–51.

44.   Fedele L, Vercellini P, Viezzoli T, et al. Intrauterine adhesions: current diagnostic and therapeutic trends. Acta Eur Fertil 1986;17:31–37.

45.   Pabuccu R, Atay V, Orhon E, et al. Hysteroscopic treatment of intrauterine adhesions is safe and effective in the restoration of normal menstruation and fertility. Fertil Steril 1997;68:1141–1143.

46. Newton JR, MacKenzie WE, Emens MJ, Jordan JA. Division of uterine adhesions (Asherman's syndrome) with the Nd-YAG laser. Br J Obstet Gynaecol 1989;96:102–104.

47. Candiani GB, Vercellini P, Fedele L, et al. Argon laser versus microscissors for hysteroscopic incision of uterine septa. Am J Obstet Gynecol 1991;164:87–90.

48. Vercellini P, Vendola N, Colombo A, et al. Hysteroscopic metroplasty with resectoscope or microscissors for the correction of septate uterus. Surg Gynecol Obstet 1993;176:439–442.

49. Bellingham FR. Intrauterine adhesions: hysteroscopic lysis and adjunctive methods. Aust N Z J Obstet Gynaecol 1996;36:171–174.

50. Chapman R, Chapman K. The value of two stage laser treatment for severe Asherman's syndrome. Br J Obstet Gynaecol 1996;103:1256–1258.

51. Salle B, Gaucherand P, de Saint Hilaire P, Rudigoz RC. Transvaginal sonohysterographic evaluation of intrauterine adhesions. J Clin Ultrasound 1999;27:131–134.

52. Karande V, Levrant S, Hoxsey R, et al. Lysis of intrauterine adhesions using gynecoradiologic techniques. Fertil Steril 1997;68:658–662.

53. Reddy S, Rock JA. Surgical management of complete obliteration of the endometrial cavity. Fertil Steril 1997;67:172–174.

54. Sanfilippo JS, Fitzgerald MR, Badawy SZ, et al. Asherman's syndrome. A comparison of therapeutic methods. J Reprod Med 1982;27:328–330.

55. Dabirashrafi H, Mohammad K, Moghadami-Tabrizi N, et al. Is estrogen necessary after hysteroscopic incision of the uterine septum? J Am Assoc Gynecol Laparosc 1996;3:623–625.

56. March CM, Israel R. Gestational outcome following hysteroscopic lysis of adhesions. Fertil Steril 1981;36:455–459.

57. Katz Z, Ben-Arie A, Lurie S, et al. Reproductive outcome following hysteroscopic adhesiolysis in Asherman's syndrome. Int J Fertil Menopausal Stud 1996;41:462–465.

58. Caspi E, Perpinal S. Reproductive performance after treatment of intrauterine adhesion. Int J Fertil 1975;20:249–252.

59. Oelsner G, David A, Insler V, Serr DM. Outcome of pregnancy after treatment of intrauterine adhesions. Obstet Gynecol 1974;44:341–344.

10 *Congenital Absence of the Uterine Cervix*

All varieties and degrees of gynatresia may result . . . failure of canalization may be limited in extent and localized to the cervical or vaginal segments of the mullerian tracts
— *R.G. Maliphant, 1948*

Congenital cervical atresia is a rare anomaly of the mullerian tract. It is characterized by failure of canalization of the cervical tissue and may be associated with both vaginal agenesis and uterine duplication abnormalities. An initial report in 1900 by Ludwig described this abnormality and an attempt at the creation of a uterine/vaginal fistula by the use of dilators. No follow-up was given in that report. In one of the earliest detailed descriptions, Napoleao in 1931 described congenital atresia of the cervix in a woman of 37 years. In this patient, recurrent abdominal pain had been present since age 15.[1] The report described marked abdominal swelling with a normal vagina. At the time of surgery, partial cervical atresia was noted. In a second case in 1936, Mongaardin operated on a patient who had a partial atresia of the cervix. In this case a supracervical hysterectomy was performed. Isolated case reports continued to appear in the literature. In 1948, Maliphant used the expression *gynatresia* to denote the absence of a cervix in specific and any obstruction of congenital origin of menstrual flow in general.[2] Early reports of attempts to form a fistula between the uterus and vagina with a variety of techniques were unsuccessful. Reports of significant postoperative morbidity and isolated cases of mortality led to the abandonment of organ-sparing reconstruction. The general recommendation in the literature through the 1960s and 1970s was a hysterectomy for congenital absence of the cervix.[3] Added to this was a growing concern for infection. Several deaths from sepsis were reported further entrenching the opinion of the necessity for hysterectomy. These recommendations were also made at a time prior to effective assisted reproductive technologies such as in vitro fertilization, zygote intrafallopian transfer, and transmyometrial embryo transfer techniques. These technologies forced a re-evaluation of treatment options.

Management recommendations continue to vary considerably, ranging from unequivocal recommendations for hysterectomy to attempts at establishing a fistula in all patients to suggestions that management should be tailored based on the presence or absence of functional cervical stroma.[4] The objective of this chapter is to review techniques for surgical correction of congenital absence of the cervix (and if present, absence of the vagina) and the role of assisted reproductive technologies in maximizing reproductive potential.

Etiology

The development of the cervix may be viewed as a continuum from the early process of elongation to the late process of canalization. The term *atretic* refers to the complete absence of any cervical tissue and *dysgenetic* to the failure of canalization of varying amounts of cervical stroma.[5] Congenital absence of the cervix (both atretic and dysgenetic) arises from a failure of the downward-growing uterus and lower uterine segment to appropriately elongate and specialize. This fusion process is incomplete. The differentiation of the uterine cervix is a complex process involving both mesoderm and endoderm. This process involves initial thickening of the caudal aspect of the mullerian duct in proximity to the urogenital sinus.[6] Abnormalities in either elongation or canalization may lead to either complete absence (atretic) or to the development of cervical stroma but failure to canalize (dysgenetic). Perturbations in mesodermal development as the etiology are suggested by the association of uterine and vaginal malformations with congenital absence of the cervix.[7–9]

Clinical Correlates

The initial presenting symptom of congenital absence of the cervix is amenorrhea. The majority of these patients may also have complaints of cyclic abdominal pain progressing in intensity depending on both the degree of endometriosis (if present) and the presence or absence of significant hematometra. There is frequently a delay in diagnosis in these patients of months to years. Initial complaints of pain are frequently diagnosed as gastrointestinal or a prodrome to menarche and treated medically without further evaluation.

The true incidence of congenital absence of the cervix is unknown. Approximately 80 cases have been reported in the world's literature. Various classification schemes have been described depending on the degree of cervical stromal development and canalization.[10] It is associated with abnormalities in vaginal development and complete absence of the vagina in approximately half of the cases. In addition, bicornuate and septate uterine abnormalities have also been described.

Congenital absence of the cervix may be divided into two types, depending on the presence or absence of cervical stroma and the presence or absence of the vagina (Table 10-1). There is some suggestion in the literature that patients with a normal vagina and presence of cervical stroma have the best prognosis for continued patency after surgery. However, because of the broad spectrum of these abnormalities, it is recommended that a conservative approach be taken for *all* patients regardless or presence or absence of cervical stroma. Hysterectomy should be postponed until appropriate evaluation and consideration is given to creating a cervical fistula. Careful

Table 10-1. Classification of Congenital Absence of Cervix	
Type I:	Normal uterus; normal vagina
Type IA:	Cervical stroma absent (atresia)
Type IB:	Noncanalized cervical stroma present (dysgenetic)
Type II:	Normal uterus; absent vagina
Type IIA:	Cervical stroma absent (atresia)
Type IIB:	Noncanalized cervical stroma present (dysgenetic)

counseling of the patient and family regarding surgical outcomes and reproductive options is absolutely essential. Previous recommendations for hysterectomy have been largely on the grounds of the need for repeated operations to maintain patency, the high failure rate, and the unlikely occurrence of pregnancy.[11,12] Assisted reproductive technologies have completely changed these circumstances with the availability of both gamete and zygote intrafallopian tube transfers and transmyometrial embryo transfers well described as successful techniques.[13-17] For patients requiring a hysterectomy as the only treatment, gestational surrogacy is an option to achieve reproductive potential as ovarian function is usually normal.

Differentiation between congenital absence of the cervix and high transverse vaginal septum in a patient presenting with cyclic abdominal pain caused by outlet obstruction is essential.[18,19] Management has changed dramatically since early recommendations for hysterectomy.[3,11] Congenital absence of the cervix in the presence of a functioning uterus may be approached conservatively. If the cervix is absent, consideration may be given to creation of a cervical–vaginal fistula.[20,21] A variety of techniques have been described for this purpose to connect the lower uterine cavity and upper vagina.[22] The assisted reproductive technologies has led to a more conservative and organ-sparing approach. Several case reports have described pregnancies after zygote intrafallopian transfer (ZIFT), making a compelling case for conservative management of congenital absence of the cervix.[15-17,20]

Diagnosis

Reports describing congenital cervical atresia emphasize the extreme difficulty in diagnosis. The typical clinical description involves a delay in diagnosis of 1 to 4 years from the onset of symptoms to diagnosis.[23] Differential diagnosis includes a high transverse vaginal septum and cervical atresia when the vagina is present. When the vagina is absent differential diagnosis includes vaginal agenesis, transverse vaginal septum, testicular feminization and congenital absence of the cervix. Delineation of pelvic anatomy is essential. In this setting, physical examination may be difficult at best and emotionally and physically traumatic at worst. In circumstances where a pelvic examination is difficult or potentially traumatic, the clinical exam should be postponed. Diagnosis should rely on imaging – transabdominal ultrasound or MRI. In any patient with amenorrhea and a blind vaginal vault, pelvic ultrasound examination should be the first study performed.[24-26] Transabdominal and, if possible, transvaginal ultrasound examination should be considered. The goal of ultrasound imaging is to evaluate the uterus and endometrial cavities, to rule out a hematometrium and secondarily assess the cervix and ovaries. The presence of normal pelvic anatomy should suggest either a transverse vaginal septum or absent cervix. Further refinement of the lower uterine segment and cervix may be obtained with magnetic resonance imaging. MRI has the added advantage of a more sensitive evaluation of the uterus to rule out any duplications and to assess for the presence or absence of ovarian endometriomas. Magnetic resonance imaging is a second technique that is a noninvasive means of diagnosing absence of the cervix and of planning surgery more precisely (Figure 10-1).[79] In select circumstances, micro-hydrovaginoscopy has been useful in evaluating young adolescents and virginal adults in whom clinical examination is impossible or difficult

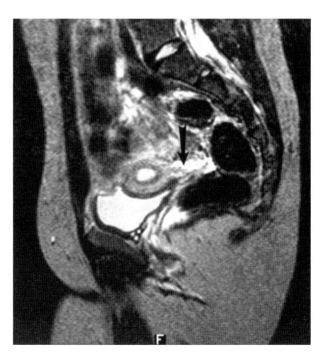

Figure 10-1   Congenital absence of the cervix. Sagittal T2-weighted magnetic resonance imaging demonstrating an absence of signals in the region of the cervix (arrow) at the junction of the uterus (to the left) and the vagina (immediately beneath the arrow).

and in whom imaging techniques have been equivocal.[28] Multiple surgical procedures are often required, usually first for the diagnosis and then for reconstruction. It is not unusual to have a history of an exploratory laparotomy for diagnosis at one center and subsequent referral to subspeciality care for corrective surgery.

Management

The aim of any surgery for the correction of congenital absence of the cervix in the presence of a functioning vagina should be the creation of a conduit for menstrual flow and conservation of the uterus for future pregnancies. When the vagina is absent, a staged procedure may be necessary to first create a neovagina and then a utero-vaginal fistula (Table 10-2). Hysterectomy should not be the first line of management. Recommendation for hysterectomy has been made on grounds of the possible need for reoperation, lack of cervical mucus and poor reproductive potential. Assisted reproductive technologies have changed that recommendation.

Treatments have ranged from pushing iodoform packs bluntly through the solid cervical remnant from the uterus into the vagina to the creation of a fistulous tract using a variety of stents. Every effort should be made to avoid hysterectomy and conserve reproductive potential. A uterovaginal fistula may be created in one- or two-stage procedures, depending on the length of the vagina (Figure 10-2). In circumstances in which the vagina is either absent or minimally developed, a neovagina should be formed by techniques

Table 10-2.
Treatment of Congenital Absence of Cervix
Surgical Options

• Laparotomy, hysterotomy, and uterovaginal anastomosis
  o Rubber stent
  o Graft with full thickness skin or bladder mucosa
• Stent placement under fluoroscopic guidance
• Laparoscopic-assisted full thickness skin graft
• Hysterectomy

ART Options
• IVF with transcervical embryo transfer if fistulous tract adequate • ZIFT/GIFT • Transmyometrial embryo transfer • Gestational surrogacy

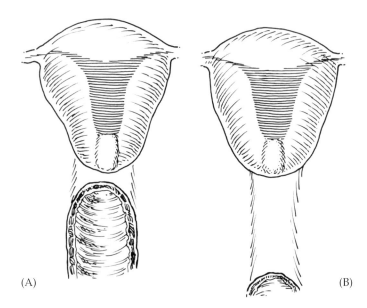

Figure 10-2   Congenital absence of the cervix in a patient with complete vaginal development (A) and in a patient with vaginal agenesis (B). Depending on the extent of vaginal development, creation of a neovagina may be necessary before attempts at forming a uterine vaginal fistula.

described for the management of vaginal agenesis. In circumstances in which there is adequate vaginal depth or after formation of a neovagina, a uterovaginal fistula may be formed with a variety of catheters and stents.[16,20] The advantage of a skin graft surrounding the stent has been suggested in several one reports.[21]

Operative Technique

In cases where there is a normal vagina, the procedure should be started with a combined vaginal and abdominal approach. A transverse incision should be made into the superior aspect of the vagina at which point a rudimentary cervix or remnant may be identified. The remnant may be of varying diameters and lengths. In rare circumstances, there may be sufficient cervix to attempt reconstruction. In this setting, failure to canalize is the appropriate diagnosis. After excision, or if no cervix is identified the space should be developed digitally to the lower uterine segment, and a Hegar dilator inserted into the space. A laparotomy is then performed. A vertical hysterotomy is made into the anterior wall of the uterus. The Hegar dilator in the vagina may be used to exert gentle upward pressure and facilitate downward dissection (Figure 10-3). The vaginal dilator is useful to define the upper limit of the vagina. The tissue and distance between the lower-most segment of the uterus and the upper-most segment of the vagina, may then be delineated. A tract is dissected between these two structures, dissecting

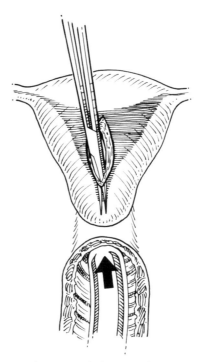

Figure 10-3   Correction of congenital absence of the cervix. Using a Hegar dilator (arrow) and gentle upward pressure at the apex of the vagina, the dissection superiorly may be carried out sharply through a hysterotomy incision. The dissection should be taken through the interval of tissue between the apex of the vagina and the inferior-most portion of the uterine cavity. A stent should then be sutured in place through the dissected tract, drawn through the vagina into the uterus.

from within the endometrial cavity downward. Tissues may vary from fibrous to a thickened cord suggestive of a rudimentary, noncanalized cervix. A polyethylene stent or tube may then be placed in the uterine body and tract and drawn into the vagina. A variety of appliances have been described for use as a stent including pediatric Foley catheters and feeding tubes, to specially designed stents. Split thickness skin grafts have also been used. The goal is to assure patency during healing, and granulation. The stent should be secured with a series of absorbable sutures to the endometrial cavity. The hysterotomy incision is then closed in two or three layers. Closure of the vagina mucosa in proximity to the stent may then be accomplished.

In addition to transabdominal approaches with hysterotomy, variations have been described. Placement of a series of guide wires under fluoroscopic guidance using a C-arm fluoroscope as a less invasive, more precise technique has been described. Laparoscopic management of congenital absence of the cervix has also been described with recanalization successfully performed.[29–32] However, the mainstay for management continues to be a combined vaginal and abdominal approach.

Extreme care must be directed toward appropriate antibiotic coverage and postoperative monitoring for any signs of infection. Two deaths have been reported secondary to postoperative sepsis. In each of these cases, patients underwent a combined simultaneous construction of a neovagina and cervical canalization procedures. Appropriate intraoperative antibiotic coverage with broad-spectrum antibiotics and postoperative monitoring are recommended. The duration for maintaining the stent in place has ranged from 1 week to 4 months in the literature. Two weeks should be adequate.

Assisted Reproductive Technologies

Given clinical awareness, sensitive imaging techniques and conservative surgical options, hysterectomy is no longer first-line management. A variety of surgical techniques to preserve uterine function make pregnancy a distinct possibility through assisted reproductive technologies. Though the likelihood of spontaneous conception is low (two cases have been reported), assisted reproductive technologies have been successful in, and hold the best prospect for, achieving live births.[33] In vitro fertilization with either transmyometrial embryo transfer, gamete intrafallopian tube transfer or zygote intrafallopian tube transfer have been described resulting in live births. In one case, transmyometrial embryo transfer was performed after in vitro fertilization in a patient in whom no surgical correction of the cervical atresia had been attempted. In this case, reconstruction of the lower uterine segment and fistulization to the vagina was accomplished using an amniotic membrane graft at the time of cesarean section.

Evaluation Prior to ART

Patients in which reconstruction of cervical and/or vaginal has been successful are candidates for ART (Table 10-3). In any patient anticipating in vitro fertilization, an attempt should be made to cannulate the reconstructed

---

Table 10-3.
Evaluation Prior to ART: Congenital Absence of the Cervix

- Vaginal assessment if there is a history of vaginal agenesis and creation of a neovagina

- Technique of embryo transfer: Trial embryo transfer for passage of catheter through the fistulous tract. Though this is unlikely to be possible, this option should be considered

- Consideration of transmyometrial embryo transfer or tubal embryo transfer (TET)/zygote intrafallopian transfer (ZIFT) if fistula is stenotic

- Prior to TET/ZIFT: Laparoscopic assessment of pelvic and tubal anatomy to guarantee access to distal tubal segments (hysterosalpingography is usually not possible)

- Evaluation for pelvic anatomy prior to in vitro fertilization and laparoscopic transfer

---

cervix with an embryo transfer catheter. Previous surgical correction for the congenital absence of the cervix should not automatically be assumed to preclude transcervical and conventional embryo transfer. If the trial or mock embryo transfer is successful with catheter placement into the endometrial cavity, a provision should be made for simultaneous sonohysterography for evaluation of the endometrial cavity. At the time of the trial transfer, transvaginal ultrasound examination should be undertaken to assure adequate imaging of the ovaries transvaginally and accessibility for transvaginal oocyte retrieval.

In the more common circumstances in which it is impossible to pass a catheter conventionally, study of pelvic anatomy is essential by laparoscopy. Laparoscopy is required to assess the accessibility of the tubes and ease of passage of the tubal catheter for gamete intrafallopian tubal transfer. Laparoscopy and chromotubation should be performed by transmyometrial injection of either indigo carmine or methylene blue to assure proximal patency. Chromotubation is particularly relevant as this approach may be the only opportunity to verify unimpeded flow through both proximal and fimbriated ends of the tube. Care should be taken to assess the lower uterine segment during laparoscopy. A detailed description of this should be included in the operative note. Reference to this detail may be made by maternal-fetal specialists should a transabdominal cerclage by considered.

Outcomes Analysis

Normal menstrual function is the goal following creation of cervical–vaginal fistula. Spontaneous pregnancies have been reported after vaginoplasty and cervical stenting for partial cervical atresia. In addition, successful pregnancies have been described through assisted reproductive technologies. However, congenital absence of the cervix is a clinically complex condition with a high likelihood of failure. The reobstruction rate is high, requiring reoperation, and the risk–benefit ratio must be carefully considered and discussed with the patient and family. Repeated attempts to form a fistula usually fail, and total hysterectomy with ovarian conservation becomes the procedure of choice.[22] In this circumstance, gestational surrogacy provides the opportunity to fulfill reproductive potential.

Summary and Recommendations

Literature describing the diagnosis and management of congenital absence of the cervix is primarily in the form of case reports. Recommendation in this circumstance had previously been hysterectomy as the only option. The availability of assisted reproductive technologies has changed this recommendation. Every attempt should be made to preserve reproductive potential. This suggestion is not to imply that reproductive potential takes precedence over well-being. Accumulated case reports and surgical experience suggest a conservative approach is feasible and appropriate first line managment. On the basis of case reports in the literature and the trend in reproductive technologies, the following recommendations may be made:

- In any patient suspected of having congenital absence of the cervix, consideration should be given to both pelvic ultrasound examination to define pelvic anatomy and to magnetic resonance imaging to make a deliberate search for the presence or absence of the cervix.
- Preoperative planning is of the utmost importance. Preoperative diagnosis is essential to adequately counsel the patient and family regarding options for management.
- A fistulous tract may be created between the uterine cavity and the vagina by using a variety of stents. Stents have ranged from simple pediatric Foley catheters to specially constructed and designed hardware.
- In rare circumstances, congenital absence of the cervix may also be accompanied by congenital absence of the vagina. In this circumstance, a two-stage procedure may be necessary, first, to form a neovagina, and second, to create a fistulous tract between the normal uterine corpus and the neovagina. In this circumstance, suppression with gonadotropin-releasing hormone (GnRH) analogs throughout the treatment may be advisable.
- Adequate preoperative counseling regarding spontaneous closure of the fistulous tract and the possibility of need for reoperation is essential.
- Aggressive postoperative antibiotic use and monitoring is essential.
- Reproductive potential has been achieved through spontaneous conception GIFT and ZIFT in circumstances in which the creation of a fistulous tract has been successful. Placement of a cervicoisthmic cerclage may be advisable in individual cases when pregnancy occurs. In circumstances in which reobstruction necessitates hysterectomy, reproductive potential may be achieved through gestational surrogacy.
- Spontaneous pregnancies have been reported. Patients undergoing successful surgery should be counseled regarding contraceptive needs if immediate pregnancy is not planned.

References

1. McIndoe, A. Treatment at congenital absence and obliterative conditions of the vagina. Br J Plast Surg 1950;2:254–260.

2. Sherwood M, Speed T. Congenital atresia of the cervix. Tex J Med 1941;37:215–219.

3. Rock JA, Schlaff WD, Zacur HA, Jones HW. Clinical management of congenital absence of the uterine cervix. Int J Gynaecol Obstet 1984;22:231–235.

4. Zarou GS, Acken HS, Brevetti RC. Surgical management of congenital atresia of the cervix. Case report and review of the literature. Am J Obstet Gynecol 1961;82:923–928.

5. Lee CL, Jain S, Wang CJ, et al. Classification for endoscopic treatment of mullerian anomalies with an obstructive cervix. J Am Assoc Gynecol Laparosc 2001;8:402–408.

6. Ulfelder H, Robboy SJ. The embryologic development of the human vagina. Am J Obstet Gynecol 1976;126:769–776.

7. Monks P. Uterus didelphys associated with unilateral cervical atresia and renal agenesis. Aust NZ J Obstet Gynaecol 1979;19:245–246.

8. Bakri YN, al-Sugair A, Hugosson C. Bicornuate nonfused rudimentary uterine horns with functioning endometria and complete cervical-vaginal agenesis: magnetic resonance diagnosis. Fertil Steril 1992;58:620–621.

9. Yang CC, Tseng JY, Chen P, Wang PH. Uterus didelphys with cervical agenesis associated with adenomyosis, a leiomyoma and ovarian endometriosis. A case report. J Reprod Med 2002;47:936–938.

10. Fujimoto VY, Miller JH, Klein NA, Soules MR. Congenital cervical atresia: report of seven cases and review of the literature. Am J Obstet Gynecol 1997;177:1419–1425.

11. Rotter CW. Surgical correction of congenital atresia of the cervix. Am J Obstet Gynecol 1958;76:643–646.

12. Jacob JH, Griffin WT. Surgical reconstruction of the congenitally atretic cervix: two cases. Obstet Gynecol Surv 1989;44:556–569.

13. Anttila L, Penttila TA, Suikkari AM. Successful pregnancy after in-vitro fertilization and transmyometrial embryo transfer in a patient with congenital atresia of cervix: case report. Hum Reprod 1999;14:1647–1649.

14. Lai TH, Wu MH, Hung KH, et al. Successful pregnancy by transmyometrial and transtubal embryo transfer after IVF in a patient with congenital cervical atresia who underwent uterovaginal canalization during Cesarean section: case report. Hum Reprod 2001;16:268–271.

15. Thijssen RF, Hollanders JM, Willemsen WN, et al. Successful pregnancy after ZIFT in a patient with congenital cervical atresia. Obstet Gynecol 1990;76:902–904.

16. Fraser IS. Successful pregnancy in a patient with congenital partial cervical atresia. Obstet Gynecol 1989;74:443–455.

17. Zarou GS, Esposito JM, Zarou DM. Pregnancy following the surgical correction of congenital atresia of the cervix. Int J Gynecol Obstet 1973;11:143.

18. Dillon WP, Mudaliar NA, Wingate MB. Congenital atresia of the cervix. Obstet Gynecol 1979;54:126–129.

19. Scott JR, Galask R, Yannone ME. Congenital atresia of the uterine cervix. Int J Gynecol Obstet 1971;9:249–252.

20.   Hampton HL, Meeks GR, Bates GW, Wiser WL. Pregnancy after successful vaginoplasty and cervical stenting for partial atresia of the cervix. Obstet Gynecol 1990;76:900–901.

21.   Bates GW, Wiser WL. A technique for uterine conservation in adolescents with vaginal agenesis and a functional uterus. Obstet Gynecol 1985;66:290–294.

22.   Cukier J, Batzofin JH, Conner JS, Franklin RR. Genital tract reconstruction in a patient with congenital absence of the vagina and hypoplasia of the cervix. Obstet Gynecol 1986;68(3 Suppl):32S–36S.

23.   Farber M, Marchant DJ. Congenital absence of the uterine cervix. Am J Obstet Gynecol 1975;121:414–417.

24.   Valdes C, Malini S, Malinak LR. Sonography in the surgical management of vaginal and cervical atresia. Fertil Steril 1983;40:263–265.

25.   Markhan SM, Parmley TH, Murphy AA, et al. Cervical agenesis combined with vaginal agenesis diagnosed by magnetic resonance imaging. Fertil Steril 1987;48:143–145.

26.   Letterie GS. Combined congenital absence of the vagina and cervix. Diagnosis with magnetic resonance imaging and surgical management. Gynecol Obstet Invest 1998;46:65–67.

27.   Reinhold C, Hricak H, Forstner R, et al. Primary amenorrhea: evaluation with MR imaging. Radiology 1997;203:383–390.

28.   Parker JD, Hibbert ML, Dainty LD, et al. Micro-hydrovaginoscopy in examining children. Obstet Gynecol 2000;96:772–774.

29.   Deffarges JV, Haddad B, Musset R, Paniel BJ. Utero-vaginal anastomosis in women with uterine cervix atresia: long-term follow-up and reproductive performance. A study of 18 cases. Hum Reprod 2001;16:1722–1725.

30.   Hovsepian DM, Auyeung A, Ratts VS. A combined surgical and radiologic technique for creating a functional neo-endocervical canal in a case of partial congenital cervical atresia. Fertil Steril 1999;71:158–162.

31.   Rock JA, Carpenter SE, Wheeless CR, Jones HW Jr. The clinical management of maldevelopment of the uterine cervix. J Pelv Surg 1995;1:129–133.

32.   Bugmann P, Amaudruz M, Hanquinet S, et al. Uterocervicoplasty with a bladder mucosa layer for the treatment of complete cervical agenesis. Fertil Steril 2002;77:831–835.

33.   Pilkington JW. Pregnancy and spontaneous delivery following operation for congenital atresia of the vagina. Am J Obstet Gynecol 1959;78:804–805.

11 *Cervical Stenosis and Techniques of Embryo Transfer*

The best way of studying the phenomenon of their movements is to take a drop of mucus from the canal of a perfectly normal cervix uteri some 15 or 20 hours after intercourse. . .
— Marion Sims, 1866

Introduction

Since the initial description of postcoital testing and suggestion that cervical mucus was essential to sperm migration, cervical anatomy and function has been a focus of infertility evaluations. Early descriptions characterized the cervix as a mere conduit for the movement of sperm and seminal plasma. Later studies suggested a complex interaction of sperm and mucus with fertility predicated on the quality of this interaction.[1] Postcoital testing evolved into an integral step in the early literature describing infertility evaluation and treatment. With the advent of evidence-based medicine and assisted reproductive technologies, emphasis has changed. The importance of cervical anatomy has come full circle. Assessment of cervical function by examining the interaction of cervical mucus and sperm as described by Sims and Huhner is no longer a core test. Though a subset of patients may benefit from this test, contemporary infertility evaluations focus instead on cervical anatomy and its impact on ease of passage of a variety of catheters. Easy, atraumatic access to the endometrial cavity transcervically for either intrauterine insemination or embryo transfer has emerged as the significant issue. Multiple factors may impact the process and ultimately the success of assisted reproductive technologies.[2]

The goal of any embryo transfer is to place precisely, and atraumatically, embryos within the endometrial cavity in the area with the greatest receptivity and the highest likelihood of implantation without causing any uterine contractions (Figure 11-1 A and B).[3] Careful atraumatic passage of the catheter is the goal. The ease or difficulty of transcervical embryo transfer has come under increasingly tighter focus as the impact of the transfer on outcome has become clearer. Though isolated reports to the contrary exist, difficult embryo transfers adversely affect outcomes.[4] In those reports suggesting no impact of transfer difficulty on success, techniques of transfer for all groups studied were less than ideal possibly impacting even the successful groups.[5,6] A threefold

(A)

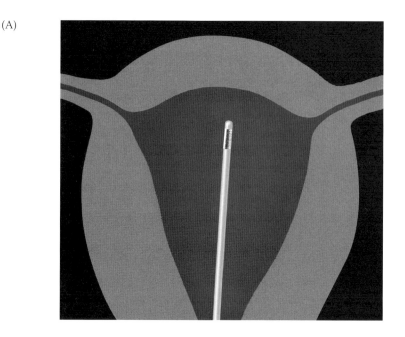

(B)

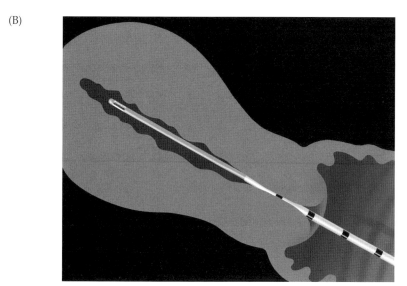

Figure 11-1   A and B: Coronal (A) and longitudinal (B) representation of transcervi-
                cal catheter placement.

difference in pregnancy rates exists between embryo transfers that are difficult
versus those that are uncomplicated. Difficult embryo transfers are associated
with damage to the endometrium and uterine contractions, both factors that
impact implantation and lower pregnancy rates. The intuition that the less
trauma to the endometrium and more precise, careful handling of the embryos
results in better outcomes is well established in clinical care.[7,8]

The technique of embryo transfer has remained relatively unchanged since the initial description by Edwards 30 years ago.[9] At the inception of IVF, embryo transfers were performed with a curved metal cannula with an inner diameter of 1.7 mm and an olive tip 3 mm in diameter. This system was passed through the endocervical canal and internal os with varying degrees of ease and difficulty.[10,11] A nylon inner sheath loaded with the embryos was then passed through the metal cannula to the uterine fundus using only tactile feedback for placement. The mere size and rigidity of the system usually resulted in some degree of cramping and bleeding. The nylon of the inner sheath posed a separate issue of embryotoxicity. Unlike the evolution of laboratory techniques and culture media that has been characterized by manifold improvements, no modifications had been introduced in the technique and materials for embryo transfer for two decades. However, over the past five years, increasing emphasis has been placed on the technique of and hardware for embryo transfer. Improved catheter types and ultrasound guidance have emerged as influential variables to achieve this goal. The objective of this chapter is to discuss the techniques of embryo transfer, variables that impact the outcome, and options to improve the ease of transfer in the presence of cervical stenosis or irregular endocervical canals that pose difficulties for embryo transfers.

Etiology

Few topics are more provocative in IVF than factors impacting pregnancy rates.[12,13] Multiple variables are integral parts of the success rate equation (Table 11-1). Subtle variations in the clinical and laboratory techniques can dramatically influence success rates. Prominent among these crucial steps are embryo transfer techniques. The significance of embryo transfer techniques

Table 11-1.
Variables of Embryo Transfer Techniques

Technical Variables

- Embryologist and clinician interface
- Ease of catheter movement
- Catheter type
- Activity after transfer
- Catheter guidance: ultrasound vs tactile
- Cervical and vaginal bacteriologic environment
- Catheter contamination

Performance Variables

- Clinician skill level
- Comparative performance among clinicians

as a variable with a defining impact on the success of the IVF cycle has only recently been appreciated. Once felt to be a simple task of relocating embryos from culture media to endometrial cavity, the process has emerged as a make-or-break process.

Various factors impact the likelihood of success. The governing paradigm for embryo transfer should be gentle, atraumatic handling of the embryos with every consideration given to a transfer from laboratory to the uterus with or without the absolute minimum of trauma to both the embryos and the endometrium. There are multiple factors that distinguish a successful embryo transfer from an unsuccessful or difficult transfer. Though interdependent, these factors may be divided into three categories: cervical anatomy, technical variables, and performance variables. These factors should be assessed and controlled as much as possible prior to the actual transfer.[14]

Cervical Anatomy as a Variable

Embryo transfer is a blind procedure. The catheter is passed through the endocervical canal with either ultrasound visualization or tactile feedback. There are no definitive techniques to determine whether the embryos have been successfully transferred intact from catheter to endometrial cavity, where in the cavity they were transferred or whether they remained in the intended area after transfer. After the embryos are loaded into the transfer catheter, no direct observation of their fate occurs. What happens on the course through the endocervical canal to final site within the endometrial cavity is speculative. It is clear however that cervical anatomy has the potential to impact the success or failure of the transfer. The catheter tip may be observed and examined after the transfer for retained embryos or contamination with blood or mucus but the embryos remain hidden, hopefully, within the cavity. The cervical factors that contribute to difficult embryo transfers include cervical stenosis, an irregularly shaped or convoluted endocervical canal, and extreme angulations between the lower uterine segment and the endocervical canal. Cervical stenosis though rare may result from an aggressive cone biopsy, trauma, cryosurgery, or a LEEP procedure. In these circumstances, easy passage of a catheter through the cervix into the endometrial cavity may be difficult or impossible and require an alternate access to the cavity, either transmyometrial or transtubal. In some circumstances, pretreatment with laminarial tents 2 months before the actual transfer or surgical correction may be required to achieve the goal of an easy (see below), transfer.

Technical Variables

Embryo transfer has traditionally been viewed simplistically (Table 11-2). Fertilization and growth of the embryos was the major goal and the simple task of transfer was viewed as an afterthought. The contemporary paradigm

---

Steps

**Table 11-2.
Essential Techniques of Successful Embryo Transfer**

- Identification of complex cervical anatomy prior to actual transfer

- Transabdominal ultrasound guidance

- Bladder filling to reduce/eliminate any angle between endometrial cavity, lower uterine segment, and cervical canal

- Soft-tipped, flexible coaxial catheter systems

- Passage of both inner and outer catheters either together or separately under ultrasound guidance

- Absolute atraumatic, gentle forward movement of the inner soft catheter into the endometrial cavity

- Transfer 1.5 to 2.0 cm from fundus

- Gentle slow withdrawal of catheter after transfer

---

and guiding principles are that the transfer is an extension of the culture conditions and embryo handling in the laboratory. This approach demands the care and craft that characterize all high-quality laboratory techniques in handling the embryos. This handling should be as precise and delicate as that governing their handling in the lab. Seven variables relating to the technique of embryo transfer and their effect on success are discussed.

The Interface Between the Embryologist and Clinician

Loading the catheter by the embryologist and passage to the clinician requires a coordinated team effort. Considerable cooperation between the embryology team and the clinical staff is necessary for successful embryo transfer. A set protocol that affords predictable movements from lab to catheter to uterus is essential. Three variables that may impact this process are volume of media in loading the catheter, the fluid–air interface and expulsion of the embryos. An adequate volume of culture media is essential to facilitate transfer of the embryos. An air–media–air interface localizes the embryos after transfer on ultrasound imaging. There is a suggestion that a reduction in the amount of air and total transfer volume to 20–40 μL may improve pregnancy rates.[15] Transfer volumes between 50 and 70 μL and a large air interface have been associated with lower pregnancy rates, possibly because of movement of the embryos into the lower uterine segment.[16] After the placement of the catheter through the cervix, *gentle* thumb pressure on the syringe plunger sustained after transfer is essential in expelling the embryos to minimize trauma to the embryos and their migration from the intended site of placement. Overly aggressive pressure may result in rupture of the blastomeres as the embryos move away from the catheter to the transfer site. Though retained embryos may be a function of this interaction (how the embryos were loaded, suspended and expelled, how the cervix was

How a cx was prepared and the catheter passed, and the amount of pressure used to expel the embryos), retained embryos do not negatively impact outcome.

Ease of Catheter Movement

Most studies demonstrate a relationship between ease of catheter passage and pregnancy rates.[17–19] The catheter should pass unimpeded through the cervix into the endometrial cavity. Difficulty or resistance especially of sufficient intensity to bend the catheter back against itself should be avoided. In one study a three times higher pregnancy rate was associated with an easy transfer than a difficult one. The presence of blood or mucus on the catheter tip does not appear to negatively impact success rates. However, the point is debatable, aggressive intervention at the time of transfer does. Need for tenaculum application to the cervix or repeated attempts at catheter passage negatively impact pregnancy rates. The use of a tenaculum may cause junctional contractions that impact the likelihood of implantation or serve as an identifier of a transfer that is intrinsically difficult and hence associated with lower pregnancy rates.[20]

Catheter Type

In 1981, the Tomcat catheter was introduced for embryo transfer.[21] This system had gained popularity in animal studies and was successfully used in the transfer of goat embryos. Its design and simplicity made it easily adaptable to embryo transfer in humans. The catheter was a significant advance over the nylon catheter and stainless steel system in use until that time.[22] Catheters have improved considerably since the initial descriptions of the rigid Tomcat catheter. Though still used successfully by some centers, there has been a trend toward soft, atraumatic, coaxial systems. Progressive improvement in the design, quality, and consistency of the catheters has characterized the current generation of catheters.[23,24] Single catheters and coaxial systems are available. Catheter systems are made from polyethylene or polyurethane with various lengths and diameters ranging from 12 to 23 cm in length. Narrow inner diameters (range 0.022 to 0.19 inches) enable a reduced volume of culture media for the transfer. Various obturators may be inserted into the outer sheath and may be adapted to form any angle to suit the cervical and uterine anatomy. In addition to soft coaxial systems, echogenic tips are now available to enhance identification with ultrasound guidance.[25] An advantage in soft catheters over a more conventional rigid Tomcat catheter is a reduction in endometrial damage. In one study evaluating the impact of catheter type on disruption of the endometrium, 50% of women with a rigid catheter versus 13% with a soft catheter were found to have endometrial disruption.[26,27] Soft, flexible catheters in a coaxial system have the intrinsic value of minimal endometrial disruption during passage through the internal cervical os into the lower uterine segment.[28]

Despite improved design and a trend toward softer, atraumatic catheters, and more precise placement, it is controversial whether any consistent improvement in pregnancy rates occurs when one system is compared with another.[29] Although soft-tipped catheters result in less endometrial disruption, it is open to question whether or not they enhance pregnancy rates. This debate may be related to study design and patient selection criteria and the multitude of variables that impact the outcome of an IVF cycle. There are no clear-cut benefits of one soft-catheter system over another in several comparative studies.[2,27,30] However, improvement in pregnancy rates was noted in one clinic changing from a Tomcat to a soft-tipped Wallace catheter.[23,31] In addition to this, there was less contamination with blood, mucus, and fewer retained embryos in using a soft-tipped catheter. The guiding principle should be to use a catheter that works well for an IVF team and yields consistently excellent outcomes. When multiple catheter systems are used, pregnancy rates should be compared for any variation between catheters to prevent any drift for a given type.

Activity After Transfer

At the inception of IVF, rigid rules dictated hospitalization and strict bed rest after the embryo transfer for at least 24 hours. Variations have evolved in clinical practice influenced more by tradition than clinical study. Little data support strict bed rest requirements. The rationale for this reduced activity was to maximize the likelihood that the embryos would remain stationary and not move from the site of transfer.[32] Clinical observations and data from a model suggest little movement occurs regardless of activity.[33] Standing and activity are unlikely to result in movement of the embryo(s) from the area of transfer. In a model using an air bubble as an embryo surrogate to study movement after trial embryo transfers, no movement of an air bubble upon standing was noted.[34] Even when it did move (6% of the subjects) it moved less than 5 mm. When extreme, (2% of the subjects), movement was 4 cm and the bubble still remained in the uterine cavity. The clinical correlate to these observations is that standing and activity are unlikely to result in movement of the embryo(s) from the area of transfer. Gravity is also unlikely to impact the position of the embryos within the cavity. The endometrial cavity is a potential space with two apposing surfaces, not a true cavity. Large volumes of media (greater than 60 µl) may result in downward migration of the embryos. A gradual transition to shorter and shorter observation intervals after a transfer is the trend in clinical practice without a negative impact on pregnancy rates. In one trial, immediate activity versus bed rest resulted in no difference in pregnancy rates.[35] Overall broad practice patterns exist ranging from complete bed rest to normal daily activities and depend on the preferences of individual practice. A steady decline in the time that patients remain supine appears to be the trend.

Catheter Guidance: Ultrasound vs Tactile

Accurate and atraumatic placement of the embryos are the goals of the transfer. Ultrasound as a guide in embryo transfer to fulfill these goals was initially suggested in 1985.[36] Ultrasound guidance provides an objective

objective method of assessing the exact position of the catheter as it passes into the cavity and final position within the endometrial cavity.[37] Two goals are facilitated with ultrasound guidance. This first observation assures that the catheter tip has not abutted against either the lateral uterine walls or the fundus and assurance that the catheter has not curled upon itself reducing the accuracy of placement and disrupting the endometrium. The second observation assures accurate positioning of the embryos in an area most likely to result in implantation. Placement is best at a distance of 1.5 to 2.0 cm from the uterine fundus when imagined in two dimensions (Figure 11-2 A and B). Ultrasound placement allows a degree of precision over a blind insertion or a "touch" technique. Ultrasound guidance also provides a means of avoiding contamination of the catheter tip against either the lateral cavity walls or the fundal region. Real-time imaging also adds a degree of patient satisfaction and enhances the confidence of a patient or couple regarding precision of placement and where the embryos are transferred. There may be a differential positive impact with ultrasound guidance for day 3 versus day 4 or 5 embryo transfers.

Ultrasound monitoring is intended to guide the movement of the catheter, avoid any impact on the endometrial lining, and cavity walls and place the embryos in a location of maximum receptivity.[38,39] Though this rationale appears self-evident, the issue has not been without controversy as not all studies clearly demonstrate an improvement in pregnancy rates. Both transvaginal and transabdominal ultrasound guidance for embryo transfer have been studied and provide clear monitoring of catheter movement.[40–44] Using transvaginal techniques in early studies, higher pregnancy rates were achieved versus a "blind" or tactile placement of the catheters; however, data are conflicting regarding definitive improvements in pregnancy rates for transabdominal guidance. A second important variable of ultrasound guidance may be in avoiding any contact with the endometrial walls. Such contact may induce contractions and impact the ultimate place of the embryos within the cavity. When carefully placed, embryos do not migrate far from the site of the placement. In a study assessing the movement of microspheres placed during a mock transfer and before hysterectomy, the microspheres were identified within 1 cm of their placement when the specimen was examined.[45] Uterine contractions as might result with abutment of a transfer catheter within the endometrial cavity are capable of dislodging the embryos. Mechanical activity of the uterus such as occurs with contractions could relocate the embryos and that activity is related to physical stimulation of the uterus. There is a connection between ease of transfer, endometrial wavelike contractions or movements, and the motility of mock embryos (30 µl of Echovist). These movements may persist for up to 45 minutes after impact of the catheter against the endometrial cavity walls. Hence, ultrasound guidance may be one technique to avoid induction of these contractions.

Precise placement of the catheter may be enhanced with three-dimensional ultrasound, placing the position of the catheter in three dimensions instead of the usual two dimensions used (Figures 11-3 and 11-4). Thus far, all

(A)

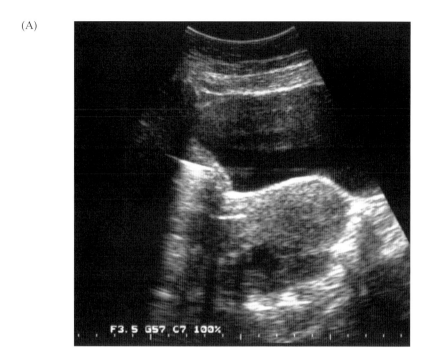

(B)

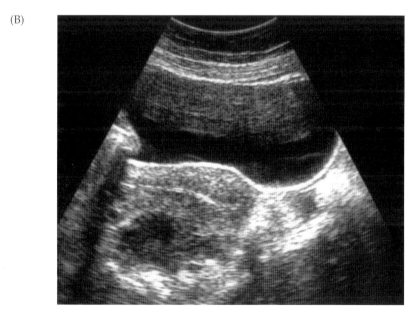

Figure 11-2   A and B: Longitudinal transabdominal ultrasound image of catheter placement at lower uterine segment (A) and final placement 2 cm from fundus of uterine cavity (B).

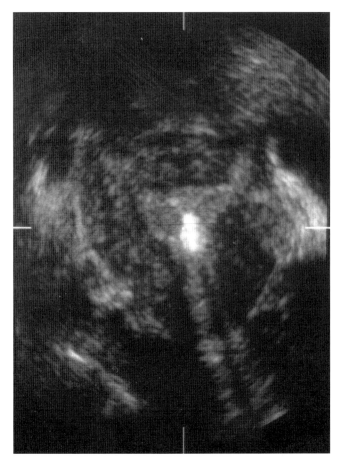

Figure 11-3   Three-dimensional coronal view of the endometrial cavity after place-
                   ment of the catheter at lower uterine segment. Note echogenic catheter
                   in the center of the cavity.

studies evaluating ultrasound guidance have used two-dimensional ultrasound, evaluating the catheter tip in relationship to the longitudinal and
coronal planes of the endometrial cavity. More precise guidance may be
obtained using three-dimensional ultrasound. In a limited series, a three-
dimensional ultrasound transvaginal probe was used as a check on catheter
placement after two-dimensional ultrasound suggested accurate placement.[46]
The three-dimensional images in some circumstances suggested that the
catheter tip was more lateral and superior than initially suspected (Figure
11-5). Further study and its impact on pregnancy rates are warranted.

In the tactile technique, the catheter is advanced into the uterine cavity until the
fundus is touched and then withdrawn 5 mm, or it is advanced to a fixed
distance of 4 to 5 cm or predetermined by uterine sound during a mock
transfer.[46] Uterine contractions negatively impact on pregnancy rates. These
contractions facilitate the dislodgement of the embryos from the implantation

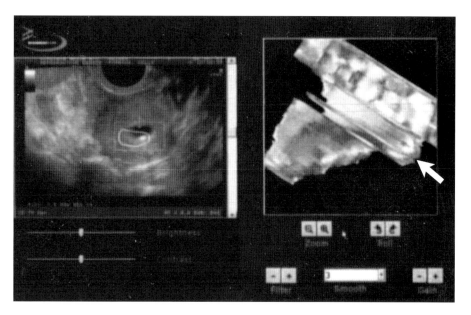

Figure 11-4   Three-dimensional ultrasound reconstruction of catheter placement through lower uterine segment into the mid-uterine cavity (arrow).

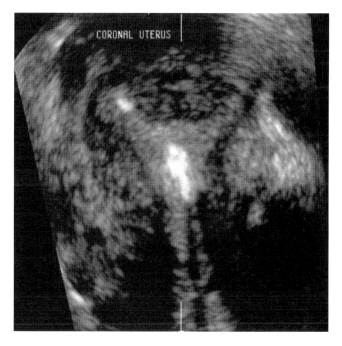

Figure 11-5   Transabdominal ultrasound image of an anteflexed uterus and partially filled bladder. Compare with Figure 11-2 in which there is zero degree angle between the cervical canal and the uterine cavity.

site. Ultrasound guidance has the theoretical advantage of avoiding the contractions associated with placement of the catheter by clinical feel. Tactile placement regardless of technique is associated with increased uterine contractions that reduce pregnancy rates and implantation rates as the contractions increase. Twenty percent of the catheters passed by clinical touch to a so-called safe, predetermined distance will abut on the fundus and 10% on the internal tubal ostia.

Cervical and Vaginal Bacteriologic Environment

Vaginal microflora, regardless of transfer technique, catheter type, or ultrasound guidance, has emerged as a significant though poorly understood variable potentially impacting the likelihood of pregnancy.[48,49] Several studies suggest that the vaginal microbiologic environment may impact the outcome of in vitro fertilization, first trimester loss, preterm delivery, and the likelihood of a live birth. Two observations are of significance. The first is that contamination of the embryo transfer catheter tip with *Streptococcus viridans* is associated with decreased clinical pregnancy rates, increased first-trimester loss rates, and ultimately a decrease in live birth rates.[49–53] The second observation is that a shift in the dominance of the vaginal flora away from *Lactobacillus* to increased concentrations of anaerobes and *Gardneralla vaginalis* (as occurs with bacterial vaginosis) is associated with decreased rates of success also.[54] Isolation of hydrogen peroxide-producing *Lactobacillus* was associated with a significantly higher live birth rate. Hydrogen peroxide-producing *Lactobacillus* dominates healthy vaginal microenvironments and the presence of this organism on a catheter tip suggests a normal vaginal flora. An altered vaginal environment as occurs in bacterial vaginosis results in dimunition in *Lactobacillus* with an increase in anaerobes, *G. vaginalis*, and genital mycoplasmas.[55] These data suggest that vaginal microflora may be an important variable in success.

The picture is further complicated by a failure to improve success rates with doxycycline therapy, suggesting a complex microbiologic environment requiring further study. These findings suggest that the cervical and vaginal environment could potentially significantly influence the success of transcervical embryo transfers. A reduction in pregnancy rates with IVF in this setting is in keeping with the picture that bacterial vaginosis is associated with increased first trimester loss rate and obstetric complications including preterm delivery.[56]

Altered vaginal concentration of bacteria is associated with an increased likelihood of isolating organisms from the catheter tip and contamination of the endometrial cavity. Bacterial contamination of the catheter tip is associated with decreased pregnancy rates. Approximately 30% of women undergoing in vitro fertilization will have bacteria recovered from the catheter tip. In these studies, significantly higher pregnancy rates were observed when the culture of the catheter tip was negative versus positive. Treatment of bacterial vaginosis with appropriate antibiotics may provide a more favorable environment.[57] The type, duration and timing of this treatment is open to question. In all previous studies evaluating embryo transfer techniques and comparing success rates, the vaginal microenvironment has been a poorly controlled variable.[58]

Catheter Contamination

Cervical mucus may be a negative factor because of two possible effects. First, the mucus may occlude the catheter tip or form a bubble in which the embryos become entrapped. Second, the mucus may contaminate the endometrial cavity. Contamination of the catheter tip and endometrial cavity by vaginal flora may adversely impact outcome. Pregnancy rates are 37 and 24% when the cultures of the catheter tip are positive or negative, respectively.[53] The likely source of the contamination is through cervical mucus (and secondarily vaginal micro-flora). A vigorous attempt to remove all cervical mucus and contamination by lavage of the endometrial canal is appropriate. The results, however, in one large comparative study were equivocal.[59] In one study, improvement of pregnancy rates by vigorous cervical lavage was demonstrated.[60] Whether the improvement in this setting was secondary to reduced bacterial contamination of the catheter tip and endometrial cavity or by reduction in the likelihood of mechanical plugging of the catheter and entrapment of the embryos is unclear. Cervical mucus may also increase the likelihood of expulsion of the embryos from the site of transfer into the lower uterine segment. Using methylene blue instillation during a trial embryo transfer, downward migration of the dye to the cervix was noted in 23% of cases when aspiration of the cervical mucus was performed and 57% of cases without aspiration.[61] These data suggest that, in this model, cervical mucus may facilitate loss of the embryos into the endocervical canal after transfer. These data may also explain the observation that 9% of patients undergoing supposedly routine, uncomplicated embryo transfers without lavage had embryos either within the cervix or on the speculum.[16] Irrigation of the cervical canal to eliminate as much mucus as possible is a simple step with the potential to positively impact pregnancy rates and should be part of the standard protocol of embryo transfer and comparitive performance among clinicians.

Performance Variables

Among the important performance variables are the clinicians' skill. The factors of retained embryos, catheter contamination, uterine contractions and catheter collision as listed in Table 11-1 have been discussed in the sections above. This section addresses the issue of clinical skill and its impact on pregnancy rates.

The technical skills among clinicians performing the transfers can impact the likelihood of success.[62,63] Embryo transfer has the potential for the greatest technical variability among clinicians of all clinical procedures in IVF. Depending on diversity among clinicians, these variations may contribute to variable success rates in the same IVF lab. Significant differences do exist between clinicians despite standardization of techniques and protocols. These performances tend to remain constant over time, suggesting that technique does in fact matter. There is also a relationship that clinicians with the lowest pregnancy rates have higher ectopic rates. It is extremely important that all participants in embryo transfers perform the embryo transfer in an identical fashion to eliminate any inter-clinician variables. Minimal inter-physician variability can be tolerated. Close tracking of the outcomes among various clinicians performing the transfers is essential. A technique that is acceptable to all participants and avoids initiation of uterine contractions will result in consistent pregnancy rates within a team. Sharing knowledge among clinicians regarding techniques and establishing a consistent, shared, one-size-fits-all protocol and technique is essential.

Standard procedures to maximize pregnancy rates mandate that all clinicians performing transfers have their pregnancy rates monitored and an internal protocol is in place for evaluating and instructing those with suboptimal pregnancy rates. When significant differences exist, patient populations should be reviewed to assure that comparable patients are within each group for individual clinicians (for example, a clinician's rate may be favorably or unfavorably influenced by the inclusion of a large number of donors or poor responders, respectively). When necessary, clinician's with lower pregnancy rates should be withdrawn (or withdraw) from the rotation temporarily. Repeat training may be necessary for the standardization of technique and improved performance. Tracking of the embryologist–clinician combination is also essential to identify if a particular team has a negative impact on outcomes. Thirty-five embryo transfers appears to be the lower limit required for basic skill acquisition in the techniques of embryo transfer.

Diagnostic Studies

Several diagnostic studies are useful in improving ease of transfer and identifying patients who require either specific and exceptional planning or who need further evaluation and intervention prior to transfer.

Physical Examination

All patients undergoing IVF and transcervical embryo transfer should have a careful speculum examination, assessment of the level of comfort that the patient has with this examination, and mock or trial embryo transfer. Specific speculum size that maximizes both patient comfort and accessibility to the cervix should be noted. If there is any suggestion that the patient is uncomfortable during the examination, a mild oral sedative should be offered. Diazepam or a similar drug prior to embryo transfer may be considered for the dual purpose of enhanced patient comfort and to reduce any uterine contractions. NSAIDs, however, are controversial in early pregnancy and may have a deleterious effect on the endometrium. Sonohysterography, hysterosalpingography, or hysteroscopy are essential studies to assess the endocervical canal and endometrial cavity. Cervical cultures may identify patients with unfavorable vaginal flora who may benefit from treatment prior to transfer. However, the exact role of cultures and the type and timing of treatment is open to discussion and requires further study for definitive guidance.

Trial or Mock Embryo Transfer

All patients should undergo a trial embryo transfer to make certain that the catheter passes without difficulty into the endometrial cavity. The goal of a mock transfer should be to anticipate the needs at the time of actual embryo transfer, assess any special needs, and define anatomy. The trial transfer should be performed with the bladder full and with ultrasound guidance. Ease of passage through the endocervical canal should be verified. The relationship between the cervix and lower uterine segment should be assessed and the catheter curved to conform to the normal anatomy. These details should be recorded for reference at the time of transfer. It is also to identify patients who are most likely to have a difficult transfer. Precise planning will improve outcomes.

Management – Techniques of Embryo Transfer

Uncomplicated Embryo Transfer

The cardinal tenet of an embryo transfer is the atraumatic, gentle placement of high-quality embryos within the endometrial cavity (Table 11–2). These goals are best achieved using a soft tipped, catheter to assure accurate placement of the embryos, avoiding any contact of the catheter tip against the endometrial lining and uterine fundus, thereby avoiding any uterine contractions.

Ultrasound-guided embryo transfer is performed as follows. Ultrasound monitoring may be performed using transabdominal and transvesical imaging with 2D and 3D probes. The bladder should be filled with the intention to both enhance imaging of the uterus and endometrial lining and to straighten any uterine flexion that may be present (Figure 11-6). There should be as small an angle as possible between the endocervical canal and

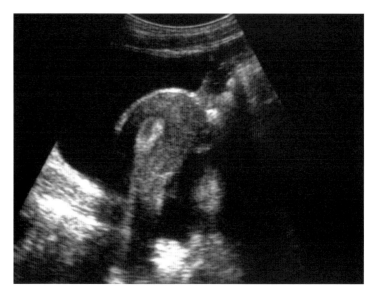

Figure 11-6   Three-dimensional ultrasound image of catheter placement. Note the
                     body of the catheter within the middle of the endometrial cavity and
                     the tip displaced into the right cornual region.

the endometrial lining. Scout imaging of the pelvis is then carried out trans-
vesically and the uterus and fundal region of the endometrium brought into
focus. This scanning may be performed by any assistant or nursing personnel available and does not require an ultrasonographer or clinician. A
bivalve speculum is then inserted into the vagina and the vaginal vault carefully swabbed with sterile culture medium to clear the area of any mucus or
debris. The endocervical canal is gently prepped by both swabbing it with
cotton-tipped applicators soaked in the medium, and by vigorously irrigating the canal using a 10-µl ringed syringe attached to a flexible catheter.
Special catheters with side ports are designed for this purpose. The guide
catheter of the coaxial system is also ideal for this purpose. Reflux of the
culture medium into the endometrial cavity during this phase of irrigation
may be observed during ultrasound imaging (Figure 11-7). This reflux has
not been shown to adversely impact outcomes. Fluid in the cavity may also
prevent any subendometrial injection of the embryos by providing slight
separation of the endometrial walls and provide a nutrient environment for
the transition from culture medium to the endometrial environment. Higher
pregnancy rates have been observed in association with this reflux.

After the irrigation process, the vaginal vault should be carefully dried of
any remaining mucus or media that may have collected. The coaxial system,
loaded with the embryos in the transfer catheter, is then brought into the
field. Both transfer and guide catheter may be advanced as a unit or individually. The guide catheter should serve to stabilize the softer and more flexible transfer catheter. The transfer catheter should be kept well within the

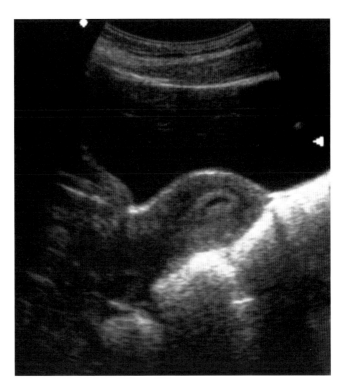

Figure 11-7   Intrauterine reflux of media at the time of irrigation of the endocervical
                   canal. Note collection of fluid throughout the endometrial cavity.

rigid guide catheter to reduce any unintended movement of the transfer catheter tip. An alternative to this is to pass the outer sheath transcervically apart from the inner flexible catheter. Care should be taken to restrict the movement of the catheter through the cervix only, avoiding any entry into the endometrial cavity or damaging the endometrial lining. In some circumstances, any minor difficulties will be encountered without exposing the embryos to this movement or trauma. Once in place, the outer sheath provides a conduit for safe, atraumatic passage of the inner catheter.

Care should be taken not to advance the guide catheter into the depth of the endometrial cavity as its rigid structure may disrupt the endometrial lining. The guide catheter is advanced just beyond the external os, a distance of approximately 1 to 2 cm into the cervical canal. Under direct transabdominal ultrasound guidance, the transfer catheter is then advanced through the endocervical canal into the lower uterine segment. Immediate identification of the catheter tip is essential to minimize motion of the catheter and avoid any impact on the endometrium. The tip of the transfer catheter will facilitate this aspect. An echo-dense tip may improve visualization of the catheter tip on ultrasound examination. In difficult cases, identification of the catheter tip may be facilitated by movement of the ultrasound probe a few degrees in the longitudinal and transverse planes. Alternatively, small changes in the brightness, contrast, and gain of the ultrasound unit may enhance identification of the catheter tip. Movement of the scanner is more advantageous than to and fro movement of the catheter for identification, as any excessive motion of the catheter may disrupt the endometrium. The transfer catheter may then be advanced to a distance of 1.5 to 2.0 cm from the uterine fundus. This measurement may be easily verified by using the calipers prior to injection of the embryos. After transfer, the catheter may be held in place for 45 to 60 seconds to permit the embryos to settle away from the catheter tip, though no prospective data support this practice. Immediate withdrawal is also an option. Both techniques are used successfully at several clinics. The transfer and guide catheters are then slowly withdrawn as a unit and inspected for any retained embryos.

In cases when an apparent obstruction is encountered or by personal preference, it is possible to bring the guide catheter into the field independent of the transfer catheter and to advance only the guide catheter through the endocervical canal. This maneuver permits more aggressive tailoring of the curve of the guide catheter to the specific cervical anatomy. The transfer catheter loaded with the embryos may then be brought independently into the field after the guide catheter is securely and safely placed in the canal. In this circumstance, the guide catheter provides a guidance and shelter for the safe passage of the embryos. This approach will avoid any possible damage to the embryos due to a difficult passage through the endocervical canal. In addition, when the passage of the guide catheter is difficult, only the transfer catheter should be removed after transfer of the embryo and inspected for any retained embryos. The guide catheter should be in place should any retained embryos be detected. This maneuver will avoid a second difficult passage should there be retained embryos.

In occasional cases, the delivery catheter of this system, due to its soft and flexible nature, will pass through the guide catheter and endocervical canal with difficulty. Resistance may be encountered as the transfer catheter is advanced through the curvature of the guide catheter. The delivery catheter may bend back on itself due to its extremely pliable nature. In this circumstance, a modified transfer catheter that incorporates a fine wire guide in the proximal two-thirds of the transfer catheter and maintains the soft, pliable nature of the distal one-third is available. This modification lends rigidity to the transfer catheter and prevents the transfer catheter from bending back on itself but maintains the extremely soft character of the catheter tip entering the uterine cavity. Care is required in its use. Gentle forward pressure should be used. Excessive pressure may provide entry into the cavity but at the risk of simultaneously damaging the embryos.

In cases of unanticipated difficulty in spite of precise planning, there are three options. Stabilizing the cervix with a fine-toothed tenaculum and gently dilating the cervix with small Pratt dilators may be useful. In select circumstances, a rigid guide may be placed in the guide catheter to maintain curvature and lend more rigidity to the system. The third technique is placement of laminaria. Laminaria may be placed at the time of oocyte retrieval if clinical exam suggests that embryo transfer may be problematic. This option however identifies patients late in the process. The placement of the laminaria may result in cramping and adversely impact pregnancy rates. These techniques are to be avoided and considered a last resort only for extreme and difficult circumstances. These clinical circumstances may be anticipated and planned for through a careful trial or mock embryo transfer well in advance of the IVF cycle. If easy passage of the catheter cannot be assured, conversion to ZIFT (if tubal access is possible) or postponement of the transfer and cryopreservation of the embryos may be considered.

Complicated Embryo Transfer

A complicated or difficult transfer is defined as one requiring long periods of time to accomplish, when blood contaminates the catheter, when excessive cramping is encountered, or when resistance is met and force is needed. In circumstances where there is a difficult transfer, there is a greater frequency of uterine contractions and lower pregnancy rate. A well-defined relationship exists between the ease of a transfer, endometrial contractions and movement of "mock embryos" (30 µl of Echovist). These contractions may persist for up to 45 minutes after transfer. These contractions and resultant movement are most commonly caused by impact of the catheter against the lateral walls and fundus of the uterus and is the most frequent type of stimulation associated with embryo transfers. These cases are identified at the trial transfer and appropriate intervention initiated to improve the ease of embryo transfer prior to the IVF cycle. In cases in which the catheter passes with extreme difficulty or is impossible to pass, two options exist. First, manipulation of the cervical canal to improve ease of passage and, second, when no improvement can be achieved, a surgical transfer may be considered. In extreme cases, options of cryopreservation and either surgery to improve the cervical canal or surrogacy may be entertained. The need for cervical dilatation is a poor prognostic sign, especially if performed in any proximity to the actual transfer.

Cervical Stenosis

In circumstances where the endocervical canal is stenotic, constricted, and inaccessible, four techniques are available (Table 11-3). The first involves placement of laminaria. A laminaria may be placed 2 months ahead of the planned transfer with a reevaluation and repeat mock transfer 1 month after placement.[64] In select circumstances, a stem pessary has been used for cervical dilatation when a laminaria does not improve access.[65] There is questionable benefit to performing a dilatation one or two days prior to transfer, but as noted above, this may be required in cases of unexpected stenosis. The second option is a variation of the first and consists of transvaginal uterine cervical dilatation using fluoroscopic guidance in circumstances where placement of a laminaria is impossible.

Table 11-3.
Evaluation Prior to ART: Cervical Stenosis
• Two options to improve transcervical embryo transfer: dilatation 2 months prior to embryo transfer and/or surgical reconstruction of the endocervix
• Evaluation of pelvic factors prior to in vitro fertilization if a tubal transfer of gametes or zygotes is an option
• If transcervical transfer is impossible, gamete or zygote intrafallopian transfer is an option
• If tubal access or tubal damage is present, transmyometrial transfer may be considered

The third option is resectoscopic reconstruction of the endocervical canal.[66–69] In this procedure, a single pass is made with a resectoscope providing a renewed endometrial canal. This procedure involves passing the operative loop along the posterior cervix in the midline creating a trough approximately 10 mm in width and 5 mm in depth. Postoperatively a pediatric Foley catheter is placed and removed 2 weeks after the procedure.

A fourth method of dilatation involves transcervical placement of a Malecot catheter.[70] This catheter is left in place for an average of 10 days with the mushroom tip of the Malecot catheter in the endometrial cavity. In this technique, hysteroscopic evaluation of the endocervical canal and uterine cavity is performed with subsequent placement of a 16 to 22 F Malecot catheter. In circumstances where none of the above techniques are considered options or possible, a transmyometrial embryo transfer may be considered.

Angulated Cervical Canal

In circumstances where there is a marked degree of anteversion between the uterus and the endocervical canal, bladder filling to the maximum is useful in reducing this angle and may improve the relationship of cervix and uterus (Figure 11-5).[71–73] In select circumstances, overfilling of the bladder may be facilitated by instillation of saline through a Foley catheter. Gentle traction with a tenaculum or placement of a #4-0 silk suture has been described, but should be avoided because of the possibility of uterine cramping.

Surgical Embryo Transfer

In cases where a transcervical approach is impossible or poses significant risk to the embryos, there are two approaches: transmyometrial/transvaginal (so-called Towako method) and transvesical/transmyometrial.[74–79] Early attempts with this technique were largely unsuccessful. However, improvement in guidance and needle design has resulted in more favorable outcomes. Precise ultrasound monitoring is required. This technique is routine for domestic and laboratory animals including horses, cows, and sheep. In these species, the transmyometrial transfer has proven to be far superior to the transcervical method in achieving pregnancies. The advantages in humans are related to the avoidance of bacterial contamination of the cavity with vaginal or cervical microorganisms, avoidance of reflux of the embryos, and lack of a cervical canal to navigate and the associated trauma to the embryos. In this technique, an 18-gauge 25 cm in length needle is advanced under ultrasound guidance through the myometrium at the level of the uterine fundus. A polyethylene catheter is then advanced through the needle into the endometrial cavity and the embryos transferred. There is no clear-cut advantage over transcervical techniques in cases where the transcervical approach is feasible.

Complications

Few complications are associated with embryo transfer regardless of technique. The greatest complication is uterine cramping and trauma to the embryos. The likelihood of an infection from transcervical embryo transfer is extremely low. Pelvic abscesses have been described.[80] Ectopic pregnancies have been described but appear to be independent of the amount of fluid or placement of the embryos.[81–84] Reflux of media into the uterine cavity at the time of cervical flushing has also been noted.[85] There is no adverse effect of this and, in fact, there appears to be some enhancement of pregnancy rates in this circumstance.

Summary and Recommendations

- Atraumatic, precise handling of embryos: the transfer should be viewed as an extension of the laboratory.
- Ultrasound guidance.
- Soft, coaxial catheter system that works well for a given IVF team.
- Track clinician and embryologist–clinician team outcomes with attention to the patient populations.
- Anticipate needs at the time of transfer: identify potential complex cases and plan ahead with either intervention to improve the cervical anatomy or appropriate instruments at the time of transfer and surgical transfer.
- Reconstruction of the cervix when needed.
- In extreme cases, consider the option of postponing the transfer or surgical embryo transfer (tubal transfer or transmyometrial).

References

1. Moghissi KS. Postcoital test: physiologic basis, technique, and interpretation. Fertil Steril 1976;27:117–129.

2. al-Shawaf T, Dave R, Harper J, et al. Transfer of embryos into the uterus: how much do technical factors affect pregnancy rates? J Assist Reprod Genet 1993;10:31–36.

3.   Englert Y, Puissant F, Camus M, et al. Clinical study on embryo transfer after human in vitro fertilization. J In Vitro Fertil Embryo Transfer 1986;3:243–246.

4.   Mansour R, Aboulghar M, Serour G. Dummy embryo transfer: a technique that minimizes the problems of embryo transfer and improves the pregnancy rate in human in vitro fertilization. Fertil Steril 1990;54:678–681.

5.   Tur-Kaspa I, Yuval Y, Bider D, et al. Difficult or repeated sequential embryo transfers do not adversely affect in-vitro fertilization pregnancy rates or outcome. Hum Reprod 1998;13:2452–2455.

6.   Nabi A, Awonuga A, Birch H, et al. Multiple attempts at embryo transfer: does this affect in-vitro fertilization treatment outcome? Hum Reprod 1997;12:1188–1190.

7.   Tomas C, Tapanainen J, Martikainen H. The difficulty of embryo transfer is an independent variable for predicting pregnancy in in vitro fertilization treatments. [Abstract] Fertil Steril 1998;70 Suppl 1: S433.

8.   Lesny P, Killick SR, Tetlow RL, et al. Embryo transfer–can we learn anything new from the observation of junctional zone contractions? Hum Reprod 1998;13:1540–1546.

9.   Lopata A. Success and failures in human in vitro fertilization. Nature 1980;288:642–643.

10.   Craft I, McLeod F, Edmonds K. Human embryo transfer technique. Lancet 1981;ii:1104–1105.

11.   Biggers JD. In vitro fertilization and embryo transfer in human beings. N Engl J Med 1981;304:336–342.

12.   Kovacs GT. What factors are important for successful embryo transfer after in vitro fertilization? Hum Reprod 1999;14:590–592.

13.   Edwards RG, Fishel SB, Cohen J, et al. Factors influencing the success of in vitro fertilization for alleviating human infertility. J In Vitro Fertil Embryo Transfer 1984;1:3–23.

14.   Glatstein IZ, Pang SC, McShane PM. Successful pregnancies with the use of laminaria tents before embryo transfer for refractory cervical stenosis. Fertil Steril 1997;67:1172–1174.

15.   Meldrum DR, Chetkowski R, Steingold KA, et al. Evolution of a highly successful in vitro fertilization-embryo transfer program. Fertil Steril 1987;48:86–93.

16.   Poindexter AN 3rd, Thompson DJ, Gibbons WE, et al. Residual embryos in failed embryo transfer. Fertil Steril 1986;46:262–267.

17.   Goudas VT, Hammitt DG, Damario MA, et al. Blood on the embryo transfer catheter is associated with decreased rates of embryo implantation and clinical pregnancy with use of in vitro fertilization-embryo transfer. Fertil Steril 1998;70:878–882.

18.   Lass A, Abusheikha N, Brinsden P, Kovacs GT. The effect of a difficult embryo transfer on the outcome of IVF. Hum Reprod 1999;14:2417.

19.   Visser DS, Fourie FL, Kruger Hightops Farm. Multiple attempts at embryo transfer: effects on pregnancy outcome in an in vitro fertilization and embryo transfer program. J Assist Reprod Genetics 1993;10:37–43.

20. Lesny P, Killick SR, Robinson J, et al. Junctional zone contractions and embryo transfer: is it safe to use a tenaculum? Hum Reprod 1999;14:2367–2370.

21. Kerin JF, Jeffrey R, Warnes GM, et al. A simple technique for human embryo transfer into the uterus. Lancet 1981;ii:726–727.

22. Leeton J, Trounson A, Jessup D, Wood C. The technique for human embryo transfer. Fertil Steril 1982;38:156–161.

23. Penzias A, Harris D, Barrett C, et al. Outcomes oriented research in an IVF program: transfer catheter type affects IVF outcome [Abstract]. In: Proceedings of the 53rd annual meeting of the American Society for Reproductive Medicine. 1997:S163.

24. Hesla J, Stevens J, Schlenker T. Comparison of malleable stylet Wallace catheter to Tomcat catheter for difficult embryo transfers. [Abstract] Fertil Steril 1998;70 Suppl 1:S222.

25. Letterie GS, Marshall L, Angle M. A new coaxial catheter system with an echodense tip for ultrasonographically guided embryo transfer. Fertil Steril 1999;72:266–268.

26. Marconi G, Vilela M, Bello J, et al. Endometrial lesions caused by catheters used for embryo transfers: a preliminary report. Fertil Steril 2003;80:363–367.

27. Wisanto A, Janssens R, Deschacht J, et al. Performance of different embryo transfer catheters in a human in vitro fertilization program. Fertil Steril 1989;52:79–84.

28. Lavie O, Margalioth EJ, Geva-Eldar T, Ben-Chetrit A. Ultrasonographic endometrial changes after intrauterine insemination: a comparison of two catheters. Fertil Steril 1997;68:731–734.

29. Prapas Y, Prapas N, Hatziparasidou A, et al. The echoguide embryo transfer maximizes the IVF results. Acta Eur Fertil 1995;26:113–115.

30. Wood EG, Batzer FR, Go KJ, et al. Ultrasound-guided soft catheter embryo transfers will improve pregnancy rates in in-vitro fertilization. Hum Reprod 2000;15:107–112.

31. Rosenlund B, Sjoblom P, Hillensjo TP. Pregnancy outcome related to the site of embryo deposition in the uterus. J Assist Reprod Genet 1996;13:511–513.

32. Baba K, Ishihara O, Hayashi N, et al. Where does the embryo implant after embryo transfer in humans? Fertil Steril 2000;73:123–125.

33. Botta G, Grudzinskas G. Is a prolonged bed rest following embryo transfer useful? Hum Reprod 1997;12:2489–2492.

34. Woolcott R, Stanger J. Ultrasound tracking of the movement of embryo-associated air bubbles on standing after transfer. Hum Reprod 1998;13:2107–2109.

35. Sharif K, Afnan M, Lenton W, et al. Do patients need to remain in bed following embryo transfer? The Birmingham experience of 103 in-vitro fertilization cycles with no bed rest following embryo transfer. Hum Reprod 1995;10:1427–1429.

36. Strickler RC, Christianson C, Crane JP, Curato A, Knight AB, Yang V. Ultrasound guidance for human embryo transfer. Fertil Steril 1985;43:54–61.

37.   Woolcott R, Stanger J. Potentially important variables identified by transvaginal ultrasound-guided embryo transfer. Hum Reprod 1997;12:963–966.

38.   Lesny P, Killick SR, Tetlow RL, Robinson J, Maguiness SD. Uterine junctional zone contractions during assisted reproduction cycles. Hum Reprod Update 1998;4:440–445.

39.   Fanchin R, Righini C, Olivennes F, Taylor S, de Ziegler D, Frydman R. Uterine contractions at the time of embryo transfer alter pregnancy rates after in-vitro fertilization. Hum Reprod 1998; 13:1968–1974.

40.   Hurley VA, Osborn JC, Leoni MA, Leeton J. Ultrasound-guided embryo transfer: a controlled trial. Fertil Steril 1991;55:559–562.

41.   Kan AK, Abdalla HI, Gafar AH, et al. Embryo transfer: ultrasound-guided versus clinical touch. Hum Reprod 1999;14:1259–1261.

42.   Leong M, Leung C, Tucker M, et al. Ultrasound-assisted embryo transfer. J In Vitro Fertil Embryo Transfer 1986;3:383–385.

43.   Lindheim SR, Cohen MA, Sauer MV. Ultrasound guided embryo transfer significantly improves pregnancy rates in women undergoing oocyte donation. Int J Gynaecol Obstet 1999;66:281–284.

44.   Coroleu B, Carreras O, Veiga A, et al. Embryo transfer under ultrasound guidance improves pregnancy rates after in-vitro fertilization. Hum Reprod 2000;15:616–620.

45.   Liedholm P, Sundstrom PO, Wramsby H. A model for experimental studies on human egg transfer. Arch Androl 1980;5:92.

46.   Letterie GS. Three-dimensional ultrasound guided embryo transfer. Am J Obstet Gynecol (in press).

47.   Waterstone J, Curson R, Parsons J. Embryo transfer to low uterine cavity. Lancet 1991;337:1413.

48.   Gaudoin M, Rekha P, Morris A, et al. Bacterial vaginosis and past chlamydial infection are strongly and independently associated with tubal infertility but do not affect in vitro fertilization success rates. Fertil Steril 1999;72:730–732.

49.   Liversedge NH, Turner A, Horner PJ, Keay SD, Jenkins JM, Hull M. The influence of bacterial vaginosis on in-vitro fertilization and embryo implantation during assisted reproduction treatment. Hum Reprod 1999;14:2411–2415.

50.   Egbase PE, al-Sharhan M, al-Othman S, et al. Incidence of microbial growth from the tip of the embryo transfer catheter after embryo transfer in relation to clinical pregnancy rate following in-vitro fertilization and embryo transfer. Hum Reprod 1996;11:1687–1689.

51.   Gorbach SL, Menda KB, Thadepalli H, Keith L. Anaerobic microflora of the cervix in healthy women. Am J Obstet Gynecol 1973;117:1053–1055.

52.   Moore DE, Soules MR, Klein NA, et al. Bacteria in the transfer catheter tip influence the live-birth rate after in vitro fertilization. Fertil Steril 2000;74:1118–1124.

53.   Fanchin R, Harmas A, Benaoudia F, et al. Microbial flora of the cervix assessed at the time of embryo transfer adversely affects in vitro fertilization outcome. Fertil Steril 1998;70:866–870.

54. Ralph SG, Rutherford AJ, Wilson JD. Influence of bacterial vaginosis on conception and miscarriage in the first trimester: cohort study. BMJ 1999;319:220–223.

55. Agnew KJ, Hillier SL. The effect of treatment regimens for vaginitis and cervicitis on vaginal colonization by lactobacilli. Sex Transm Dis 1995;22:269–273.

56. Morales WJ, Schorr S, Albritton J. Effect of metronidazole in patients with preterm birth in preceding pregnancy and bacterial vaginosis: a placebo-controlled, double-blind study. Am J Obstet Gynecol 1994;171:345–349.

57. Kurki T, Sivonen A, Renkonen OV, Savia E, Ylikorkala O. Bacterial vaginosis in early pregnancy and pregnancy outcome. Obstet Gynecol 1992;80:173–177.

58. Letterie GS, Eckert LO. How homogeneous are groups in studies comparing embryo transfer techniques? Hum Reprod 2003;18:1110.

59. Glass KB, Green CA, Fluker MR, Schoolcraft WB, McNamee PI, Meldrum D. Multicenter randomized trial of cervical irrigation at the time of embryo transfer [Abstract]. Fertil Steril 2000;74 Suppl 1:S31.

60. McNamee P, Huang T, Carwile A. Significant increase in pregnancy rates achieved by vigorous irrigation of endocervical mucus prior to embryo transfer with a Wallace catheter in an IVF-ET program [Abstract]. Fertil Steril 1998;70 Suppl 1:S228.

61. Mansour RT, Aboulghar MA, Serour GI, Amin YM. Dummy embryo transfer using methylene blue dye. Hum Reprod 1994;9:1257–1259.

62. Karande VC, Morris R, Chapman C, Rinehart J, Gleicher N. Impact of the "physician factor" on pregnancy rates in a large assisted reproductive technology program: do too many cooks spoil the broth? Fertil Steril 1999;71:1001–1009.

63. Hearns-Stokes RM, Miller BT, Scott L, et al. Pregnancy rates after embryo transfer depend on the provider at embryo transfer. Fertil Steril 2000;74:80–86.

64. Abusheikha N, Lass A, Akagbosu F, Brinsden P. How useful is cervical dilatation in patients with cervical stenosis who are participating in an in vitro fertilization-embryo transfer program? The Bourn Hall experience. Fertil Steril 1999;72:610–612.

65. Frishman GN. The use of the stem pessary to facilitate transcervical embryo transfer in women with cervical stenosis. J Assist Reprod Genet 1994;11:225–228.

66. Dickey KW, Zreik TG, Hsia HC, et al. Transvaginal uterine cervical dilation with fluoroscopic guidance: preliminary results in patients with infertility. Radiology 1996;200:497–503.

67. Noyes N, Licciardi F, Grifo J, et al. In vitro fertilization outcome relative to embryo transfer difficulty: a novel approach to the forbidding cervix. Fertil Steril 1999;72:261–265.

68. Noyes N. Hysteroscopic cervical canal shaving: a new therapy for cervical stenosis before embryo transplant in patients undergoing in vitro fertilization. Fertil Steril 1999;71:965–966.

69. Groutz A, Lessing JB, Wolf Y, et al. Cervical dilatation during ovum pick-up in patients with cervical stenosis: effect on pregnancy outcome in an in vitro fertilization-embryo transfer program. Fertil Steril 1997;67:909–911.

70. Yanushpolsky EH, Ginsburg ES, Fox JH, Stewart EA. Transcervical placement of a Malecot catheter after hysteroscopic evaluation provides for easier entry into the endometrial cavity for women with histories of difficult intrauterine inseminations and/or embryo transfers: a prospective case series. Fertil Steril 2000;73:402–405.

71. Lewin A, Schenker JG, Avrech O, Shapira S, Safran A, Friedler S. The role of uterine straightening by passive bladder distension before embryo transfer in IVF cycles. J Assist Reprod Genet 1997;14:32–34.

72. Mitchell JD, Wardle PG, Foster PA, Hull MG. Effect of bladder filling on embryo transfer. J In Vitro Fert Embryo Transf 1989;6:263–265.

73. Sundstrom P, Wramsby H, Persson PH, Liedholm P. Filled bladder simplifies human embryo transfer. Br J Obstet Gynaecol 1984;91:506–507.

74. Groutz A, Lessing J, Wolf Y, et al. Comparison of transmyometrial and transcervical embryo transfer in patients with previously failed in vitro fertilization-embryo transfer cycles and/or cervical stenosis. Fertil Steril 1997;67:1073–1076.

75. Kato O, Takatsuka R, Asch RH. Transvaginal-transmyometrial embryo transfer: the Towako method; experiences of 104 cases. Fertil Steril 1993;59:51–53.

76. Khalifa Y, Redgment CJ, Yazdani N, Taranissi M, Craft IL. Intramural pregnancy following difficult embryo transfer. Hum Reprod 1994;9:2427–2428.

77. Nakayama T, Goto Y, Kanzaki H, et al. The use of intra-endometrial embryo transfer for increasing the pregnancy rate. Hum Reprod 1995;10:1833–1836.

78. Lenz S, Leeton J, Rogers P, Trounson A. Transfundal transfer of embryos using ultrasound. J In Vitro Fert Embryo Transf 1987;4:13–17.

79. Sharif K, Afnan M, Lenton W, et al. Transmyometrial embryo transfer after difficult immediate mock transcervical transfer. Fertil Steril 1996;65:1071–1074.

80. Sauer MV, Paulson RJ. Pelvic abscess complicating transcervical embryo transfer. Am J Obstet Gynecol 1992;166:148–149.

81. Yovich JL, Turner SR, Murphy AJ. Embryo transfer technique as a cause of ectopic pregnancies in in vitro fertilization. Fertil Steril 1985;44:318–321.

82. Nazari A, Askari HA, Check JH, O'Shaughnessy A. Embryo transfer technique as a cause of ectopic pregnancy in in vitro fertilization. Fertil Steril 1993;60:919–921.

83. Lesny P, Killick SR, Robinson J, Maguiness SD. Transcervical embryo transfer as a risk factor for ectopic pregnancy. Fertil Steril 1999;72:305–309.

84. Bennett S, Waterstone J, Parsons J, Creighton S. Two cases of cervical pregnancy following in vitro fertilization and embryo transfer to the lower uterine cavity. J Assist Reprod Genet 1993;10:100–103.

85. Letterie GS, Marshall L, Angle M. Intrauterine reflux of media during cervical irrigation at embryo transfer. Fertil Steril 2003;79:1444–1446.

12 *Distal Tubal Obstruction: surgery and ART*

The plastic procedure on the tubes to overcome sterility is not worthwhile. . . .
— *J. P. Greenhill, 1936*

Tubal surgery to relieve obstruction dates to the 1880s. In 1895, Martin reported 62 cases of distal salpingostomies. The procedure entailed a fenestration at the distal obstruction. Two pregnancies and two deaths from postoperative peritonitis were described in this series.[1] Pregnancy rates in early reports after repair for distal obstruction were uniformly poor and ranged from 0 to 15%.[2] Poor pregnancy rates, however, were not the only cause for concern. The most sinister complication was an ectopic pregnancy, a clinical event associated at the time with appreciable mortality.[3] From the 1930s, various techniques for tubal repair appeared in the literature. In 1932, the first description of a distal salpingostomy with eversion of the distal tubal segment was reported, providing practitioners with a reliable and reproducible technique of exposing the distal tubal segment.[4]

Concern over poor pregnancy rates and the possibility of an ectopic pregnancy contributed to a consensus in 1936 that recommended tubal surgery be abandoned.[5] This position held sway until the 1950s when surgical technique and management of ectopic pregnancy improved. Subsequently, advances in both techniques and instrumentation, especially in microsurgery during the 1970s, led to the recommendation of tubal surgery for *all* tubal obstructions. Reports of success through the 1970s and early 1980s were variable because of the wide spectrum of tubal disease treated and methods of reporting results. The paradigm in effect held that regardless of extent of damage, distal obstruction was considered repairable. This approach was appropriate for the time. In vitro fertilization (IVF) was on the horizon – the potential discussed but not yet realized. The advent of several staging schemes, advanced endoscopy, and improved success rates for IVF led to the selective use of tubal surgery for only mild distal tubal obstructions.[6,7] Contemporary management reflects a posture somewhere between these two views by selecting patients who may best benefit from tubal surgery and referring all others for IVF.[8] The trend in contemporary practice reflects a tendency to recommend IVF in most patients with distal obstruction. There are clearly patients, however, who will benefit from surgery.[9] This group has present mild obstruction amenable to endoscopic repair. This chapter reviews the pathophysiology of distal obstruction, the criteria for patient selection for surgery or referral for IVF, techniques for tubal repair, and the role of tubal ligation prior to IVF for cases of severe hydrosalpinx.

Etiology

Distal obstruction is occlusion distal to the isthmic segment, primarily within the ampullae and at the fimbriated end. Distal tubal obstruction accounts for approximately 30% of infertile patients, depending on the population studied.[10] The most common cause is acute and chronic pelvic inflammatory disease (PID).[11,12] Results linking the intrauterine device to increased incidences of PID and tubal damage and pelvic adhesions have not been consistent in demonstrating any increased risk.[13] Studies that demonstrated a substantial increased risk of PID with IUD were primarily case–control studies and inconsistent in their findings.[14,15] Multiple partners were associated with increased risk for PID in this population. IUD use alone does not appear to increase the risk of tubal damage or ectopic pregnancy. The only clinical circumstance associated with a slight increased risk of pelvic infection with IUD is at the time of insertion.[16] Though infection accounts for the vast majority of cases, additional causes have been described. Congenital absence of the distal tube and obstruction in association with endometriosis are less common, though well-described causes.[17]

Normal tubal physiology involves a series of complex steps that include ovum capture at the interface of the fimbriated ends of the tube and ovary and transport of the oocyte through the fimbria into the ampullary region. Both mechanisms are dependent on the interaction of the oocyte–cumulus mass with the mucosa of the distal tubal segments. Ciliary activity in this region of the tube enhances both ovum capture and transport. The ampullary mucosa creates a unique environment that fosters sperm–egg interaction, fertilization, and embryonic growth.[18] Complex interactions occur within the ampullae involving sperm, the cumulus mass, oocyte, and tubal fluid. These delicate aspects of tubal function are disturbed by any trauma, whether surgical or infectious, that results in distal obstruction and mucosal injury. Damage to the fimbria, mucosa, or both contribute to either failure of oocyte capture or compromises sperm–egg interaction and ovum/embryo tubal transport.

Tubal damage after an episode of any infection involves the ampullary mucosa and fimbriated ends. These two structures are the linchpins of tubal contributions for in vivo reproduction. Their importance is illustrated in the rabbit model.[19–21] In this model, a direct correlation exists between ovum capture and the degree of ciliation of the fimbria. In experiments in which the fimbria and ampulla were left intact, ovum capture was 85%. In this series of experiments, when the fimbria were excised ovum capture was reduced to 30%. When both fimbria and ampulla were absent, ovum capture did not occur. A second aspect of these studies investigated the character of the tubal fluid and tubal transport when the ampullary mucosa was denuded. There was inadequate tubal fluid and transport in circumstances in which the experimental mucosal damage was created.

The rabbit model correlates well with clinical findings in cases of moderate to severe hydrosalpinx. In these patients, sufficient damage to the fimbria and ampullary mucosa occurs to prevent ovum pickup and fertilization. Even after reconstructive tubal surgery for severe hydrosalpinges pregnancy rates remain low, although patency persists postoperatively in 80% of the cases.[22,23] Though patency may exist, mucosal function is not restored. This series of animal studies emphasizes the need for intact fimbria and ampulla for tubal function and provides insight into the criteria used for patient selection for tubal surgery.

Sexually transmitted diseases cause the largest percentage of tubal damage resulting in infertility. In a cohort study of women aged 35 or younger attempting pregnancy, 1309 with laparoscopically verified acute salpingitis and 451 with normal infertility, tubal damage was diagnosed in 12.1% of the salpingitis group and 0.9% of the controls.[24] In these two groups, the first pregnancy was ectopic in 7.8 and 1.3%, respectively. The number of infections, severity of the infections, treatment, contraception at the index laparoscopy, age, and delayed treatment contribute to tubal damage and the likelihood of ectopic pregnancy. Sexually transmitted diseases are preventable and hence, as an epidemiologic issue, so is tubal infertility.[25] *Chlamydia trachomatis* is the leading cause of PID. *C. trachomatis* infection often presents without symptoms but may result in long-term morbidity. Up to one-third of inadequately treated women may go on to develop PID and, of these, one-fifth may become infertile and one-tenth may have an ectopic pregnancy.[26,27] Sexually transmitted microorganisms such as gonnorrhea are common pathogens found in the genital tract of patients with acute salpingitis with a high prevalence of *C. trachomatis*.[28]

Bacterial vaginosis is a common concurrent disorder of women with acute salpingitis. Bacterial vaginosis microorganisms are commonly isolated from the upper genital tracts of patients with PID.[29] Bacterial vaginosis is present in 62% of patients with acute salpingitis. One hundred percent of anaerobes isolated from the upper genital tract of patients with acute salpingitis are bacterial vaginosis microorganisms. Hence, the initiation of acute salpingitis is predominantly due to the ascending spread of sexually transmitted organisms complicated by bacterial vaginosis microorganisms.

Infection with *C. trachomatis* and other microorganisms can induce an intense cell-mediated immune response. A lymphocyte proliferative response to chlamydial heat-shock proteins (HSP) is a common feature of the pathogenesis of upper tract infections.[30] The association between the presence of serum IgA antibodies to C-hsp 60 and *Chlamydia*-associated chronic salpingitis with tubal occlusion appears to underlie the significance of C-hsp 60 in the pathogenesis of tubal infertility.[31,32]

PID can result in a broad spectrum of anatomic changes that compromise reproduction. Fifteen percent of women with a single episode of PID develop tubal infertility.[33] Damage by PID to the distal tube ranges from peritubal adhesions, fimbrial agglutination, and phimosis to complete tubal occlusion with or without hydrosalpinx formation. Anatomic changes caused by scarring may distort the normal tubo-ovarian relation and thus interfere with ovum pickup. The most common abnormality is closure of the distal tubal segment and concomitant damage to the tubal mucosa resulting ultimately in a hydrosalpinx of various degrees. Mucosal changes develop in part from the infectious process and in part from the hydrosalpinx itself. Histologic changes of tubal mucosa include loss of cilia, flattening of the mucosal epithelium, atrophy of the mucosa and muscularis, a decrease in estrogen and progesterone receptors, and loss of adrenergic innervation.

Cilia play a major role in tubal transport. Fimbrial microbiopsies and the calculation of a ciliation index (the percentage of ciliated cells) provide valuable insights into the prognosis of tubal surgery and lend support to surgery in select cases. No difference in ciliation index was found in biopsies from tubes with fimbrial agglutination or mild hydrosalpinx. Similar pregnancy rates after these procedures have been described. A significant decrease in ciliation index and pregnancy rates has been observed in patients with distal occlusion and tubal diameters greater than 15 mm compared with rates in patients with mild tubal obstruction. The ciliation index for tubes with diameters larger than 25 mm was extremely low. Thickness of the tubal wall is also of prognostic value. No pregnancy occurred after salpingostomy for thick-walled hydrosalpinx.[43] These findings further support the notion that assessment of the tubal mucosa is essential. In mild cases, mucosal cilia are minimally damaged suggesting a role for surgery in select cases.

The development of a hydrosalpinx is particularly ominous. The fluid of the hydrosalpinx is a transudate from tubal vasculature or from residual epithelial cell function. Studies evaluating the outcome of IVF in patients with hydrosalpinges have shown that this fluid is potentially detrimental and embryotoxic.[34–39] These studies suggest that this fluid may prevent implantation. An enhancement of success rates with IVF is noted when the hydrosalpinx is removed or a tubal ligation is performed at the uterotubal junction as described below.[40] Anatomic changes can be restored through microsurgical techniques of salpingostomy, fimbrioplasty, and salpingolysis with tubal patency rates of 79 to 90%.[41] However, there is no method to reverse the physiologic changes on the tubal mucosa, and postoperative pregnancy rates remain low when tubal damage is moderate or severe. The natural healing process may restore the tubal mucosa to some degree after a distal tubal repair for a hydrosalpinx. Restoration may require 1 to 2 years, and may be responsible for the continued first pregnancies for as long as 3 years.[42]

Clinical Correlates

Distal tubal obstruction is usually diagnosed during an evaluation of infertility. Occasionally, patients present with pelvic pain that necessitates laparoscopy. In this circumstance, tubal obstruction and, possibly, pelvic adhesive disease are discovered. The two most significant clinical abnormalities that impact reproductive outcome are degrees of hydrosalpinx and pelvic adhesive disease. Success of tubal surgery depends on the severity of tubal and adhesive disease and the selection of patients.[43,44]

Because these two factors are significant as determinants for referral to IVF or the likelihood of a pregnancy after surgical repair, there is continued clinical interest in classification systems for distal tubal obstruction. A variety of schemes have been proposed to predict the likely outcome of tubal surgery and to identify patients for referral to IVF. Classifications have included gross assessment of distal tubal damage at the time of tubal repair[45] to the development of more complicated numerical scoring systems.[46] The intention of any classification is, in part, to make possible comparison of data from various centers and guide decisions to the treatment with highest success. Clinically, classifications provide a means for determining both the efficiency of tubal microsurgery and the prognosis for patients with varying degrees of tubal damage and adhesions and should assist in selection of the optimal treatment, that is, surgery or endoscopic repair versus IVF.

Early systems of staging tubal disease were primarily retrospective, that is, an assessment of the likelihood of pregnancy was made after an intraoperative assessment of tubal damage and distal tubal repair. Despite obvious shortcomings, clinical observations and outcomes stage for stage provide a crude method for counseling.[43–48] These systems were a significant step forward in aiding selection of appropriate candidates. One practical system classified distal tubal disease according to the severity of the hydrosalpinx.[43] Tubal diameters of less than 15 mm, 15 to 30 mm and more than 30 mm were rated as mild, moderate, and severe, respectively. A strong correlation exists between the severity of tubal disease, decreasing pregnancy rates, and increasing ectopic rates. Patients with a success rate less than IVR after a proposed tubal surgery could then be referred for IVF.

In a second, more complicated system, the degree of tubal damage is divided into three prognostic categories.[46] This system attempted to categorize patients preoperatively and select patients most likely to benefit from a surgical procedure. This classification system incorporates clinical findings from HSG and laparoscopy and formulated a weighted score for tubal status and for pelvic adhesive disease. Success after tubal surgery using this system showed a downward trend in intrauterine pregnancy and an upward trend in ectopic pregnancy as scores increased. Low intrauterine and high ectopic rates in the intermediate and poor prognosis groups after tubal surgery made a compelling case for IVF referral. The outcomes from these two systems further support the concept that tubal surgery for distal obstruction should be used only under the most favorable conditions.

Pelvic adhesive disease (see Chapter 17) is an independent and additive factor influencing outcome. The nature and extent of pelvic and adnexal

	Degree	Occlusion	Rugae	IUP (%)	SAB (%)	EP (%)
	Table 12-1.					
	Classification of Distal Obstruction and Pregnancy Outcome					
Tubal status	Minimal	Partial	Normal	58	19	8
	Mild	Total	Normal	36	15	10
	Moderate	Total	Decreased	9	4	14
	Severe	Total	Absent	0	0	0
Adhesion status	Mild	Filmy	Ovary or tube	32	12	0
	Moderate	Vascular	Ovary and tube	26	10	6
	Severe	Dense	Ovary and tube	5	2	10

EP = ectopic pregnancy; IUP = intrauterine pregnancy; SAB = spontaneous abortion
References: 15, 21

adhesions are inversely related to success rate. In an attempt to incorporate the degree of tubal damage and extent of pelvic adhesions, a revised and updated numerical scoring system was devised.[49] The system was designed to be used at the time of surgery to assess the likelihood of success and, in part, to gauge the follow-up interval. Factors assigned numerical values are the extent and type of adhesions, the thickness and rigidity of the tubal wall, the distal ampullary diameter, and the extent of preservation of mucosal folds. The condition of the endosalpinx (as assessed on HSG or falloposcopy), the extent of ampullary dilatation, the thickness and rigidity of the tubal wall, and extent of pelvic adhesive disease, independently and additively influence outcome.[50–57] The worst-case scenario is either distal ampullary dilatation exceeding 3 cm or a hydrosalpinx with a rigid, thickened wall and narrowed lumen with overall outer tubal diameter unaffected (Table 12-1). When occlusion is minimal and tubal rugae are normal with no or minimal adhesive disease, surgery may be considered. When hydrosalpinx is severe with dense and vascular adhesions involving ovary and tube, and no rugal markings are present on HSG, IVF is recommended. Similar classifications have been proposed for fimbrial occlusion.[50] Only in exceptional cases of mild tubal occlusion should surgery be considered. For patients with moderate or severe hydrosalpinx and any degree of pelvic adhesive disease, IVF is recommended.[51,52]

Diagnosis

The most common complaint associated with distal tubal obstruction is infertility.[10] Secondary presentations may be a palpable mass detected on routine clinical examination or incidental adnexal cystic mass detected on pelvic ultrasound examination performed for unrelated indications. Proper investigation is the key to selecting the primary treatment modality. Accurate diagnosis and classification of degree of tubal damage are essential in referral for surgery or IVF. Counseling for patients with tubal disease is a complex process and relies on the results of a careful clinical questionnaire and a few well-chosen diagnostic studies.

Clinical history provides insight into the likelihood of tubal obstruction as the etiology of infertility. A history of previous episodes of PID places the patient at risk for tubal obstruction. Risk increases with the number of episodes of gonorrhea or trichomoniasis.[12] A history of any sexually transmitted disease, an ectopic pregnancy, or PID multiplies the risk of tubal factor infertility by a factor of 4, 5, and 7, respectively.[11] Antibodies to *C. trachomatis* are useful to identify those patients at risk for tubal occlusion.[58–60] An enzyme-linked immunosorbent assay for *C. trachomatis* has shown a strong correlation between salpingitis, tubal occlusion, and pelvic adhesions.[61] Serum chlamydial antibody testing by ELISA provides a useful method of assessing the degree of tubal damage in selecting patients for IVF. Definitive diagnosis is made by HSG with characteristic obstruction of the distal tube (Figures 12-1, 12-2, and 12-3). Further refinement of the diagnosis of hydrosalpinx may be made by classifying the degree of tubal dilatation into mild, moderate, or severe and making a diligent search of the distal

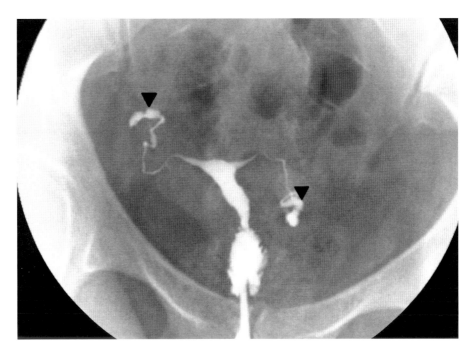

Figure 12-1   Hysterosalpingogram showing mild hydrosalpinx bilaterally. Note rugal markings (arrowheads).

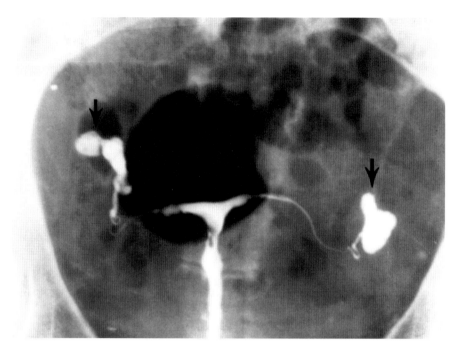

Figure 12-2   Hysterosalpingogram showing moderate hydrosalpinx bilaterally (arrows).

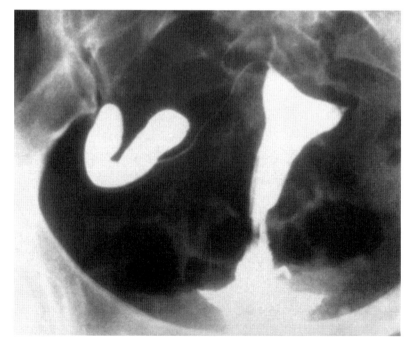

Figure 12-3   Hysterosalpingogram demonstrating left proximate tubal obstruction and a right severe hydrosalpinx. Note complete loss of rugal markings.

segments for rugal markings. Careful inspection of the HSG for contrast in loculations suggests adhesions. Such assessment assists in deciding which patients are surgical candidates and which patients should be referred for IVF.

Using HSG, a reliable diagnosis and an appropriate referral for IVF may be made if a severe hydrosalpinx is noted. However, should equivocal results be noted, further evaluation is warranted to evaluate the distal tubal segments and possible additional adnexal pathology such as pelvic adhesive disease.[62] This search is essential given the adverse impact untreated hydrosalpinges have on IVF outcome.

Ultrasound

Ultrasound examination may detect a characteristic linear sonolucency in the adnexae (Figure 12-4). However, the procedure is secondary to HSG for detection of tubal obstruction and quality of the tubal anatomy. Transvaginal ultrasound (TVS) images tubal structures poorly unless they are fluid-filled. As a sole diagnostic study, TVS has poor sensitivity for diagnosing tubal obstruction.[63] However, when a hydrosalpinx is present, TVS detects a characteristic fluid-filled, convoluted linear structure in 50% of cases. Its accuracy depends on the degree of fluid distension and location of the tube.[64]

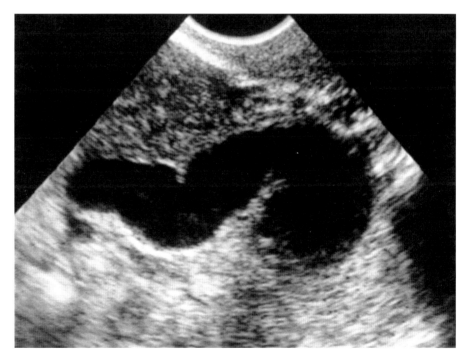

Figure 12-4   Transvaginal ultrasound image demonstrating a curvilinear sonolucency consistent with a severe hydrosalpinx.

Magnetic Resonance Imaging

Magnetic resonance imaging (MRI) may demonstrate fallopian tubes. The signal intensity of a normal fallopian tube appears intermediate on T2-weighted images, with a lower signal intensity at the muscularis. There is not sufficient fluid within a normal tube to allow identification of the lumen on T2-weighted images. The tubal lumen is filled with interdigitating plicae lined by tubal epithelium.[65,66] The epithelium and submucosa of the tube have intermediate signal intensities on T2-weighted images.[67] These structures may not be reliably demonstrated on MRI and depend on the plane of sections. However, pathologic conditions will render the tube visible on MRI. A tubal lumen filled with fluid may be visualized and its appearance may depend on whether it is T1- or T2-weighted (Figure 12-5 A and B).

Laparoscopy

Diagnostic laparoscopy should be performed for any equivocal findings on HSG to further assess the extent of tubal damage, pelvic adhesive disease, and any additional pelvic pathology such as endometriosis. Laparoscopy may be chosen as the initial diagnostic study, depending on the patient's history and clinical circumstances. HSG and laparoscopy are complementary procedures for the diagnosis of tubal obstruction and for planning therapy.[68] Definitive diagnosis of severe and inoperable tubal obstruction and recommendation for IVF may be made by HSG. However, laparoscopy may be needed in cases in which HSG findings are equivocal or to identify the most favorable cases for repair or for tubal ligation in cases of severe hydrosalpinges.[69–71] If laparoscopy reveals, for example, that the hydrosalpinx is mild with otherwise normal architecture, laparoscopic salpingostomy and lysis of adhesions may be performed.[72]

The reproductive surgeon should be prepared at the time of diagnostic laparoscopy to proceed with an operative laparoscopy and distal tubal repair or tubal ligation versus salpingectomy in candidates not for surgical repair and who have been adequately counseled for IVF. If the tubal condition is favorable enough to warrant a distal tubal repair, repair should be undertaken endoscopically. The purpose of the laparoscopy is to identify any patient with a poor prognosis not evident on HSG. Laparoscopic salpingostomy for mild hydrosalpinx is the first step in surgical repair. Inspection of the tubal lumen to identify intratubal adhesions and to assess the tubal wall thickness is the second step. If extensive intraluminal adhesions are present or the tubal wall is thickened or mucosa denuded, the procedure should be abandoned and the patient referred for IVF.[73–77] Any patient undergoing laparoscopy for distal obstruction should be counseled of the role of tubal ligation or salpingectomy prior to IVF if the conditions are unfavorable for tubal repair.

Any scoring system is intended to provide a prognosis for patients who are candidates for surgical repair. Inspection of the interior of tubes and assessing

(A)

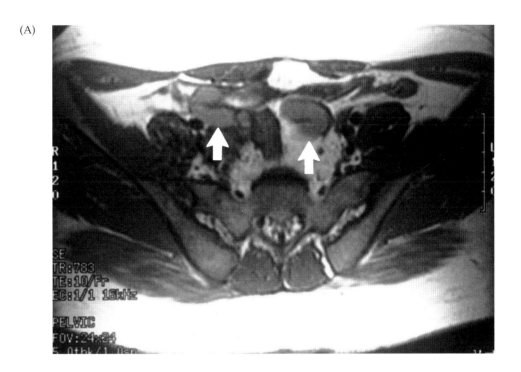

(B)

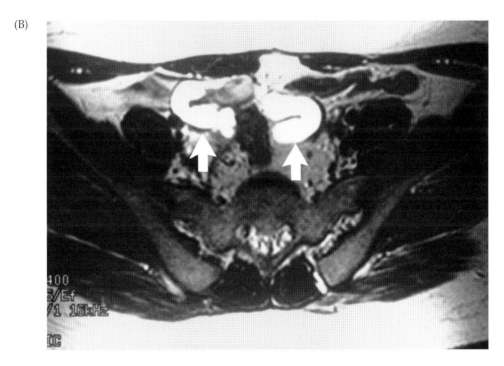

Figure 12-5   Bilateral hydrosalpinges; low signal intensity is demonstrated on T1-weighted images (A) and high signal intensity is demonstrated on T2-weighted images (B) of bilateral fallopian tubes and hydrosalpinges (arrows).

the character and quality of the tubal mucosa at laparoscopy provide insight regarding laparoscopy which patients should be referred for surgery or IVF. Patients with any significant mucosal damage regardless of tubal diameter have a uniformly low pregnancy rate and are best referred for IVF.[78] Investigation of tubal mucosa is an integral part of the evaluation and may be performed during diagnostic laparoscopy.[79–81] Falloposcopy is a second technique to evaluate this tubal lumen. There is a significant correlation between the appearance of the fallopian tubes on falloposcopy and term pregnancies after adhesiolysis and on neosalpingostomy. Inspection of the interior of the fallopian tube and tubal mucosa by falloposcopy may be a more precise method of classifying the likelihood of term pregnancy.[82] Falloposcopy using a linear everting catheter system may be used to diagnose and to stage tubal damage and possibly treat specific tubal factors in infertility.[83]

Evaluation Prior to ART

Management of tubal disease focused on surgical repair of hydrosalpinges prior to the early 1980s (Table 12–2). With the advent of in vitro fertilization, and especially with improved success that ranges from 30 to 60% depending on age of patient and number of IVF cycles, the decision regarding management options for tubal disease is more complicated. At one extreme, any patient with any degree of tubal obstruction should proceed directly to IVF, especially for those patients over age 35. A more moderate approach selects patients based on the degree of tubal obstruction and tubal dilatation, reserving surgery only for those patients with mild hydrosalpinges and no evidence of tubal dilatation and adhesions, with an age of less than 35 years, and a normal male factor.

The final question that should be answered regarding the management of the patient is whether or not hydrosalpinges should be removed or the tube ligated at the uterotubal junction.[84] IVF outcomes in patients with hydrosalpinges appear to be improved after salpingectomy or tubal ligation for moderate and severe hydrosalpinges. The possible adverse influence of a hydrosalpinx during in vitro fertilization may result from either a direct embryotoxic effect of the fluid contained within the hydrosalpinx changes in

Table 12-2. Evaluation Prior to ART: Distal Tubal Factor
o Assessment of tubal mucosa and degree of dilatation of the distal tubal via hysterosalpingography
o Verification of HSG findings through laparoscopy in questionable cases
o Tubal ligation at the cornual insertion of the tube versus salpingectomy
o Discussion and counseling regarding the quality of the literature supporting salpingectomy/tubal ligation and its impact on the outcome of IVF

the endometrial function and microenvironment or a mechanical backwashing of the fluid into the uterus.[83–86] The clinical trend suggests an improvement in IVF success rates when the tube is removed or ligated. This approach may have a role only in those patients who have a demonstrable hydrosalpinx on ultrasonography or in any patient with any degree of tubal dilatation and fluid contained within the hydrosalpinx.

The Impact of Hydrosalpinx on the Likelihood of Outcome with in vitro Fertilization

Two treatment options are available for patients with hydrosalpinges. Distal tubal repair is appropriate only for patients with preserved tubal mucosa. Because of an unacceptably low pregnancy rate and a risk of ectopic pregnancy in other circumstances, this is the only setting in which tubal surgery should be considered. The alternative of in vitro fertilization in cases of hydrosalpinges not amenable to surgery is impacted by fluid contained within the hydrosalpinges. This adverse impact may be due to backwash of fluid into the endometrial cavity causing a mechanical displacement or a true embryo toxic effect of this fluid on embryo expansion and development.[34–76] There is also a definitive impact of the fluid contained within a hydrosalpinx on the endometrium. In one study, there is a decreased expression of $\alpha_v\beta_3$ integrin, one of the endometrial receptivity markers for implantation. The expression of this essential integrin is increased when the hydrosalpinx is removed or obstructed. In addition, recent evidence of the adverse impact of the hydrosalpinx on the endometrium suggest an increased transformating growth factor-β_1 expression in the endometrium of women with a hydrosalpinx during the implantation window. The impact of hydrosalpinx fluid on the endometrium is also demonstrated in donor cycles of recipients who had significantly lower implantation rates and first-trimester loss rates than did controls. These findings collectively suggest that the fluid contained within a hydrosalpinx has an adverse effect on implantation during in vitro fertilization. These data make a compelling case for either removal of the tube or tubal ligation. In addition, chronic chlamydial infections in patients with hydrosalpinx may also impair implantation and embryo development. A salpingectomy or tubal ligation is recommended as a method to overcome the negative influence of the hydrosalpingeal fluid on implantation and development.

Salpingectomy was found to be an effective therapy in many retrospective studies. A prospective study was published in 1998 suggesting that pregnancy rates increased per cycle and per embryo transfer in patients after a salpingectomy, compared with those who were not treated and whose hydrosalpinges were left in situ. A randomized, prospective control data described delivery rates of 30% in patients undergoing a salpingectomy prior to IVF versus 17% in patients who did not undergo a salpingectomy. This is a 72% improvement in pregnancy rates in those patients who had a salpingectomy. A meta-analysis also demonstrated improved trends in favor of salpingectomy groups. However, these did not reach statistical significance with an odds ratio of 1.74 (95% confidence interval 0.96–3.16) and 1.36 (CI

0.82–2.23). Improved pregnancy rates occur after either removal of a hydrosalpinx or tubal ligation from the perspective of an evidence-based approach.

In a Cochrane database review, the odds ratio of pregnancy (OR 1.75, 95% CI 1.07–2.86) and of ongoing pregnancy and live birth (OR 2.13, 95% CI 1.24–3.65) were increased with laparoscopic salpingectomy for hydrosalpinges prior to IVF. A laparoscopic salpingectomy, based upon this Cochrane database review, should be considered for all women with hydrosalpinges prior to IVF treatment. Unilateral salpingectomy for unilateral hydrosalpinx is also recommended, though the data for this are less compelling.

Care should be exercised when removing a tube. The circumstance is frequently encountered when the tube is firmly adhered to the ovary, precluding dissection of the tube away from the ovary. In this setting, rather than risking any compromise to ovarian responsiveness and ovarian blood supply, a tubal ligation should be performed. An alternative to this is aspiration of the hydrosalpinges at the time of oocyte retrieval. This does improve pregnancy rate and may be an alternative to salpingectomy or tubal ligation for the treatment of patients with moderate to severe salpinges who did not have the hydrosalpinx repaired prior to surgery. A hysteroscopic obstruction at the cornual insertion of the tube has not been evaluated.

Management

Surgery vs IVF: the Possible Role of Tubal Surgery

The success of surgical management of distal tubal obstruction must be weighed against the success of IVF (Table 12-3). If the expectancy from tubal surgery is inferior to that from IVF, then referral should be made for IVF. This is especially true in the 35- to 39-year age group, in whom each year may influence ultimate success with IVF.[89–93] Except in rare circumstances, patients older than 36–38 years should be referred for IVF.[94,95] In those patients younger than 35 years with minimal tubal damage, normal tubal mucosa, and absence of pelvic adhesive disease, surgical management of distal tubal obstruction is an option.[96] This decision should be reached only after careful and thorough counseling.

Several factors affect this decision. The two most important are monthly fecundity rates and cost considerations. Surgery for mild tubal obstruction of any degree results in a monthly fecundity of 3.5%. This is compared with the fecundity rate in the general population of 20% and a per cycle success rate for IVF ranging from 20 to 50% in some clinics. The success of in vitro fertilization calls into question the role of tubal surgery in the current algorithm for the management of tubal factors. In addition to this, the relative risk of having an ectopic pregnancy is also increased with tubal surgery, with one study prescribing the relative risk at 4.5 (95% CI, 1.5–3.9), which was increased in the presence of pelvic adhesions to 5.6 (95% CI 2.3–13.8).

Table 12-3. Selection Criteria: Tubal Surgery versus In Vitro Fertilization		
Surgical candidates	o	Mild hydrosalpinx
	o	Fimbrial damage only
	o	Absent or minimal adhesions
	o	Age < 35
	o	Normal male factor
	o	Preference of couple
IVF candidates	o	Moderate to severe hydrosalpinx
	o	Moderate to severe adhesions
	o	Reocclusion after surgery
	o	Age $\geq$ 36
	o	No conception 6 to 12 mo after surgery
	o	Prior ectopic pregnancy
	o	Abnormal male factor
	o	Preference of couple

Cost considerations become of paramount important in balancing the economic impact of the possibility for a repeat ectopic pregnancy in these patients against the likelihood of success.[97,98] The cost of ectopic pregnancies in 1995 was estimated to be over $1 billion, with direct costs for hospitalization contributing 77% of the total costs. Balanced against this cost and the risk of an ectopic pregnancy is the economic impact of pregnancy outcomes after in vitro fertilization. These costs are particularly impacted by the incidence of multiple gestation after IVF.

The comparison of these technologies to the incidence of multiple pregnancies and the potential impact for that on the family must also be considered in making a decision regarding the option for tubal surgery in patients in the above restricted category. Two cost analyses are noteworthy: cost of delivery and cost of achieving a pregnancy. The cost of a successful delivery after in vitro fertilization also increases from $66,000 for the first cycle of IVF to $140,000 by the sixth cycle. For more complicated cases in which the female partner is older than 35 years with a diagnosis of male factor, costs may rise from $160,000 for the first cycle to $800,000 for the sixth. The success rate of in vitro fertilization with this indication, and the reduced incidence of ectopic pregnancies after in vitro fertilization, make a compelling case for proceeding with in vitro fertilization in any patient with moderate or severe hydrosalpinges.[99] When all cost factors are taken into consideration, including costs of surgery and potential costs for ectopic pregnancy, the calculated cost per pregnancy after tubal surgery is approximately $17,000 compared with $17,000–20,000 after one cycle in vitro fertilization.[100] Life-table analyses also demonstrate a highly significant increased rate of delivery after IVF treatment (72% per patient) compared with tubal surgery (23%) when surgery is considered for *any* patient regardless of degree of tubal damage. When patient selection criteria are more rigorous and surgery restricted only to patients with minimal tubal damage, no pelvic adhesive disease, and normal male factor, pregnancy rates are comparable with in vitro fertilization. In this restricted setting, surgery also offers the advantage of avoidance of ovarian-stimulating drugs, ovarian hyperstimulation syndrome, and reduced multiples pregnancy rates and reduced cost per delivery.

Surgical Management

Definitions of distal repair vary, depending on the location of the obstruction. The surgical procedures for repair of distal tubal obstruction include fimbrioplasty (for partial obstruction), distal salpingostomy, or salpingoneostomy. Fimbrioplasty is dissection and lysis of bands of adhesive disease or phimosis that surround and partially occlude the fimbriated end of the tube. The procedure is performed by incising the serosal or constrictive ring on the distal tubal wall. In these circumstances, the fimbria beneath the adhesive bands are usually normal. A distal salpingostomy or salpingoneostomy is classified as either terminal, ampullary, or isthmic. A terminal or distal salpingostomy or neosalpingostomy is incision of an occluded distal tubal segment and reconstruction of the distal, fimbriated end of the tube. In these circumstances, the ampullary portion of the tube is preserved. Ampullary and isthmic salpingostomies are procedures involved in opening up tubal segments in the respective anatomic areas. The outcomes of these procedures have been consistently poor and have been abandoned with the advent of IVF. IVF should not be considered as the last option. It should be placed on the list of alternatives for the couple that has to make important decisions about future management, especially when the female partner is older than 35 years. *Proper patient selection is essential.*

Laparoscopic Distal Salpingostomy

The decision to proceed with any surgical procedure in the management of distal tubal obstruction depends on the degree of tubal damage and the extent of pelvic adhesive disease. Considerations include the probability of success (defined as a term delivery), avoidance of ectopic complications, and the financial costs of each method. There continues to be a distinct role, though restricted, for endoscopic distal salpingostomy for patients with mild tubal obstruction, as noted above. Endoscopic salpingostomy offers improved pregnancy rates over microsurgery, based on better patient selection, provided that surgical skill, equipment, and personnel are available.[101,103] Improved rates for endoscopic salpingostomy are secondary to patient selection. Patients with more favorable tubal architecture and limited tubal damage should be selected for an endoscopic procedure and those patients with more extensive damage referred for IVF. The endoscopic objective is the eversion and exposure of distal tubal mucosa and fixation of the serosa to maintain exposure.

Operative Technique

Chromotubation is first performed transcervically to gently distend the tube and better define the distal-most point of the occlusion. This maneuver frequently illustrates potential lines of dissection and cleavage at the distal point of occlusion. With this demonstration, the tube is gently grasped with laparoscopic grasping forceps at a 3 o'clock and 9 o'clock position, placing the tube on traction. A dilute vasopressin solution of 20 units in 20 mL of normal saline may be injected, and the point of convergence of the radial scars (i.e., clubbing) is identified. An incision is then made in the distal portion of the tube with either needle-tip cautery or a laser. The tube should be immobilized by using the countertraction of two opposing grasping forceps.

The distal portion of the tube is grasped with forceps and with use of a laser fiber, fine needle-tip cautery, or scissor tips, a cruciate incision is made to create an opening on the distal tubal segment. Inspection of the tubal lumen as described above should be carried out. If this mucosa is denuded or the tubal wall thickened, the procedure should be abandoned. If the mucosa and walls are normal, each flap is then folded over and, with use of a low-power setting, tacked to the underlying serosa at a distance of approximately 1 to 1.5 cm proximal to the original incision. Alternatively, the flaps may be sutured in place using fine absorbable suture.

Laparoscopic salpingostomy by an intussusception technique is a second, alternative endoscopic approach.[104] With use of gentle traction along the initial incision, the scissors may be inserted into the incision and the incision extended distally. Gentle traction should demonstrate the interior of the tube and intraluminal mucosa. The lateral portions of the distal tube may then be grasped and the incisions extended. With completion of the incisions on the distal tubal segments, the mucosa is gently grasped with one set of forceps and the distal edge of the incised tube grasped with the second. Gentle traction is placed to draw the serosa proximally and evert the mucosa. Further stabilization of the everted tubal mucosa may be achieved by placing isolated 6–0 polyglactin sutures through the flap.

339

Fimbrioplasty

At times, tubal damage may be limited to the fimbriae. Minimal damage to the ampulla and adhesive disease may involve only the very most distal portion of the tube and fimbria.[105–107] Minimal degrees of fimbrial damage in the form of fimbrial agglutination, encapsulation, or phimosis provide the most favorable clinical circumstances. These conditions are particularly amenable to repair by an endoscopic approach.

Operative Technique

Chromotubation and careful observation of the flow patterns at the distal segment may give important clues to the location of the adhesive bands. The distal portion of the tube should be grasped with fine atraumatic graspers. Gentle traction and countertraction using a second grasper is necessary to expose the adhesions and define the underlying fimbria. With use of a low-power cautery or laser, the bands of tissue adhesions may be lysed using two to four radial incisions on the mesosalpinx. Eversion of these flaps is then undertaken if necessary. Alternatively, the distal tubal lumen may be gently probed with laparoscopic scissors. The lumen is stretched with two grasping forceps gently exerting traction in opposite directions. This maneuver should provide immediate identification of scarred areas and adhesive areas in the distal tubal segments. The segments are then incised to allow eversion of the fimbria.

Repeated Tuboplasty

There is no role for a second tubal surgery. In patients who have undergone one distal repair, a second tuboplasty is not recommended. Intrauterine pregnancy rates of 8% to 10% apply.[108] In these circumstances, the most likely determining factor is the character of the distal tube. Patients who do not conceive after one surgery for mild tubal obstruction should be referred to IVF.

Postoperative Follow-Up

Depending on their ages, patients should be followed for 6 to 18 months. The longer follow-up interval in some studies led to an increased pregnancy rate.[109] The pregnancy rates do not fall to zero until after 36 to 72 months postoperatively (Figure 12-6). The duration of follow-up depends on the patient's age. For patients aged 35 years or younger, an interval of follow-up of 6 months is probably advisable. For patients aged 36 and older who elect surgery over IVF, a briefer follow-up interval is warranted, and the appropriate steps for using other assisted reproductive technologies should be made if the patient is not pregnant after 6 months.

Postoperative HSG reveals direct information only about tubal patency and rugal patterns and indirect information about adnexal adhesions. As an

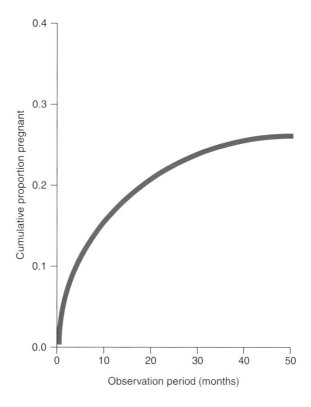

Figure 12-6   Cumulative pregnancy rates after distal salpingostomy.

assessment of postoperative status of the tubes, HSG has proven unreli-able,[110] and postoperative laparoscopy may be considered in select circumstances. Postoperatively, 60% of patients who undergo laparoscopy 4 to 16 weeks after tubal surgery have filmy avascular adhesions. Lysis of adhesions at this point has resulted in higher pregnancy rates. Sixty-three percent of patients who undergo laparoscopy more than 18 months after the original tubal operation have thicker neovascular adhesions. Laparoscopy or HSG after tubal surgery should be considered only in exceptional circumstances. If a patient is not pregnant after surgery and an appropriate follow-up interval, referral for IVF is appropriate.

Outcomes Analysis

The most critical aspect in the management of distal tubal obstruction is the decision regarding who is a surgical candidate and who is best referred for IVF (see Table 12-3).[93] Factors to be considered in deciding whether IVF or tubal surgery is appropriate include the condition of the tubes, the extent of pelvic adhesive disease, the age of the patient, the status of other fertility factors, and financial considerations.[91] For example, a couple with a mild hydrosalpinx and a favorable surgical profile but also with severe male factor would be best served by IVF and intracytoplasmic sperm injection (ICSI). Similarly, the couple with a mild hydrosalpinx, normal male factor, and neither the interest nor the financial means to pursue IVF should be managed surgically. Intrauterine pregnancy rates depend on the type of tubal damage repaired and, additional factors impacting fertility and the duration of follow-up.[43,108]

Pregnancy rates after distal salpingostomy vary considerably. These figures vary widely secondary to heterogeneous populations studied, failure to control for additional anatomic and endocrine factors that may contribute to success, and variable follow-up intervals. The greater number of variables considered, the more refined the prediction for any given patient. Studies in which no stratification of tubal disease is made describe success rates of 0 to 31%. Ectopic rates range from 30 to 18% and are similar regardless of the operative technique.[110,111] When additional factors are considered and controlled, a more clinically accurate picture emerges and a useful strategy may be developed. When the two factors of tubal diameter and extent of adhesions are considered, pregnancy rates range from 30 to 58%.[43,46,112] When these two factors plus condition of tubal mucosa and thickness of tubal wall are considered, pregnancy rates range from 30 to 47%. In both settings, when multiple factors were present, success was in very low single digits. By considering additional factors, therapy may be optimized and appropriate referral made (see Table 12-2). When the most favorable circumstances prevailed, for example, mild hydrosalpinx without adhesions, intrauterine pregnancy rates ranged from 50 to 80%.[46] Pregnancy rates for mild hydrosalpinx repaired by either endoscopic or microsurgical techniques are similar. A meta-analysis revealed no differences in pregnancy rates in patients matched for tubal damage and pelvic adhesive disease and for approach, that is, microsurgical versus laparoscopic repair.[54] Given the excellent results and cost-savings, any distal repair should be performed by laparoscopy. If the repair is complex, requiring laparotomy, surgery should not be performed. If complete tubal occlusion is not present but a small degree of impairment of the distal aspect is present, laparoscopic fimbrioplasty has been shown to result in cumulative pregnancy rates of 22, 35, and 58% at 6, 12, and 24 months, respectively.[106]

A 1- to 2-year follow-up may be required to determine the likelihood of success for distal tubal repair. Pregnancies continue to occur over as long as 5 years postoperatively. In clinical practice however, observation should be 6 months for patients older than 35 years. A follow-up interval of 1 year should be reserved for young patients with optimal tubal conditions and for whom IVF is not an option. In circumstances that are less than ideal, patients should be referred for IVF, especially when the patient's age exceeds 35 years.[112]

The role of tubal surgery is a debated point in contemporary management of distal tubal occlusion. Despite a distinct slant to assisted reproductive technologies, laparascopic repair is a cost-effective treatment for patients with mild tubal disease. The risks of ectopic pregnancies must be balanced against the risk of multiple pregnancies, ovarian hyperstimulation cost, and the complexity of ART.[113,114] In assessing the costs attendant to these procedures, focus should not only be on the likelihood of achieving success but also on the likelihood of achieving a complicated costly outcomes, such as an ectopic pregnancy or multiple pregnancy. Distal tubal repair is appropriate in the setting of mild distal obstruction/mild hydrosalpinx and when tubal obstruction is the only cause for the infertility. In circumstances where there are multiple factors contributing to infertility, IVF is the treatment. Unsuccessful surgery for tubal disease does not adversely impact the likelihood of success with in vitro fertilization, provided a limited postoperative observation is enforced and care is used in selecting patients based on age. The role of microsurgery and laparoscopic repair of distal tubal obstruction in any contemporary management paradigm is a debated point. In well-selected cases, outcomes with either surgical technique may achieve outcomes similar to IVF. Performed by skilled endoscopists and with proper patient selection, pregnancy rates of 40–60% (and as high as 80%) may be achieved. Because of this, the option of tubal surgery should be offered to all patients with favorable distal tubal obstruction.

Summary and Recommendations

Patients with distal tubal obstruction should be offered options tailored to their clinical unique circumstances. Any discussion with a couple should include consideration of the age of the female partner, the extent of tubal disease, previous surgical therapy, and the presence of any other associated factors that could influence outcome. Two additional factors that should be taken into consideration are the financial aspects of the assisted reproductive technologies, and the couple's personal attitudes regarding these technologies. On the basis of outcomes after distal tubal surgery and success rates for IVF, the following recommendations may be made.

- Factors that influence the success of a salpingostomy include the diameter of the hydrosalpinx, the appearance of the fimbria and tubal mucosa after eversion, and the degree of pelvic adhesive disease and rugal pattern on HSG.
- In the case of distal tubal occlusion, patients aged 35 and younger with mild tubal disease and minimal or no pelvic adhesive disease may be treated with operative laparoscopy and distal repair.
- Patients who are not candidates for surgery and patients who have reocclusion and have failed to conceive within 6 to 12 months postoperatively *or* have had an ectopic pregnancy after surgery should be referred for IVF.
- Surgery should not be considered for patients who have moderate or severe hydrosalpinx and moderate or severe pelvic adhesive disease. Care and counseling are essential in these circumstances.

- Surgery in any patient older than 36 years should be considered only after extensive counseling regarding outcomes, influence of age on fertility, IVF success, and cost.
- Removal of tubes or tubal ligation at the cornual junction should be considered for any patient with moderate to severe hydrosalpinx prior to referral for IVF.
- Considerations guiding any decision-making process are the probability of success (i.e., take home baby, live birth); the possible side effects attendant to tubal surgery or IVF, such as ectopic pregnancy, multiple births; complexity of ART; financial costs of each method; and the personal attitudes of the patient/couple regarding ART.

References

1. Martin A. Die krankenheiten der eileiter. Leipzig: Karger Press, 1895.

2. Seigler AM. Surgical treatments for tuboperitoneal causes of infertility since 1967. Fertil Steril 1977;28:1019–1032.

3. Marchetti AA, Kudger K, Kudger A. A clinical evaluation of ectopic pregnancy. Am J Obstet Gynecol 1946;10:544–555.

4. Holden FC, Sovak FW. Reconstruction of the oviducts: an improved technique with reports of cases. Am J Obstet Gynecol 1932;24:684–690.

5. Greenhill JP. Evaluation of salpingostomy and tubal implantation for treatment of sterility. Am J Obstet Gynecol 1937;33:39–45.

6. DeCherney AH. "The leader of the band is tired. . . . Fertil Steril 1985;44:299–302.

7. Holst N, Maltau JM, Forsdahl F, Hansen LJ. Handling of tubal infertility after introduction of in vitro fertilization: changes and consequences. Fertil Steril 1991;55:140–143.

8. Penzias AS, DeCherney AH. Is there ever a role for tubal surgery? Am J Obstet Gynecol 1996;174:1218–1221.

9. Lilford RJ, Watson AJ. Has in-vitro fertilization made salpingostomy obsolete? Br J Obstet Gynaecol 1990;97:557–560.

10. Bateman BG, Nunley WC Jr, Kitchin JD 3rd. Surgical management of distal tubal obstruction–are we making progress? Fertil Steril 1987;48:523–542.

11. Thonneau P, Quesnot S, Ducot B, et al. Risk factors for female and male infertility: results of a case-control study. Hum Reprod 1992;7:55–58.

12. Grodstein F, Goldman MB, Cramer DW. Relation of tubal infertility to history of sexually transmitted diseases. Am J Epidemiol 1993;137:577–584.

13. Kessel E. Pelvic inflammatory disease with intrauterine device use: a reassessment. Fertil Steril 1984;51:1–11.

14. Kirshon B, Poindexter AN 3rd, Spitz MR. Pelvic adhesions and intrauterine device users. Obstet Gynecol 1988;71:251–254.

15. Vessey MP, Yeates D, Flavel R, McPherson K. Pelvic inflammatory disease and the intrauterine device: findings in a large cohort study. Br Med J (Clin Res Ed) 1981;282:855–857.

16. Maqueo MT, Calderon JJ, Guerra AZ. Salpingitis associated with the presence of nonmedicated IUDs. Contraception 1979;19:539–542.

17. McBean JH, Brumsted JR. Pregnancy after laparoscopic neosalpingostomy in a patient with atresia of the distal fallopian tubes. Fertil Steril 1994;61:1163–1164.

18. Okamura H, Morikawa H, Oshima M, et al. A morphological and physiological study of mesotubarium ovarica in humans. Int J Fertil 1977;22:179–183.

19. Halbert SA, McComb PF, Patton DL. Function and structure of the rabbit oviduct following fimbriectomy. I. Distal ampullary salpingostomy. Fertil Steril 1981;35:349–354.

20. Odor DL, Blandau RJ. EGG transport over the fimbrial surface of the rabbit oviduct under experimental conditions. Fertil Steril 1973;24:292–300.

21. Halbert SA, Patton DL. Ovum pick-up following fimbriectomy and infundibular salpingostomy in rabbits. J Reprod Med 1981;26:299–304.

22. Hull MG. Epidemiology of tubal infertility: how to judge results. Ref Gynecol Obstet 1995;2:14–19.

23. Canis M, Mage G, Pouly JL, et al. Laparoscopic distal tuboplasty: report of 87 cases and a 4-year experience. Fertil Steril 1991;56:616–621.

24. Bevan CD, Johal BJ, Mumtaz G, et al. Clinical, laparoscopic and microbiological findings in acute salpingitis: report on a United Kingdom cohort. Br J Obstet Gynaecol 1995;102:407–414.

25. Westrom LV. Sexually transmitted diseases and infertility. Sex Transm Dis 1994;21(suppl):S32–S37.

26. Czerwenka K, Heuss F, Hosmann J, et al. Salpingitis caused by *Chlamydia trachomatis* and its significance for infertility. Acta Obstet Gynecol Scand 1994;73:711–715.

27. Patton DL, Askienazy-Elbhar M, Henry-Suchet J, et al. Detection of *Chlamydia trachomatis* in fallopian tube tissue in women with postinfectious tubal infertility. Am J Obstet Gynecol 1994;171:95–101.

28. Bevan CD, Johal BJ, Mumtaz G, et al. Clinical, laparoscopic and microbiological findings in acute salpingitis: report on a United Kingdom cohort. Br J Obstet Gynaecol 1995;102:407–414.

29. Soper DE, Brockwell NJ, Dalton HP, Johnson D. Observations concerning the microbial etiology of acute salpingitis. Am J Obstet Gynecol 1994;170:1008–1014.

30. Witkin SS, Jeremias J, Toth M, Ledger WJ. Cell-mediated immune response to the recombinant 57-kDa heat-shock protein of *Chlamydia trachomatis* in women with salpingitis. J Infect Dis 1993;167:1379–1383.

31. Dieterle S, Wollenhaupt J. Humoral immune response to the chlamydial heat shock proteins hsp60 and hsp70 in *Chlamydia*-associated chronic salpingitis with tubal occlusion. Hum Reprod 1996;11:1352–1356.

32. Witkin SS, Jeremias J, Toth M, Ledger WJ. Proliferative response to conserved epitopes of the *Chlamydia trachomatis* and human 60-kilodalton heat-shock proteins by lymphocytes from women with salpingitis. Am J Obstet Gynecol 1994;171:455–460.

33. Westrom L. Incidence, prevalence and trends of acute pelvic inflammatory disease and its consequences in industrialized countries. Am J Obstet Gynecol 1980;138:880–892.

34. Fleming C, Hull MG. Impaired implantation after in vitro fertilisation treatment associated with hydrosalpinx. Br J Obstet Gynaecol 1996;103:268–272.

35. Sharara FI, Scott RT Jr, Marut EL, Queenan JT Jr. In-vitro fertilization outcome in women with hydrosalpinx. Hum Reprod 1996;11:526–530.

36. Voss E, Boldes R, Stark M. Impaired implantation after in vitro fertilisation treatment associated with hydrosalpinx [letter]. Br J Obstet Gynaecol 1996;103:851.

37. Chen CD, Yang JH, Lin KC, et al. The significance of cytokines, chemical composition, and murine embryo development in hydrosalpinx fluid for predicting the IVF outcome in women with hydrosalpinx. Hum Reprod 2002;17:128–133.

38. Blazar AS, Hogan JW, Seifer DB, et al. The impact of hydrosalpinx on successful pregnancy in tubal factor infertility treated by in vitro fertilization. Fertil Steril 1997;67:517–520.

39. Oehninger S, Scott R, Muasher SJ, et al. Effects of the severity of tubo-ovarian disease and previous tubal surgery on the results of in vitro fertilization and embryo transfer. Fertil Steril 1989;51:126–130.

40. Strandell A. How to treat hydrosalpinges: IVF as the treatment of choice. Reprod Biomed Online 2002;3:37–39.

41. Gauwerky JF, Forssmann WG, Kurz M, et al. Hydrosalpinx formation and its regeneration after microsurgical reconstruction – a functional and morphological study on rabbits. Human Reprod 1994;9:2090–2102.

42. Larsson B. Late results of salpingostomy combined with salpingolysis and ovariolysis by electromicroscopy in 54 women. Fertil Steril 1982;37:156–160.

43. Rock JA, Katayama KP, Martin EJ, et al. Factors influencing the success of salpingostomy techniques for distal fimbrial obstruction. Obstet Gynecol 1978;52:591–596.

44. Johnson NP, Sadler L, Merrilees M. IVF and tubal pathology – not all bad news. Aust N Z J Obstet Gynaecol 2002;42:285–288.

45. Shirodkar VN. Factors influencing the results of salpingostomy. Int J Fertil 1966;11:361–365.

46. Boer-Meisel ME, te Velde ER, Habbema JD, Kardaun JW. Predicting the pregnancy outcome in patients treated for hydrosalpinx: a prospective study. Fertil Steril 1986;45:23–29.

47. Aboulghar MA, Mansour RT, Serour GI. Controversies in the modern management of hydrosalpinx. Hum Reprod Update 1998;4:882–890.

48. Mage G, Pouly JL, de Joliniere JB, et al. A preoperative classification to predict the intrauterine and ectopic pregnancy rates after distal tubal microsurgery. Fertil Steril 1986;46:807–810.

49. American Fertility Society. The American Fertility Society classification of adnexal adhesions, distal tubal occlusion, tubal occlusions secondary to tubal ligation, tubal pregnancies, Müllerian abnormalities, and intrauterine adhesions. Fertil Steril 1988;49:944–955.

50. Donnez J, Casanas-Roux F. Prognostic factors of fimbrial microsurgery. Fertil Steril 1986;46:200–204.

51. Loy RA, DeCherney AH. The impact of assisted reproductive technologies on surgery of the fallopian tube. Semin Reprod Endocrinol 1990;8:304–312.

52. Singhal V, Li TC, Cooke ID. An analysis of factors influencing the outcome of 232 consecutive tubal microsurgery cases. Br J Obstet Gynaecol 1991;98:628–636.

53. Winston RM. Microsurgery of the fallopian tube: from fantasy to reality. Fertil Steril 1980;34:521–530.

54. Schlaff WD, Hassiakos DK, Damewood MD, Rock JA. Neosalpingostomy for distal tubal obstruction: prognostic factors and impact of surgical technique. Fertil Steril 1990;54:984–990.

55. Verhoeven HC, Berry H, Frantzen C, Schlosser HW. Surgical treatment for distal tubal occlusion. A review of 167 cases. J Reprod Med 1983;28:293–304.

56. Kitchin JD 3rd, Nunley WC Jr, Bateman BG. Surgical management of distal tubal occlusion. Am J Obstet Gynecol 1986;155:524–531.

57. Scudamore IW, Dunphy BC, Cooke ID. Outpatient falloposcopy: intra-luminal imaging of the fallopian tube by trans-uterine fibre-optic endoscopy as an outpatient procedure. Br J Obstet Gynaecol 1992;99:829–835.

58. Hu D, Hook EW, Goldie SJ. Screening for *Chlamydia trachomatis* in women 15 to 29 years. Ann Intern Med 2004;141:501–513.

59. Veenemans LM, van der Linden PJ. The value of *Chlamydia trachomatis* antibody testing in predicting tubal factor fertility. Hum Reprod 2002;17:695–698.

60. Mouton JW, Peeters MF, van Rijssort-Vos JH, Verkooyen RP. Tubal factor pathology caused by *Chlamydia trachomatis*: the role of serology. Int J STD AIDS 2002;13 Suppl 2:26–29.

61. Minassian SS, Wu CH. *Chlamydia* antibody by enzyme-linked immunosorbent assay and associated severity of tubal factor infertility. Fertil Steril 1992;58:1245–1247.

62. Collins JI, Woodward PJ. Radiological evaluation of infertility. Semin Ultrasound CT MR 1995;16:304–316.

63. Atri M, Tran CN, Bret PM, et al. Accuracy of endovaginal sonography for the detection of fallopian tube blockage. J Ultrasound Med 1994;13:429–434.

64. Mitri FF, Andronikou AD, Perpinyal S, et al. A clinical comparison of sonographic hydrotubation and hysterosonography. Br J Obstet Gynaecol 1991;98:1031–1036.

65. Chenn YM, Zagoria RJ. Normal radiographic anatomy. In: Ott DJ, Fayez JA, eds. Hysterosalpingography: a text and atlas. Baltimore, MD: Urban and Schwarzenberg 1991:33–46.

66. Edelman RR, Warach S. Magnetic resonance imaging (2). N Engl J Med 1993;328:785–791.

67. Outwater EK, Talerman A, Dunton C. Normal adnexa uteri specimens: anatomic basis of MR imaging features. Radiology 1996;201:751–755.

68. Karande VC, Pratt DE, Rabin DS, Gleicher N. The limited value of hysterosalpingography in assessing tubal status and fertility potential. Fertil Steril 1995;63:1167–1171.

69. Mol BW, Swart P, Bossuyt PM, et al. Reproducibility of the interpretation of hysterosalpingography in the diagnosis of tubal pathology. Hum Reprod 1996;11:1204–1208.

70.   Rowling SE, Ramchandani P. Imaging of the fallopian tubes. Semin Roentgenol 1996;31:299–311.

71.   Swart P, Mol BW, van der Veen F, et al. The accuracy of hysterosalpingography in the diagnosis of tubal pathology: a meta-analysis. Fertil Steril 1995;64:486–491.

72.   Soliman S, Daya S, Collins J, Jarrell J. A randomized trial of in vitro fertilization versus conventional treatment for infertility. Fertil Steril 1993;59:1239–1244.

73.   Dubuisson JB, Chapron C, Morice P, et al. Laparoscopic salpingostomy: fertility results according to the tubal mucosal appearance. Hum Reprod 1994;9:334–339.

74.   Strandell A, Lindhard A, Waldenstrom U, Thorburn J. Hydrosalpinx and IVF outcome: cumulative results after salpingectomy in a randomized controlled trial. Hum Reprod 2001;16:2403–2410.

75.   Johnson NP, Mak W, Sowter MC. Laparoscopic salpingectomy for women with hydrosalpinges enhances the success of IVF: a Cochrane review. Hum Reprod 2002;17: 543–548.

76.   Strandell A, Lindhard A. Why does hydrosalpinx reduce fertility? The importance of hydrosalpinx fluid. Hum Reprod 2002;17:1141–1145.

77.   Bontis JN, Dinas KD. Management of hydrosalpinx: reconstructive surgery or IVF? Ann NY Acad Sci 2000:900;260–271.

78.   Heylen SM, Brosens IA, Puttemans PJ. Clinical value and cumulative pregnancy rates following rigid salpingoscopy during laparoscopy for infertility. Hum Reprod 1995;10:2913–2916.

79.   Scudamore IW, Dunphy BC, Bowman M, et al. Comparison of ampullary assessment by falloposcopy and salpingoscopy. Hum Reprod 1994;9:1516–1518.

80.   Sueoka K, Asada H, Tsuchiya S, et al. Falloposcopic tuboplasty for bilateral tubal occlusion. A novel infertility treatment as an alternative for in-vitro fertilization? Hum Reprod 1998;13:71–74.

81.   Dunphy B, Pattinson HA. Office falloposcopy; a tertiary level assessment for planning the management of infertile women. Aust N Z J Obstet Gynaecol 1994;34:189–190.

82.   Marana R, Rizzi M, Muzii L, et al. Correlation between the American Fertility Society classifications of adnexal adhesions and distal tubal occlusion, salpingoscopy, and reproductive outcome in tubal surgery. Fertil Steril 1995;64:924–929.

83.   Watrelot A, Dreyfus JM, Cohen M. Systematic salpingoscopy and microsalpingoscopy during fertiloscopy. J Am Assoc Gynecol Laparosc 2002;9:453–459.

84.   Andersen AN, Lindhard A, Loft A, et al. The infertile patient with hydrosalpinges – IVF with or without salpingectomy ? Hum Reprod 1996;11:2081–2084.

85.   Ajonuma LC, Ng EH, Chan HC. New insights into the mechanisms underlying hydrosalpinx fluid formation and its adverse effect on IVF outcome. Hum Reprod Update 2002;8(3):255–264.

86.   Dechaud H, Anahory T, Aligier N, et al. Salpingectomy for repeated embryo nonimplantation after in vitro fertilization in patients with severe tubal factor infertility. J Assist Reprod Genet 2000;17:200–206.

87.   Dechaud H. Hydrosalpinx and ART: hydrosalpinges suitable for salpingectomy before IVF. Hum Reprod 2000;15:2464–2465.

88.   Johnson NP, Mak W, Sowter MC. Surgical treatment for tubal disease in women due to undergo in vitro fertilisation. Cochrane Database Syst Rev 2001;CD002125.

89.   Hassiakos DK, Muasher SJ, Veeck LL, Jones HW Jr. In vitro fertilization: effective alternative to surgery for distal tubal occlusion. Va Med Q 1991;118:26–30.

90.   Jones HW Jr. The impact of in vitro fertilization on the practice of gynecology and obstetrics. Int J Fertil 1986;31:99, 102–105, 109–111.

91.   Lilford RJ, Watson AJ. Has in vitro fertilization made salpingostomy obsolete? Br J Obstet Gynaecol 1990;97:557–560.

92.   Holst N, Maltau JM, Forsdahl F, Hansen LJ. Handling of tubal infertility after introduction of in vitro fertilization: changes and consequences. Fertil Steril 1991;55:140–143.

93.   Paterson PJ. Indications for the treatment of tubal infertility patients by microsurgery or in vitro fertilization. Aust N Z J Obstet Gynaecol 1984;24:262–264.

94.   Penzias AS, DeCherney AH. Is there ever a role for tubal surgery? Am J Obstet Gynecol 1996;174:1218–1221.

95.   Benadiva CA, Kligman I, Davis O, Rosenwaks Z. In vitro fertilization versus tubal surgery: is pelvic reconstructive surgery obsolete? Fertil Steril 1995;64:1051–1061.

96.   Callahan TL, Hall JE, Ettner SL, et al. The economic impact of multiple-gestation pregnancies and the contribution of assisted-reproduction techniques to their incidence. N Engl J Med 1994;331:244–249.

97.   Neumann PJ, Gharib SD, Weinstein MC. The cost of a successful delivery with in vitro fertilization. N Engl J Med 1994;331:239–243.

98.   Winston RM, Margara RA. Microsurgical salpingostomy is not an obsolete procedure. Br J Obstet Gynaecol 1991;98:637–642.

99.   Washington AE, Katz P. Ectopic pregnancy in the United States: economic consequences and payment source trends. Obstet Gynecol 1993;81:287–292.

100.   Koivurova S, Hartikianen AL, Gissler M, et al. Health care costs resulting from IVF. Human Reprod 2004;23:1141–1149.

101.   Fayez JA. An assessment of the role of operative laparoscopy in tuboplasty. Fertil Steril 1983;39:476–479.

102.   Daniell JF, Herbert CM. Laparoscopic salpingostomy utilizing the CO_2 laser. Fertil Steril 1984;41:558–563.

103.   Gomel V, Swolin K. Salpingostomy: microsurgical technique and results. Clin Obstet Gynecol 1980;23:1243–1258.

104.   McComb PF, Paleologou A. The intussusception salpingostomy technique for the therapy of distal oviductal occlusion at laparoscopy. Obstet Gynecol 1991;78:443–447.

105.   Dlugi AM, Reddy S, Saleh WA, et al. Pregnancy rates after operative endoscopic treatment of total (neosalpingostomy) or near total (salpingostomy) distal tubal occlusion. Fertil Steril 1994;62:913–920.

106.   Saleh WA, Dlugi AM. Pregnancy outcome after laparoscopic fimbrioplasty in nonocclusive distal tubal disease. Fertil Steril 1997;67:474–480.

107.   Audebert AJ, Pouly JL, Von Theobald P. Laparoscopic fimbrioplasty: an evaluation of 35 cases. Hum Reprod 1998;13:1496–1499.

108.   Thie JL, Williams TJ, Coulam CB. Repeat tuboplasty compared with primary microsurgery for postinflammatory tubal disease. Fertil Steril 1986;45:784–787.

109.   Russell JB, DeCherney AH, Laufer N, et al. Neosalpingostomy: comparison of 24– and 72–month follow-up time shows increased pregnancy rate. Fertil Steril 1986;45:296–298.

110.   Letterie GS, Haggerty MF, Fellows DW. Sensitivity of hysterosalpingography after tubal surgery. Arch Gynecol Obstet 1992;251:175–80.

111.   Tomazevic T, Ribic-Pucelj M. Ectopic pregnancy following the treatment of tubal infertility. J Reprod Med 1992;37:611–614.

112.   Holst N, Maltau JM, Forsdahl F, Hansen LJ. Handling of tubal infertility after introduction of in vitro fertilization: changes and consequences. Fertil Steril 1991;55:140–143.

113.   Benadiva CA, Klingman I, Davis O, Rosenwaks Z. In vitro fertilization versus tubal surgery: is pelvic reconstructive surgery obsolete? Fertil Steril 1995;64:1051–1061.

114.   Collins JA, Bustillo M, Visscher RD, Lawrence LD. An estimate of the cost of in vitro fertilization services in the United States in 1995. Fertil Steril 1995;64:538–545.

13 *Proximal Tubal Obstruction*

By means of a hollow silver tube . . . the point of the instrument was conveyed to the corner of the uterus and made to pass into the tube.
— W. Tyler Smith, 1848

Obstruction of the proximal tube has been a well-recognized entity in gynecology since the early 1800s. A technique for tubal cannulation to relieve proximal tubal obstruction (PTO) was described in the mid-1800s. Forward thinking and insightful, Smith attempted to cannulate proximally obstructed fallopian tubes by using a whale bone bougie in 1849.[1] The procedure was described as "a new uterine operation" (Figure 13-1) and, ironically, is an early, rudimentary form of selective salpingography and transcervical cannulation. Smith's procedure relied on tactile feedback as the bougie was advanced through the cervix and uterus. Though not widely used, its importance was in the concept of mechanical dilatation of proximally obstructed tubes. Management for PTO varied considerably as surgical techniques evolved but remained problematic and frustrating for clinicians. In 1896, the first tubal implantation was performed by Watkins in a patient with a myoma blocking the uterotubal junction. After the procedure, a pregnancy was reported but ended in a miscarriage.[2] In 1921, a case report described a uterotubal implantation that resulted in the first living child after this procedure.[3] However, success after surgical repair remained uniformly poor, prompting investigations to bypass the tube entirely. With this intent, Estes

---

THE NEW UTERINE OPERATION.

ON A
NEW METHOD OF TREATING STERILITY, BY THE REMOVAL OF OBSTRUCTIONS OF THE FALLOPIAN TUBES.
By W. TYLER SMITH, M.D.,
LECTURER ON OBSTETRICS AND THE DISEASES OF WOMEN IN THE HUNTERIAN SCHOOL OF MEDICINE.

Figure 13-1   Announcement of a new uterine operation, the initial description of fallopian tube cannulation in 1849.

described a procedure for direct approximation of the ovary into a uterine window (Estes' operation). It was abandoned because of poor outcomes. A similar procedure involved placement of the ovary into the uterine cavity (Tuffier's procedure) and had similar poor results.[4]

Despite poor outcomes and pregnancy rates ranging from 0% to 30%, the lack of alternative therapies prompted a continued interest in tubal implantation procedures through the 1940s.[5] This technique consisted of implantation of the ampullae directly into the uterus. In 1961, van Ikle described an isthmic implantation into a small cornual aperture.[6] In 1965, Ehrler found that in proximal tubal obstruction the intramural segment is rarely affected and usually patent.[7,8] These findings, along with the concept that as much tube as possible should be preserved, led to the suggestion that tubocornual anastomosis was the optimal procedure.

Advances in microsurgery led to the abandonment of implantation procedures in favor of the less invasive anastomosis. Descriptions of several different techniques, understanding of tubal physiology, and the success of in vitro fertilization (IVF) have significantly changed the approach to diagnosis and therapy for PTO. Transcervical fallopian tube cannulation and selective salpingography for diagnosis and treatment of proximal tubal disease have become well-established tools. The procedures are clinically effective, minimally invasive, and cost-effective. Furthermore, continued improvements in equipment and methodology improve technique and outcomes. Assisted reproductive technologies have led to the abandonment of microsurgical procedures for PTO after failed canalization or recurrent obstruction. If obstruction persists after a canalization, IVF is the next step. This chapter discusses patient selection for intervention, defines the role that fallopian tube cannulation has in the management of PTO, and describes populations most likely to benefit from IVF.

Etiology

PTO is the cause of infertility in 20% of women with tubal disease.[9] PTO is the blockage of the intramural, isthmic, or both portions of the fallopian tube. The obstruction may extend for a variable distance and include a portion of or the entire intramural segment and, in some circumstances, a portion of proximal isthmic tube. The extent of obstruction has important clinical implications. The intramural portion of the tube has crucial functions and is divided into a proximal 1-cm segment and a distal 1.5-cm segment. These two portions of the intramural tube are clearly distinct from the isthmic portion of the fallopian tube.

A crucial aspect of PTO was proposed in 1954 by Ruben, who described the potential differences between tubal obstruction and tubal occlusion in an article on uterotubal insufflation.[10] Tubal occlusion may be secondary to complete obliteration of the tubal lumen, as may occur with fibrosis and is not amenable to conservative therapy. Tubal obstruction may be reversible and secondary to the presence of debris in the lumen or tubal spasm. The architecture of the tubal lumen is preserved. Differentiation between occlusion and obstruction is important for clinical management: patients with true occlusion or blockage are best managed with IVF; those with obstruction secondary to intraluminal debris are best managed with fallopian tube cannulation as first-line therapy.[11] Contemporary use of these terms may be confusing. Proximal tubal obstruction or occlusion are frequently used interchangeably to denote any blockage of the proximal tube despite having different clinical implications. The more traditional term proximal tubal obstruction is used throughout this chapter.

Proximal tubal obstruction is not a homogeneous condition. Causes of PTO are diverse and include spasm in the cornual portion of the tube, technical difficulties resulting in underfilling of the uterine cavity and insufficient intrauterine pressure during hysterosalpingography (HSG), obstruction of the intramural portion of the tube by debris or occlusive plugs, adhesions at the tubal ostia, and salpingitis isthmica nodosa (SIN).[12] These are potentially reversible. True occlusion of the proximal tube occurs because of fibrosis and obliteration of the tubal lumen. This entity is not reversible.

The histology of obstruction is unique in that in 40 to 60% of patients with clinical PTO, the tubal lumen is patent when studied histologically.[13] There is no evidence of the chronic inflammation characteristic of distal tubal obstructions. In specimens demonstrating a histologic basis for the obstruction, the spectrum of histologic changes is broad. Data on the histology of the proximal tubal segment in these patients describe inflammation involved in 25%, SIN in 25 to 30% (see Chapter 14), and endometriosis in 10 to 15%.[12,13] The prevalence of a discrete plug of amorphous material resulting in proximal tubal obstruction is as high as 75%.[14,15] The debris is of unknown etiology and often appears as casts (Figure 13-2). Such plugs may have no clearly established clinical origin. Such obstruction may be treatable by selective salpingography or cannulation. There is also the phenomenon of tubal spasm or pseudo-obstruction. This spasm may explain the presence of histologically normal tubes despite a patient's history of multiple preoperative examinations showing the obstruction. Apparent proximal tubal obstruction has been associated with a 60% incidence of histologically normal proximal segments.[13] This finding is significant and has important clinical implications.

The concept that proximal tubal obstruction may be artifactual and secondary to spasm and clinically insignificant is open to question based on selective salpingography and tubal perfusion pressure studies. A finding of proximal tubal obstruction on one HSG and its disappearance on subsequent studies suggests that either the tube was under spasm secondary to the HSG or that intermittent obstruction is present. The latter would suggest significant

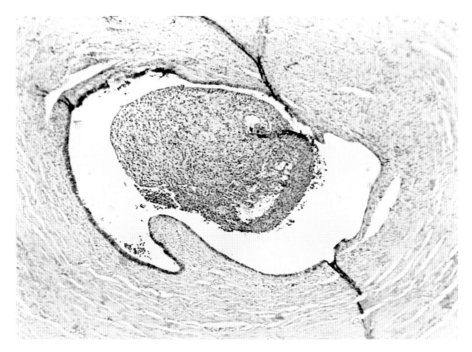

Figure 13-2   Histology of proximal tubal obstruction demonstrating amorphous material in the lumen of the proximal segment of the tube.

proximal tubal disease warranting further evaluation.[16–19] Patients who have intermittent spasm resulting in proximal tubal obstruction on one HSG with patency on another may in fact have significant underlying proximal tubal disease.[19] An assessment of the functional status of the tube with tubal perfusion pressures in this setting suggests decreased tubal wall compliance. These patients have low pregnancy rates despite successful canalization. Intermittent obstruction suggests intrinsic tubal disease. Assessment of intratubal pressure and patency status before and after transcervical canalization suggests that intratubal pressure in freely patent tubes was 0.3 ± 0.06 atmospheres, in partially obstructed tubes 1.23 ± 0.52 atmospheres and in completely obstructed tubes 2.79 ± 1.4 atmospheres. After canalization, these values are decreased in partially obstructed tubes too 0.64 ± 0.3 atmospheres and in completely obstructed tubes to 1.86 ± 1.3 atmospheres. Assessment of intratubal pressures represents one method of refining diagnosis and therapy for proximately tubal obstruction.[20,21]

Clinical Correlates

PTO is a silent process with no overt clinical manifestation. The abnormalities come to clinical attention only in the evaluation for infertility. In some cases of proximal obstruction secondary to SIN, a nodular, somewhat swollen appearance to the proximal portion of the tube may be noted at laparoscopy or as a characteristic honeycomb appearance on HSG.

Two classification systems of proximal tubal obstruction have been proposed, both intended to assist the clinician and the patient in deciding upon the appropriate therapy (catheterization/cannulation or IVF). To this end, it is important to differentiate tubal occlusion from tubal obstruction. The latter is reversible and correctable through conservative techniques. The former is far more difficult to manage and requires IVF. The first classification scheme for proximal tubal obstruction is based on the appearance of the tubal isthmus and isthmic–cornual junction.[22,23] This system is based on results of falloposcopy and laparoscopy and classifies proximal tubal obstruction into three categories. Category 1 is non-nodular or complete fibrotic occlusion resulting from an inflammatory process; category 2 is nodular obstruction such as that which results from salpingitis isthmica nodosa or endometriosis; and category 3 is tubal obstruction resulting from polyps or amorphous debris within the tubal lumen. These classifications enable the categorization of proximal tubal obstruction into entities that are best managed by tubal cannulation, or IVF (category 1); are amenable to medical management using GnRH analogs (category 2); or tubal cannulation and catheterization (category 3).

The second system is based on the anatomic site of obstruction, whether intraluminal, intramural, or extramural. Intraluminal occlusion is secondary to debris, polyps, amorphous plugs, or parasitic infections.[24] Intramural occlusion includes abnormalities in the mucosa, muscularis, and serosa, such as muscular spasm, fibrosis, salpingitis isthmica nodosa, endometriosis, and congenital atresia. Extramural abnormalities include leiomyomas, intrauterine synechiae, and osteal polyps that block the opening of the proximal tube into the uterus. This classification system also provides a means of differentiating those patients who would benefit from cannulation or IVF. Neither system has been evaluated regarding its predictive power nor been formally adopted. Entities such as mucosal agglutination, amorphous debris, or muscle spasm are most likely to respond to cannulation. Chronic salpingitis, salpingitis isthmica nodosa, and endometriosis are less likely to respond. Luminal fibrosis, leiomyomas, or any occlusion secondary to infectious processes rarely respond to cannulation techniques.

Bipolar obstruction involves blockage at both proximal and distal tubal segments. In patients who have both proximal and distal tubal disease, referral for IVF should be made. Results after combined surgery of the distal and proximal tubal segments have been uniformly poor.[25] A combination of fallopian tube catheterization for proximal obstruction and microsurgery for distal obstruction has also been poor.

Diagnosis

The most common method of diagnosis of PTO is HSG (Figures 13-3 and 13-4). Unlike distal obstruction in which tubal dilatation might be incidentally detected on ultrasound or MRI, PTO is not detected as a finding incidental to an evaluation initiated for other indications. It is identified only as part of an evaluation for infertility. PTO is seen on 10 to 20% of hysterosalpingograms. One shortcoming of HSG is that it does not reliably differentiate potential spasm from obstruction or occlusion. Because underfilling of the tube, tubal spasm, and mechanical obstruction from a variety of causes cannot be differentiated (false positive) from obstruction or occlusion (true positive) on HSG, a false-positive finding by HSG of PTO must be considered when proximal obstruction is demonstrated. Methods to differentiate true occlusion from functional obstruction of the fallopian tubes to reduce false positives include the use of prostaglandin antagonists such as aspirin and β_2 agonists such as terbutaline in addition to diazepam, glucagon, amyl nitrate, and morphine (see Chapter 3). All remain in clinical use. None are reliable.

The difficulties in relying solely on HSG to diagnose PTO are made clear when eligibility criteria for early studies on fallopian tube cannulation are studied. The criteria for these studies included at least two previous HSG studies, chromotubation, or both at laparoscopy to fulfill the diagnosis of

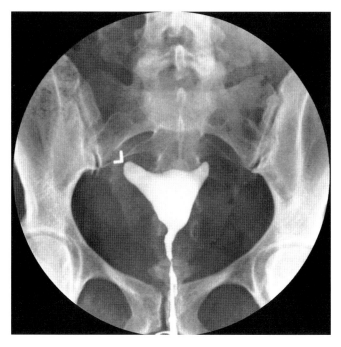

Figure 13-3   Hysterosalpingogram demonstrating bilateral proximal tubal obstruction. No filling of any segment of the proximal tube can be defined in this study.

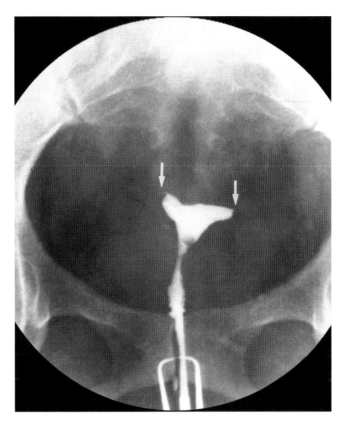

Figure 13-4   Hysterosalpingogram demonstrating complete proximal obstruction on
                     left and filling of a short portion of the intramural segment on right
                     (arrows).

PTO. In these studies, 20% of patients had at least one patent tube at the time
of HSG performed as part of transcervical balloon tuboplasty.[25] The false-
positive rate for PTO on HSG is as high as 25%. Despite several different
spasmolytic agents at the time of HSG, the false-positive rate for PTO
remains a clinical problem. Determination of tubal perfusion pressures may
reduce this incidence by identifying tubal pathology underlying intermittent
PTO.[19,20]

Excessive injection pressures may lead to the occurrence of iatrogenically
introduced cornual spasm, and to a false positive. However, using proper techniques for HSG, the presence of proximal obstruction when a subsequent
study reveals proximal patency can be considered intermittent tubal occlusion.
This may suggest significant proximal tubal disease as noted above and warrants further evaluation with more sophisticated diagnostic studies, including
selective salpingography and assessment of tubal perfusion pressures.

Selective salpingography is a technique to assess proximal patency by differentiating occlusion from obstruction (Figure 13-5).[26,27] Proximal obstruction

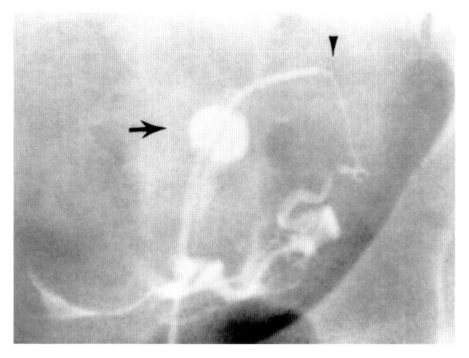

Figure 13-5   Selective salpingography with half-strength contrast media filling the intrauterine balloon (arrow) and with coaxial catheter in the proximal tubal segment (arrowhead).

diagnosed on HSG should be substantiated by repeat HSG or by laparoscopy and chromotubation. One practical approach to the patient with PTO evident by only one HSG is to evaluate the proximal segment with repeat hysteros-alpingogram with the immediate availability of selective salpingography and tubal cannulation or laparoscopy, chromotubation, and hysteroscopic cannulation if the obstruction is again demonstrated. Sonohysterography has been used to assess proximal tubal patency with an enhanced microbubble contrast medium. Injection of the contrast medium under transvaginal ultrasound guidance has a specificity of 96% and sensitivity of 68% in the evaluation of proximal tubal patency.[28–30] As an adjunct in evaluation of PTO, falloposcopy may be performed to assess the lumen and mucosa of the proximal tube segments and more accurately characterize any tubal pathology. This approach provides additional information to guide decision-making and referral for IVF.[31,32]

Management

Microsurgical tubocornual anastomosis and tubal implantation have been the mainstays of surgical management for PTO.[33,34] However, the options of tubal cannulation and IVF have nearly eliminated the need for either surgery. Management may be based upon reference to classification systems described above to provide guidance in deciding which therapy is most efficacious and cost-effective. Contemporary management should include initial attempts at establishing patency with selective salpingography and progress to cannulation with fluoroscopic, ultrasound, or hysteroscopic guidance techniques.[35] In patients with proximal obstruction successfully canalized, approximately 40% of pregnancies will occur after the first 12 months following selective salpingography and tubal catheterization. The presence of any additional causes of infertility should not be regarded as an absolute contraindication to tubal canalization. If unsuccessful, IVF is the best option and in select cases (for example, religious or ethical objections to IVF), microsurgical anastomosis. This management plan represents the most cost-effective approach for PTO, progressing from the most conservative to the most aggressive and costly options.

Despite marked changes in the spectrum of therapies and abandonment of surgery, some patients refuse IVF and do require a surgical approach. The surgical option is rarely if ever exercised. It is included in this discussion for completeness and in consideration of unique circumstances of some couples. In these rare circumstances in which IVF is not an option, tubal implantation has yielded to microsurgical tubocornual anastomosis as a primary surgical management.[35,36] For these cases two prognostic factors are tubal length at conclusion of surgery, and the histology of the excised segment.[32-34] The intent of any surgical approach to PTO should be to maximize tubal length and, most importantly, preserve as much of the intramural segment as possible. The remaining tubal length is in part a reflection of the extent to which the intramural tube is occluded, and the length of the resected tube correlates directly with subsequent fertility. The histology of the resected portions of tube also provides insight into outcome. Pregnancy rates vary from 60% for fibrosis to 17% for chronic salpingitis.[32] The most favorable surgical factors include maximized tubal length and preserved intramural portion. Favorable histology includes the absence of chronic inflammation, tubal inclusions, and tubal endometriosis.[36] Hormonal treatment for PTO has been described in very limited series without consistent success.[37,38]

Transcervical Fallopian-Tube Cannulation

A variety of terms have been used for techniques of probing the proximal tubal segment, including cannulation, recannulation, catheterization, and cannulization. These terms are similar in their clinical implications and imply the passage of a catheter, guide wire, or balloon apparatus into the proximal segment under fluoroscopic, ultrasound, or hysteroscopic control to diagnose PTO and establish proximal patency. The term cannulation is used in this text.

The technique of cannulation of the proximal tubal segment with a variety of wires, catheters, and balloons is effective therapy for PTO.[39-47] The largest series involved fluoroscopically guided tubal cannulation, but several series describe hysteroscopic and ultrasound guidance.[48] No comparative studies are available to demonstrate superiority of one approach to another. There are no data to suggest that the use of a balloon is more advantageous than a wire.[49,50]

As in distal tubal repair, the crucial factor for success may be the condition of the tube.[51] In patients in whom fallopian-tube cannulation is unsuccessful, a more severe degree of PTO may exist.[52] In patients in whom fluoroscopically guided tubal cannulation failed, the failure was secondary to severe intrinsic disease and tubal occlusion, not to the technique. Histologic examination of excised cornual and isthmic tubal segments in cases of failed canalization reveal abnormalities in 93% of the specimens. Obliterative fibrosis (61%), chronic salpingitis (57%), and salpingitis isthmica nodosa (42%) were the most commonly found histologic tubal abnormalities. The failure of the procedure may be due to severe intrinsic tubal disease and the degree of occlusion after failed cannulation (Figure 13-6). An ancillary role of fallopian-tube cannulation and selective salpingography may be to differentiate a functional obstruction from a true occlusion.

Transcervical fallopian cannulation is performed under fluoroscopic guidance using a modified angiographic technique and one of several commercially available coaxial systems. A number of catheter systems and guide wires and tubal cannulas are available (Figure 13-7). A coaxial catheter system includes a series of progressively narrower cannulas and a variety of

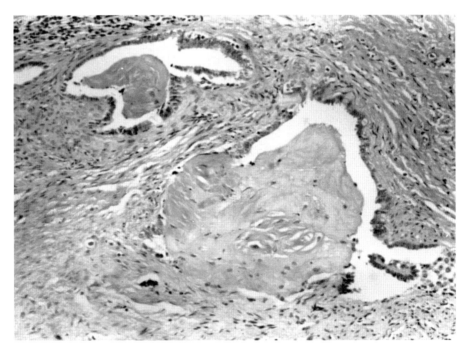

Figure 13-6   Histology of proximal tubal segment from a case of failed fallopian tube cannulation demonstrating salpingitis isthmica nodosa (SIN).

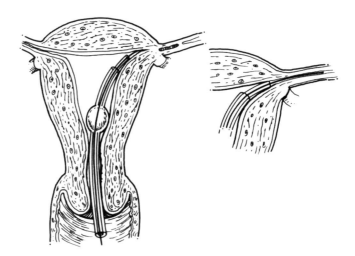

Figure 13-7   Fallopian tube cannulation. The principal catheter and balloon are placed into the uterine cavity and the coaxial catheters advanced into the region of the ostia. Once placed, the lumen may be gently probed using a variety of wires, catheters, or balloons (insert, upper right-hand side).

wires and usually meets the needs of any clinical circumstance.[53] One such catheter set consists of three coaxial catheters, 9 Fr, 5.5 Fr, and 3 Fr in diameter. The 9 Fr radiopaque polytef (Teflon) catheter is 32 cm long and has a check-flow valve. The 5.5 Fr catheter is 50 cm long, is made of braided polyethylene, and has a 3-cm nonbraided tip curved in a 45° angle. The 3 Fr catheter is 65 cm long, and two types are available, one made of radiopaque polytef and the other of nylon. Three 90-cm long guide wires complete the set. A 0.035-inch (0.089 cm) diameter tapered stainless steel guide wire with a 1.5-mm jade tip may also be used. A 0.015-inch (0.038 cm) diameter guide wire with a soft platinum tip is occasionally used for probing the proximal portion of the fallopian tube. If probing of the mid-isthmic portion of the tube is needed, a 0.015-inch (0.03 cm) guide wire with an ultrasoft platinum tip is used.

Operative Technique

The procedure is done in the early follicular phase of the menstrual cycle. The procedure should be performed in three stages to verify the obstruction and to establish patency by performing the least invasive procedure (Figure 13-8). Premedication may consist of 3 to 5 mg of intravenous midazolam and narcotics as needed during the procedure.

First, an HSG is performed to verify PTO using a water-soluble medium such as meglumine iothalamate contrast medium (Conray 60, Mallinckrodt, St. Louis, MO). (An oil-based contrast may damage the catheter systems and

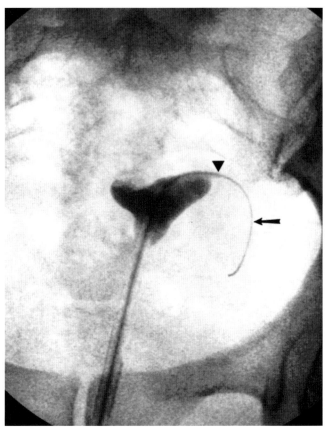

Figure 13-8   Fallopian tube cannulation. Hysterosalpingogram demonstrating bilateral proximal tube obstruction. The intramural portion of the tube may be seen, right greater than left, on the radiograph. The catheter is set into the ostia (arrowhead) and a soft-tipped wire is passed through the area of obstruction (arrow).

makes the procedure difficult and cumbersome due to its viscosity.) The cannula is advanced into the ostial region of the uterine cavity and contrast is injected. If this procedure verifies the presence of proximal tubal obstruction, a 9 Fr catheter may be advanced into the region of the distal-most portion of the cornua (see Figure 13-8) and a series of catheters or wires may be inserted. Typically, a 5.5 Fr catheter is then placed and seated into the cornua. Selective salpingography may then be performed. If the selective salpingography is unsuccessful, cannulation may be undertaken by inserting the guide wires or balloon catheters through the coaxial catheter system under fluoroscopic guidance (Figure 13-9). A 3 Fr tapered catheter and 0.015-inch soft-tip guide wire are used to advance through the area of obstruction into the isthmic portion of the tube. If the obstruction is bypassed, salpingography may be performed to delineate the entire tube, verify distal tubal patency, and attempt to assess the distal tubal segments and ampullary mucosa (Figures 13-10 and 13-11).

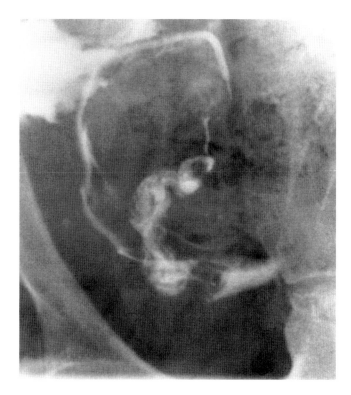

Figure 13-9   Selective salpingography after cannulation reveals a normal distal tubal segment and tubal patency.

Complications occur in 6% of cases.[54] Perforation is the most frequent and requires no intervention. Febrile morbidity and Gram-negative sepsis have been described. The total duration of radiation exposure may vary. The radiation dose absorbed by the ovaries during radiographic fallopian tube recannulation has been determined. The average fluoroscopic time is approximately 8.5 minutes (±5 min). An average of 14 (±5) 105-mm spot radiographs indicated that the average radiation dose absorbed by the ovaries was 8.5 mGy.[55,56] Tubal canalization is cost-effective therapy. Cost per live birth is approximately $7000.

All patients should be given prophylactic antibiotics (100 mg of doxycycline twice a day) administered on the day before, on the day of, and on the day after the procedure. Fluoroscopic cannulation may be performed with mild narcotic analgesia and on an outpatient basis in the angiographic suites. After the procedure, patients should be observed for 1 hour prior to discharge.

Hysteroscopic cannulation of the proximal tubal segment is an option in patients undergoing laparoscopy as part of their evaluation or as a sole procedure.[57] The procedure is identical in concept and practice to fluoroscopically guided cannulation. A cannula and guide wire may be passed through

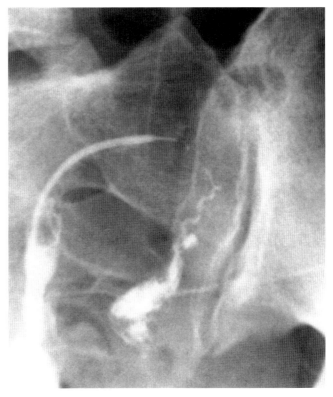

Figure 13-10   Fallopian tube cannulation successfully relieves obstruction. Injection of contrast reveals a mild distal hydrosalpinx.

the 3-mm operating channel of the hysteroscope. Under direct visualization, the cannula may be advanced into the region of the ostia, and through the catheter a series of guide wires may then be passed. Tubal cannulation may also be performed with ultrasound guidance.[62-64] This procedure has the advantages of relative ease of performance and elimination of radiation exposure during fluoroscopy, and it is cost-effective. To enhance visualization of the tubal segments, a microbubble contrast medium may be used.[65]

Microsurgical Tubocornual Anastomosis

Microsurgical tubocornual anastomosis may be a secondary approach to correct a proximal tubal obstruction in rare circumstance for those patients for whom IVF is not an option. Otherwise, any patient with failed canalization or recurrent obstruction should be immediately referred for IVF. Successful surgery for PTO depends on preservation of as much of the tubocornual segment as possible. The more of the tube preserved, the higher the pregnancy rates. In patients in whom microsurgical tubocornual anastomosis has been performed, 40 to 60% pregnancy rates have been noted.[66] For tubocornual anastomosis, high magnification is essential (20 to 25x) to allow

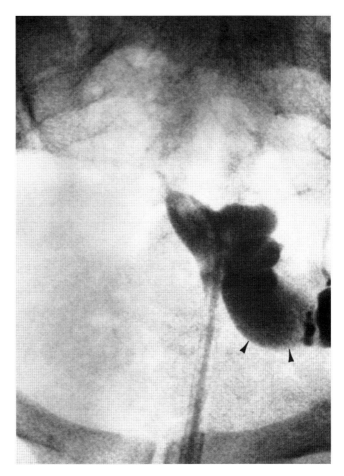

Figure 13-11   Selective salpingography reveals proximal patency and a distal severe hydrosalpinx (arrowheads).

accurate assessment of the cornual section of the tube and to identify the portion of the intramural tube that appears viable and healthy. Resection may involve only a small portion or nearly the entire segment of the intramural portion of the tube, depending on the extent of obstruction. All efforts should be taken to conserve as much of the intramural segment of the tube as possible.

The procedure is begun by injecting a dilute solution of vasopressin into the cornual region of the tube with a 25-gauge needle. The uterine cavity and proximal tubal segment are gently distended by chromotubation with a dilute methylene blue solution through a transcervical catheter system. The distal-most portion of the proximal tube is defined by exerting gentle thumb pressure on the catheter system and palpating the proximal segment. The approximate point of obstruction may be ascertained by gentle palpation of the proximal segment as dye is pulsed through the chromotubation system.

The serosa and muscularis are then incised at the isthmic–cornual junction in a region just distal to the suspected obstruction. The incision may be extended down into tubal mucosa. Care should be exercised not to divide any of the arterial supply in this region because bleeding may occur, which could compromise tubal blood supply. Small passes with the scalpel are necessary to identify viable tube as soon as possible and to minimize trauma. Serial sectioning of the tube is then carried proximally in an attempt to identify the distal-most portion of viable tube within the intramural segment. The distal-most portion may often be occluded, which necessitates resection.

After viable intramural tube has been identified, attention is directed to the distal portion of the tube. Dye is injected retrograde to identify the proximal-most segment of tubal fill. This region is then serially sectioned by beginning at the proximal segment, sectioning distally, and attempting to preserve as much of the isthmic segment of the tube as possible. The process is continued until free retrograde flow of dye is established. Approximation of the intramural and isthmic segment of the tube may be accomplished using 8-0 Vicryl suture. Four sutures are usually required for mucosal approximation; 6-0 or 8-0 Vicryl may be used on the serosa, depending on the distance between the anastomosed segments. With use of 8-0 Vicryl suture on a cutting needle, the microsurgical tubocornual anastomosis is then complete. Closure is finished in two layers.

Evaluation Prior to ART

In cases of recurrent obstruction, immediate referral for IVF is indicated (Table 13-1). In this circumstance, distal tubal segments have been evaluated and are normal (based on successful first canalization). No other evaluation is required. A more complex circumstance arises when proximal obstruction co-exists with a hydrosalpinx. The hydrosalpinx may be detected after a successful canalization enables evaluation of the distal segment, on transvaginal ultrasonography or at laparoscopy. In this setting, it is unclear what role a tubal ligation or salpingectomy has prior to IVF. A case could be made in favor of these procedures given the intermittent nature of proximal obstruction in some circumstances. Individualization of each case and extensive counseling is indicated.

Table 13-1. Evaluation Prior to ART: Proximal Tubal Obstruction
• Verification of proximal tubal obstruction with follow-up HSG/selective salpingography
• Consideration of laparoscopy to evaluate distal tubal aspects if proximal obstruction persists
• Tubal ligation if hydrosalpinx is noted regardless of persistence of proximal obstruction
• If canalization is successful, evaluation of patency with HSG 6-month follow-up

Outcomes Analysis

Proximal tubal obstruction should be thought of as a continuum, with tubal obstruction at one end and complete tubal occlusion, the most extreme form, at the other end. Tubal obstruction may be secondary to such entities as intraluminal debris or plugs and amenable to conservative measures such as selective salpingography or tubal cannulation, and tubal occlusion representing complete tubal obliteration secondary to infectious processes and requiring more extreme measures. Intermittent obstruction may be viewed as a mid-point in this continuum. The less severe forms may be amenable to more conservative therapy. Success for PTO will vary considerably depending on the entity treated and the procedure used. Hence, selection bias may influence the success rate of each modality.

By use of selective salpingography, successful catheter insertion into the tubal ostia occurs in 94% of patients, and 75% establish patency with simple selective salpingography (Table 13-2).[67-70] Tubal implantation, once the mainstay for management of proximal tubal obstruction is no longer a viable option. Cannulation of the tubes for patients who do not have patency established by selective salpingography yields 80 to 90% patency of at least one tube, and there is a 45 to 50% intrauterine pregnancy (IUP) rate and a 0 to 5% ectopic pregnancy (EP) rate after cannulation. Follow-up HSG reveals continued patency in 50 to 70% of patients when the HSG is performed 6 to 12 months after the procedure. In patients who do not achieve pregnancy 6 to 12 months after the procedure, repeat HSG is essential to rule out recurrent obstruction. Fluoroscopically guided tubal cannulation may provide a means to differentiate functional distribution (amenable to conservative management) from true occlusion (requiring management by IVF). In the rare cases in which tubocornual anastomosis is performed, IUP rates of 60% (range, 55 to 65%) and 8% EP rate have been described.

Table 13-2.
Outcomes After Cannulation for Proximal Tubal Obstruction

| Technique | N | Patency Rate | | Pregnancy Rate | | | |
		Selective Salpingography	Cannulation	IUP	EP	Coexisting Distal Tube Disease	Reocclusion
Fluoroscopic guidance	1.132	47% (44, 50)	73% (70, 75)	52% (20, 25)	4% (3, 5)	19% (17, 21)	42% (39, 45)
Hysteroscopic guidance	1.57	†	84% (77, 89)	43% (35, 51)	5% (3, 11)	20% (13, 29)	52% (42, 62)

95% confidence interval in parentheses
† Salpingogram not performed
References: 7, 14, 31, 40

salpingography, tubal catheterization and wire-guide recanalization in the treatment of proximal fallopian tube obstruction. Hum Reprod 1995;10:1423–1426.

18. Karande VC, Pratt DE, Rabin DS, Gleicher N. The limited value of hysterosalpingography in assessing tubal status and fertility potential. Fertil Steril 1995;63:1167–1171.

19. Karande VC, Pratt DE, Rao R, Balin M, Gleicher N. Elevated tubal perfusion pressures during selective salpingography are highly suggestive of tubal endometriosis. Fertil Steril 1995;64:1070–1073.

20. Hilgers TW, Yeung P. Intratubal pressure before and after transcervical catheterization of the fallopian tubes. Fertil Steril 1999;72:174–178.

21. Papaioannou S, Afnan M, Girling AJ, et al. The effect on pregnancy rates of tubal perfusion pressure reductions achieved by guide-wire tubal catheterization. Hum Reprod 2002;17:2174–2179.

22. Wiedemann R, Montag M, Sterzik K. A modern approach to the diagnosis and treatment of proximal tubal occlusion. Hum Reprod 1996;11:1823–1825.

23. Wiedemann R, Sterzik K, Gombisch V, Stuckensen J. Beyond recanalizing proximal tubal occlusion: the argument for further diagnosis and classification. Hum Reprod 1996;11:986–991.

24. Novy MJ, Thurmond AS, Patton P, et al. Diagnosis of cornual obstruction by transcervical fallopian tube cannulation. Fertil Steril 1988;50:434–440.

25. Confino E, Tur-Kaspa I, DeCherney A, et al. Transcervical balloon tuboplasty. A multicenter study. JAMA 1990;264:2079–2082.

26. Thurmond AS. Selective salpingography and fallopian tube recanalization. Am J Roentgen 1991;156:33–38.

27. Thurmond AS, Rosch J. Nonsurgical fallopian tube recanalization for treatment of infertility. Radiology 1990;174:371–374.

28. Deichert U, Schleif R, van de Sandt M, Juhnke I. Transvaginal hysterosalpingo-contrast-sonography (Hy-Co-Sy) compared with conventional tubal diagnostics. Hum Reprod 1989;4:418–424.

29. Korell M, Seehaus D, Strowitzki T, Hepp H. Radiologic (HSG) or sonograph (HKSGN) hysterosonography for evaluation of tubal patency – patient's discomfort and diagnostic accuracy. Ultraschall Med 1996;2:300–305.

30. Session DR, Lerner JP, Tchen CK, Kelly AC. Ultrasound-guided fallopian tube cannulation using Albunex. Fertil Steril 1997;67:972–974.

31. Dunphy BC. Office falloposcopic assessment in proximal tubal occlusive disease. Fertil Steril 1994;61:168–170.

32. Scudamore IW, Dunphy BC, Cooke ID. Falloposcopic comparison of unilateral and bilateral proximal tubal occlusive disease. Hum Reprod 1994;9:340–342.

33. Gomel V. Clinical results in infertility microsurgery. In: Crosignani PG, Rubin BL, eds. Microsurgery in female infertility. New York: Grune & Stratton, 1980.

34. Siegler AM. Surgical treatment of tuboperitoneal causes of infertility since 1967. Fertil Steril 1977;28:1019–1032.

35. Ransom MX, Garcia AJ. Surgical management of cornual-isthmic tubal obstruction. Fertil Steril 1997;68:887–891.

36. Papaioannou S, Afnan M, Girling AJ, et al. Diagnostic and therapeutic value of selective salpingography and tubal catheterization in an unselected infertile population. Fertil Steril 2003;79:613–617.

37. Surrey ES, Bishop JA, Surrey MW. Role of GnRH agonists in managing proximal fallopian tube obstruction. J Reprod Med 2000;45:126–130.

38. Muneyyirci-Delale O, Karacan M. Hormonal treatment of bilateral proximal tubal obstruction. Int J Fertil Womens Med 1999;44:204–208.

39. Lang EK, Dunaway HE Jr, Roniger WE. Selective osteal salpingography and transvaginal catheter dilatation in the diagnosis and treatment of fallopian tube obstruction. Am J Roentgenol 1990;154:735–740.

40. Rosch J, Thurmond AS, Uchida BT, Sovak M. Selective transcervical fallopian tube catheterization: technique update. Radiology 1988;168:1–5.

41. Ataya K, Thomas M. New technique for selective transcervical osteal salpingography and catheterization in the diagnosis and treatment of proximal tubal obstruction. Fertil Steril 1991;56:980–983.

42. Hurd WW, Randolph JF Jr, Smith YR, et al. Transcervical tubal cannulation: a comparison of two techniques. Fertil Steril 1992;58:1068–1070.

43. Hovsepian DM, Bonn J, Eschelman DJ, et al. Fallopian tube recanalization in an unrestricted population. Radiology 1994;190:137–140.

44. Platia MP, Krudy AG. Transvaginal fluoroscopic recanalization of a proximally occluded oviduct. Fertil Steril 1985;44:704–706.

45. Nakamura K, Ishiguchi T, Maekoshi H, et al. Selective fallopian tube catheterisation in female infertility: clinical results and absorbed radiation dose. Eur Radiol 1996;6:465–469.

46. Hepp H, Korell M, Strowitzki T. Proximal tubal obstruction – is there a best way to treat it? Hum Reprod 1996;11:1828–1831.

47. Hayashi M, Hoshimoto K, Ohkura T. Successful conception following Fallopian tube recanalization in infertile patients with a unilateral proximally occluded tube and a contralateral patent tube. Hum Reprod 2003;18:96–99.

48. Bloechle M, Schreiner T, Gouma E, Lisse K. Comparison between hysterosalpingo-contrast sonography and sonographically controlled selective tubal catheterization. Hum Reprod 1996;11:1423–1426.

49. Gleicher N, Redding L, Parrilli M, et al. Wire guide cannulation alone is no treatment of proximal tubal occlusion. Hum Reprod 1994;9:1109–1111.

50. Gazzera C, Gallo T, Faissola B, Zanon E. Tubal catheterization and selective salpingography. Rays 1998;23:735–741.

51. Letterie GS, Sakas EL. Histology of proximal tubal obstruction in cases of unsuccessful tubal canalization. Fertil Steril 1991;56:831–835.

52. Gazzero C, Gallo T, Faissola B, Zanon E. Tubal catheterization and selective salpingography. Rays 1998;4:735–741.

53. Risquez F, Confino E. Transcervical tubal cannulation, past, present, and future. Fertil Steril 1993;60:221–226.

54. Lang EK, Dunaway HH. Recanalization of obstructed fallopian tube by selective salpingography and transvaginal bougie dilatation: outcome and cost analysis. Fertil Steril 1996;66:205–209.

55. Hedgpeth PL, Thurmond AS, Fry R, et al. Radiographic fallopian tube recanalization: absorbed ovarian radiation dose. Radiology 1991;180:121–122.

56. Nakamura K, Isiguchi T, Maekoshi H, et al. Selective fallopian tube catheterization in female infertility: clinical results and absorbed radiation dose. Eur Radiol 1996;6:465–469.

57. Das K, Nagel TC, Malo JW. Hysteroscopic cannulation for proximal tubal obstruction: a change for the better? Fertil Steril 1995;63:1009–1015.

58. Sulak PJ, Letterie GS, Hayslip CC, et al. Hysteroscopic cannulation and lavage in the treatment of proximal tubal obstruction. Fertil Steril 1987;48:493–494.

59. Daniell JF, Miller W. Hysteroscopic correction of cornual occlusion with resultant term pregnancy. Fertil Steril 1987;48:490–492.

60. Deaton JL, Gibson M, Riddick DH, Brumsted JR. Diagnosis and treatment of cornual obstruction using a flexible tip guidewire. Fertil Steril 1990;53:232–236.

61. Li SC, Liu MN, Hu XZ, Lu ZL. Hysteroscopic tubal catheterization and hydrotubation for treatment of infertile women with tubal obstruction. Chin Med J (Engl) 1994;107:790–793.

62. Spiewankiewicz B, Stelmachow J. Hysteroscopic tubal catheterization in diagnosis and treatment of proximal oviductal obstruction. Clin Exper Obstet Gynecol 1995;22:23–27.

63. Lisse K, Sydow P. Fallopian tube catheterization and recanalization under ultrasonic observation: a simplified technique to evaluate tubal patency and open proximally obstructed tubes. Fertil Steril 1991;56:198–201.

64. Bloechle M, Schreiner T, Gouma E, Lisse K. Comparison between hysterosalpingo-contrast sonography and sonographically controlled selective tubal catheterization. Hum Reprod 1996;11:1423–1426.

65. Session D, Lerner JP, Tchen CK, Kelly AC. Ultrasound-guided fallopian tube cannulation using Albunex. Fertil Steril 1997;67:972–974.

66. Papaioannou S, Afnan M, Girling AJ, et al. Long-term fertility prognosis following selective salpingography and tubal catheterization. Human Reprod 2002;17:2325–2330.

67. Thompson KA, Kiltz RJ, Koci T, et al. Transcervical fallopian tube catheterization and recanalization for proximal tubal obstruction. Fertil Steril 1994;61:243–247.

68. Martensson O, Nilsson B, Ekelund L, et al. Selective salpingography and fluoroscopic transcervical salpingoplasty for diagnosis and treatment of proximal fallopian tube occlusions. Acta Obstet Gynecol Scand 1993;72:458–464.

69. Thurmond AS, Machan LS, Maubon AJ, et al. A review of selective salpingography and fallopian tube catheterization. Radiographics 2000;20:1759–1768.

70. Houston JG, Anderson D, Mills J, Harrold A. Fluoroscopically guided transcervical fallopian tube recanalization of post-sterilization reversal mid-tubal obstructions. Cardio Interven Radiol 2000;23:173–176.

71. McComb PF, Lee NH, Stephenson MD. Reproductive outcome after microsurgery for proximal and distal occlusions in the same fallopian tube. Fertil Steril 1991;56:134–135.

72. Patton PE, Williams TJ, Coulam CB. Results of microsurgical reconstruction in patients with combined proximal and distal tubal occlusion: double obstruction. Fertil Steril 1987;48:670–674.

73. Letterie GS, Lutkehans M. Fluoroscopic tubal canalization and microsurgery in the management of bipolar obstruction. J Gynecol Surg 1993;27:162–163.

14 *Isthmic and Mid-Tubal Obstruction*

*Heavy suture material and large needles can all damage the tubal mucosa suffi-
ciently to cause hemorrhage and adhesions . . .*
— Louis Hellman, 1951

Tubal surgery to correct mid-segment occlusions was described in 1910 by Christian and Sanderson. The procedure gained notoriety at mid-century, however, as a method to reverse tubal ligations. Between 1948 and 1968, nine publications on the reversal of sterilizations were described.[2] The pregnancy rates ranged from 6% to a remarkable 30%. The techniques were macroscopic and used sutures of catgut and silk. Initial and isolated descriptions of microsurgical techniques can be traced to the early 1950s when Hellman described the role of fine sutures, needles and atraumatic technique and hinted at magnification in tubal surgery as a means to improve outcome.[3] Tubal anastomoses became significantly improved in the mid-1960s with the use of magnification instruments, both microscopes and operative loops, and with the evolution of microsurgical techniques. Microsurgery became the standard for repair of any mid-tubal or isthmic obstruction. This technique has yielded significantly higher pregnancy rates whether for the reversal of a tubal ligation or management of salpingitis isthmica nodosa or congenital isthmic absence.[4] This chapter describes the circumstances under which tubal anastomosis is most effective, discusses the controversy surrounding the management of salpingitis isthmica nodosa (SIN) and describes the technique of microsurgical anastomosis.

Etiology

Early reports based on reviews of hysterosalpingography (HSG) suggested that mid-tubal occlusions were responsible for 2.7 to 13.3% of all tubal occlusions.[5] These figures, however, may represent overestimates due to the various definitions of isthmic occlusion and the inclusion of true proximal tubal obstruction in some series. Isthmic occlusion is obstruction of the tube at a point beyond the intramural (cornual) portion of the tube with at least a portion of, or the entire, ampullary segment intact. Occlusion of the isthmic portion of the tube is most commonly due to surgical sterilization, a tubal pregnancy treated by segmental resection, SIN, or congenital absence of the isthmic portion of the tube. Mid-tubal occlusion secondary to infectious processes is rare.

Surgery to correct abnormalities in the mid-section of the tube (isthmus) and restore fertility evolved in contemporary practice with a focus on three clinical scenarios: after tubal ligation or segmental resection for tubal pregnancy, to correct the rare circumstances of congenital absence of the isthmic portion of the tube and to bypass a portion of the isthmia affected by SIN.

Tubal Occlusion Secondary to Tubal Ligation

The reversibility of tubal ligations is related to the type of tubal ligation and resulting anatomic distortion. Tubal anatomy after ligation ranges from nearly normal after clip application to multiple segmental defects after cautery. Clips and rings for tubal ligations provide the most favorable circumstance, with tubal damage restricted to approximately 1 cm. At the opposite extreme, electrocautery frequently places the tube beyond surgical repair, especially when the cautery is applied at multiple sites. In these circumstances, the patient is best referred for in vitro fertilization (IVF).

An estimated 650,000 female sterilization procedures are performed each year in the United States.[6] Sterilization procedures account for approximately 45% of the contraceptive techniques used by women 15 to 44 years old. The average age of sterilization is 26.7 years. Sixty-four percent of sterilizations occur immediately after a pregnancy. Analyses of patients who present for reversal detect several trends. Women between the ages of 20 and 24 years at sterilization are twice as likely to experience regret after the procedure as those sterilized between ages 30 and 34 years.[7–9] Approximately 6% of women who undergo a tubal ligation will request information about sterilization reversal within 5 years of the procedure.[10] A new partner is strongly associated with requests for the reversal. Reasons for considering a reversal of a tubal ligation include pressure from the patient's gynecologist or partner at the time of the tubal ligation, and insufficient time to decide to undergo a tubal ligation.[11,12] In one study, 75% of patients who underwent a tubal ligation were unhappily married at the time of the ligation and remarriage was the primary reason for a request for reversal.[13,14] Only 10% to 30% requesting consideration for reversal of a tubal ligation actually undergo the procedure.[15,16]

Congenital Absence of the Mid-Segment of the Tube

Segmental absence of the tube is a rare abnormality, sometimes described in association with other mullerian abnormalities. Isolated case reports describe congenital absence of the isthmic portion of the tube.[17–20] In this circumstance, usually a hypoplastic mid-tubal (isthmic) segment lies between normal proximal (cornual) and distal (ampullary) tubal segments. This condition should be evaluated in a fashion identical to that of a previous tubal ligation. The likelihood of success depends on the amount of viable proximal and distal tubal segments.

Salpingitis Isthmica Nodosa

SIN is a rare condition involving the fallopian tubes characterized radiologically and histologically by small diverticula involving the proximal two-thirds of the isthmic portion of the tube.[21] SIN is a progressive condition detected during the reproductive years. SIN is found in women between the ages of 25 and 60 years with the average age at diagnosis at 30 years. Its exact etiology is unknown, although three classic hypotheses are congenital, acquired, or postinflammatory. The condition was originally reported in 1887 by Chiari, who described epithelial occlusions within the tubal walls. The congenital theory was proposed by von Recklinghaus in 1896, who suggested that the anatomic findings of SIN resulted from wolffian arrest because embryologically the tubal isthmus is in the region where the mullerian and wolffian ducts cross.[22] In 1951, Benjamin hypothesized that SIN may be an acquired anomaly that begins as a proliferation of normal epithelium within the isthmus of the tube with subsequent cyst formation and progression in size throughout the reproductive years.[23] The third hypothesis suggests an infectious cause, though specific organisms have not been identified.

The term salpingitis isthmica nodosa suggests a process that is manifested by observable anatomic changes. The pathologic features of multiple diverticulae are well known (Figures 14-1 and 14-2).[23,24] Macroscopically, the tube may be normal in appearance and be covered by a smooth serosal surface or may have focal fusiform swellings or nodular thickening involving the entire

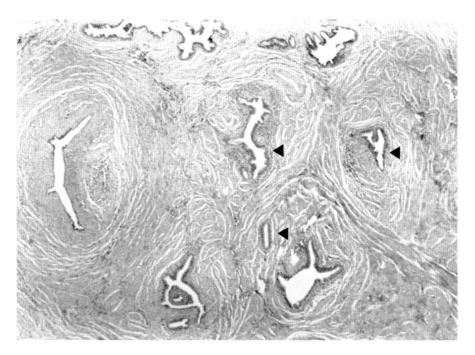

Figure 14-1   Histology of SIN. Note islands of glandular diverticulae (arrowheads) surrounding the tubal lumen.

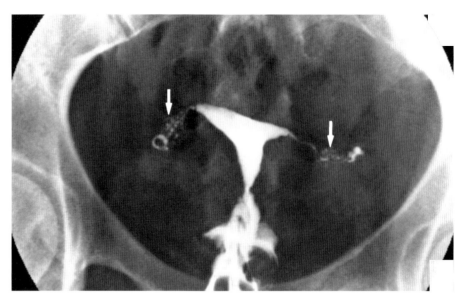

Figure 14-2   Hysterosalpingogram showing diverticula characteristic of SIN throughout the isthmic portion of the tubes bilaterally filled with contrast medium (arrows).

circumference of the isthmic portion of the tube. The presence of SIN may be suggested only after microscopic examination. The condition has distinct histologic features. Tubal epithelium lines the intramural epithelial downgrowths. These structures are without any endometrial stroma. Usually there are several foci of epithelial occlusions. In extreme cases, the whole wall may be covered with honeycombed spaces.[20] This process differs from intramural tubal endometriosis, which typically consists of one or more eccentrically located foci of ectopic endometrium in the outer myosalpinx. Numerous other designations have been put forth, such as endosalpingiosis, endosalpingoblastosis, and endoepithelial myosis. The term "salpingitis" as part of this designation is unfortunate and misleading because no direct evidence shows that an inflammatory process leads to the development of SIN. The association of pelvic and perihepatic adhesions with SIN in select cases however supports infection and inflammation as part of the process. The histologic criteria of SIN include numerous irregular benign extensions of tubal epithelium into the myosalpinx associated with reactive myohypertrophy but no inflammation.

SIN may be diagnosed by characteristic changes on HSG or on inspection of the tube (see Figure 14-2). Its incidence in fertile women ranges from 0.6 to 11%.[24,25] These findings draw into debate whether or not resection and tubal anastomosis should be performed when SIN is found on HSG. SIN is clinically significant because of a high incidence of infertility and ectopic pregnancy associated with this condition.[26–29] SIN has been described in 5 and 25% of tubal specimens obtained after tubal ligation and tubocornual anastomosis for proximal obstruction, respectively. Fifty-seven percent of tubal specimens after ectopic pregnancy manifest characteristic findings of SIN.[26] This incidence has a broad range from low values of 7 to 13% to high values of 50 to 60%, depending on the report. These observations suggest an association between ectopic pregnancy and SIN, though causality has not been proven. SIN has been detected on HSG in 38% of patients with infertility. SIN may also be a progressive disease.[30] Observations have been made by serial HSG of both the later development of SIN and the progression of the disease process after diagnosis by previous HSG. Repeated HSGs may be required to rule out its recurrence or progression of this entity.

Clinical Correlates

This anastomosis continues to have a role in contemporary fertility therapies. It is without the risk of multiple pregnancy and complex stimulation protocols. In carefully selected patients reversal of a tubal ligation offers an excellent success rate. Careful counseling is essential balancing the risks of surgery and ectopic pregnancy against the complexity and cost of ART. The decision to reverse a tubal ligation is complex (Table 14-1). Of patients presenting to discuss reversal, 30% go no further than the first consultation; 10% decide against on the basis of success rates or risk–benefit ratios after further

---

Table 14-1.
Management of Reproductive Options after Tubal Ligation

Evaluation for Reversal of Tubal Ligation (TL)

- Age: <35 and >35 years
- Operative note and pathology report
- Semen analysis (SA)
- If above normal: HSG for proximal patency

Referral for IVF if:

- TL by multiple burns or unknown technique
- Age ≥ 35 years
- Abnormal SA
- Proximal obstruction on HSG
- Preference of couple

Referral for Reversal of TL if:

- TL by Pomeroy, clip, ring, or single burn
- Age < 35 years
- Normal SA
- Proximal patency on HSG
- IVF unacceptable for personal/religious reasons

---

discussion; 30% have inoperable tubes; and 30% undergo the procedure.[13,16] Because not every woman requesting undergoes a reversal, careful counseling is required to select the appropriate candidate.

Careful screening is an integral step in successful anastomoses.[31] A few additional diagnostic studies for this selection process are warranted preoperatively. A careful history, noting the patient's age, documentation of ovulation, health before pregnancy, outcome of previous pregnancies, and the status and social disposition of the children is essential. A basic infertility evaluation should be initiated before reversal is considered. The evaluation should include a semen analysis, documentation of regular ovulatory cycles, and routine health care such as mammography and cervical cytology. In women older than 35 years, a pelvic ultrasound is essential to rule out myomas or polyps. Women older than age 38 are a special category because of the potential of age-related infertility, although several series suggest that certain patients with the most favorable surgical circumstances may proceed with the reversal.[32,33] In this group, the most important decision is how to invest time. The risk is the time required for postoperative surveillance if unsuccessful and the impact this time loss might have on IVF success.

The circumstances in which reversal of a tubal ligation are ill advised are those after cautery in which multiple burns have been placed throughout the entirety of the tube and after a fimbriectomy (Kroener procedure). Several studies suggest that attempts at surgical reversal after either procedure may be successful, but the success rates vary widely and do not exceed pregnancy rates with IVF.[34,35] Success rates with IVF make any attempt at reversal of a tubal ligation with multiple burns or fimbriectomy ill-advised.

Diagnostic Studies

Patients who present for reversal of a tubal ligation may have the procedure scheduled after a careful review of both the operative report and the histologic report of the excised tubal segments.[36] Provided that sufficient detail is included in these two reports, the patient can be taken directly to surgery with the expectation that at least one tube will be repairable (Figure 14-3). Three per cent of cases scheduled using decision tree will be inoperable. Not all operative reports are accurate – care is required in their review. Details considered crucial are: site of the ligation; if clip or ring was used, and the site of placement of the device; if cautery was used, and the site and number of burns; if a Pomeroy resection was done and the location and size of the resection. One-quarter of cases where the operative note described a favorable candidate, less than 4 cm of tube was found.[37] The final evaluation, after screening patients for the above parameters, consists of studies to assess tubal anatomy using HSG, or in select cases, diagnostic laparoscopy.

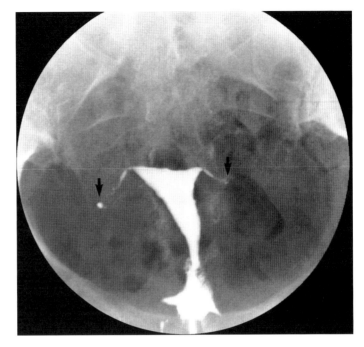

Figure 14-3   Hysterosalpingogram demonstrating a normal uterine cavity and passage of the dye through the proximal tubal segment with mid-isthmic obstruction in a patient with a previous tubal ligation.

Hysterosalpingography

When the operative report suggests that the tube was damaged in a region close to the uterine cavity, a preoperative HSG may provide guidance regarding the patency and length of the proximal tubal segment.[38] When the operative report lacks sufficient detail the HSG suggests proximal obstruction or cautery was used IVF is the best choice. Diagnostic laparoscopy should be considered when IVF is not an option.[39]

The technical and clinical success of the surgery depends on the site of the ligation. In one series of interstitial, isthmic, or ampullary obstruction by HSG correctly correlated with surgical findings in 12, 94, and 69%, respectively, of patients.[38] An anastomosis was successfully performed in 82% of patients who had tubes with interstitial obstruction, 88% with isthmic, and 72% with ampullary occlusion. When occlusion was at the distal ampullae by HSG, 10% of patients had inoperable ampullary obstruction. Dilatation of the distal fallopian tube (i.e. at the site of the ligation) was noted in 67% of x-rays. The dilatation may occur regardless of length of the proximal tubal remnants. It is not a contraindication to surgery. Most importantly, neither the length nor the degree of dilatation of the proximal segment on HSG is associated with success of the surgery or pregnancy outcome.[40]

There are no specific diagnostic studies for SIN. SIN is a condition diagnosed by HSG or during diagnostic laparoscopy when inspection shows gross morphologic changes in the isthmic portions of the tube. Both these diagnostic studies are usually performed as part of an evaluation for infertility. When SIN is discovered in these circumstances, falloposcopy may be considered.[41] Patients with falloposcopic evidence of intraluminal damage are candidates for IVF or surgery. Intraluminal damage and distal obstruction is considered bipolar tubal obstruction. These patients are not candidates for surgery and should be referred for IVF regardless of the extent of distal obstruction. The finding of SIN should prompt discussion about management options of IVF and the possibility of surgery. The discussion should be placed in the context of the patient's reproductive history, personal preferences, prior ectopic pregnancies, potentially contributory factors to reproductive failure, and her age.

Diagnostic and Operative Laparoscopy

Laparoscopic findings depend on the etiology of the isthmic obstruction. Diagnostic laparoscopy may be considered to evaluate tubal segments when inadequate details are included in the operative report. This diagnostic procedure may be combined with laparoscopic anastomosis. The ability to accurately assess tubal segments, select ideal candidates and complete the anastomosis contribute to the increasing preference for laparoscopic anastomosis in patients for whom surgery is the preferred option. Findings at laparoscopy associated with SIN include dilatation of the proximal and isthmic portions of the tube. On close inspection, sac-like structures may be noted immediately beneath the tubal serosa in the involved region.

Congenital absence of the mid-segment of tube is usually diagnosed on laparoscopy after HSG suggests either a proximal tubal or mid-tubal obstruction. Laparoscopy may be considered for any patient who has undergone segmental resection for an ectopic pregnancy. Segmental resection is frequently performed by coagulating the regions of the tube on both the proximal and distal sides of the ectopic pregnancy. Because of the variable distance of cautery damage both proximal and distal to the surgical site, a proximal obstruction may be present. These factors contribute to a variable amount of viable proximal and distal tube for anastomosis in this setting. This option is secondary to IVF for this unique group.

Management

Multiple factors influence the outcome of microsurgical reversal of a tubal ligation. One classification for reversal of tubal ligations provides a method to assess the likelihood of success based on the tubal segments to be anastomased and the final length of the tube.[42] Other important factors are the time from sterilization to reversal, the site of anastomosis, any additional tubal pathology, and the age of the patient.[43–46]

Reversals of tubal ligation are classified according to the tubal segments that are anastomosed. Three important factors influencing success are the type of tubal anastomosis performed, the length of tube at the conclusion of the procedure and type of tubal ligations. As a general rule, the closer the diameter of the segments to be anastomosed, the better the outcome and the technically easier the procedure. The most favorable circumstance is an isthmic–isthmic anastomosis. The preservation of most of the ampullary segment in this circumstance and the technically superior repair achieved when anastomosing nearly identical diameters contributes to the higher success rate. Circumstances considered less favorable are an ampullary–ampullary anastomosis, in part because a portion of the ampulla (a critical segment of the tube in which fertilization occurs) is missing. If more than 50% of the ampulla is missing, pregnancy rates approach zero. In this circumstance, if anastomosis cannot be accomplished with a more favorable repair on the opposite side, the procedure is best abandoned and the patient referred for IVF. Isthmic–cornual anastomoses are the second-most successful. Ampullary–cornual anastomoses should rarely, if ever, be performed because of the dual problem of markedly discrepant tubal diameters (which makes the procedure technically difficult) and absence of the critical ampullae.[48]

Ideal circumstances are a tubal length after repair of 6 cm or more.[48] When less than 3 cm of tube remains, pregnancy rates approach 0%. If at least 4 cm of tubal length cannot be obtained, the patient is best referred for IVF. Reversals are least favorable after coagulation and most favorable after noncoagulation techniques such as Falope rings, Hulka clips, or Pomeroy tubal ligation with limited tubal resection. Patients who undergo reversal of a coagulation procedure have an average time to conception of 13 months compared with 7 months for the patients with a noncoagulation procedure. A higher incidence of ectopic pregnancies occur after reversal of a ligation performed by coagulation. In addition, in this group tubal abnormalities including loss of mucosal folds and deciliation have been noted in approximately half the patients who have undergone reversal of tubal ligation.[49] These conditions increase in incidence the longer the time after sterilization, and they may contribute to failure of pregnancy despite a technically acceptable anastomosis. In the aggregate, These factors speak against reversals after cautery ligations.

Decisions regarding the surgical management of SIN are more problematic. The problem frequently facing the clinician is a patient with evidence by HSG of SIN and a history of infertility. A decision must be reached whether to undertake surgical resection of the involved tubal segments as surgical therapy for infertility or to undertake other more conservative (and at times empiric) therapies in hope of enhancing fertility.[50] The decision should be influenced by several factors in the patient's history and by the patient's interests and motivations. Given the progressive nature of SIN and its possible effects on reproduction, surgical resection of SIN in these circumstances though controversial has been recommended by some investigators.[29,30] Excellent results can be obtained by resection of the damaged segment of the fallopian tube and microsurgical anastomosis. Options of surgery vs ART vs observation must be carefully weighed.

Microsurgical Technique

Microsurgery involves minimal tissue trauma and precise placement of incision, suture, or cautery.[51] The technique requires a magnification system with an operating microscope or operative loops to enable accurate approximation and alignment of the segments of tube.[52,53] Delicate handling of tissue with microsurgical, lightweight instruments is essential. Fine graspers may be used to gently mobilize specific segments of tube. The tissue should be grasped at precise points without crushing or clamping, and copious irrigation is essential to maintain moisture in all tissues. Tissues should never be permitted to become desiccated or abraded. Wet sponges should be passed delicately over any serosal surface. Judicious use of needle-tip and bipolar cautery guided by magnification is necessary to limit damage to tissue. Use of nonreactive absorbable sutures (polyglycolic acid, polyglactin, polydioxanone) is essential. These sutures minimize reaction and subsequent formation of adhesions. Chromic suture should not be used in any microsurgical procedure.

Magnification can be achieved with operative loops or an operating microscope. Loops are a simple, inexpensive form of magnification. Most conventional loops provide magnification of 2.5 to 3.5x. The disadvantage, however, is the fixed magnification at a fixed distance. Loops are also somewhat uncomfortable to use because they are mounted on eyeglasses and are somewhat weighty. An operating microscope is floor mounted, has a magnification range of 2 to 40x, and is more versatile than operating loops. It has the advantage of variable magnification and variable focal lengths and can be rotated into the operative field with or without a drape after the tubes have been fully exposed and may be rotated away at completion of the microsurgical portion of the reanastomosis.

Tubal Anastomosis

Tubal anastomosis is performed with the patient in the supine position. Provision should be made to assess the patency of the segments during surgery and to assess their patency after completion of the procedure. To this end, several transcervical systems have been described. A pediatric Foley catheter or a disposable catheter system designed for HSGs may be inserted transcervically, the balloon inflated, and the catheter attached to a 30-µl syringe containing dilute methylene blue or indigo carmine. The system may be used for retrograde injection of dye to define the distal-most portion of the proximal segments at the start of the procedure and used again at the completion of the anastomosis to establish patency. The system should be placed at the start of the procedure. The syringe and extension tubing can then be drawn into the operative field.

If this system fails to operate or if a transcervical system is not elected, transfundal injection of dye may be used intraoperatively or a stent may be passed through the tubal segments. Transfundal injection of dye may be accomplished by using a Buxton clamp to occlude the lower uterine segment and then passing a 16- or 18-gauge IV set through the fundus into the uterine cavity. The needle may be withdrawn and the IV set attached to a 10-μl syringe containing methylene blue. Alternatively, a stent may be placed retrograde through the distal segment and advanced into the proximal portion of this segment and thence into the distal segment of the proximal portion of the tube to be anastomosed. The stent may be left in place during the microsurgical portion of the procedure. At the completion of the reanastomosis, the stent may be removed, thus ensuring adequate approximation of the mucosal segments.

After preoperative and sterile preparation of the patient, the operative scope should be brought to the operating field. The intraocular distance of the binocular portion of the microscope should be fixed to minimize intraoperative handling of the scope. The scope may or may not be draped with a sterile transparent plastic sheet.

A 4- to 5-cm Pfannenstiel incision may be used to enter the abdomen. The uterus should be lifted from the pelvis and placed on wet packs for support. The tubal segments should then be closely inspected for patency, which may be accomplished by defining the distal-most point of the proximal segment with chromotubation and gentle palpation of the proximal segment. The tubes should be elevated with moist packs and the proximal stump distended with dilute methylene blue solution injected through an intrauterine Foley catheter. The tube is then serially resected by beginning at the distal-most segment and working proximally until free flow of dye and normal-appearing tubal mucosa is identified. With use of retrograde chromotubation after cannulation of the fimbriated end of the tube, the proximal-most portion of the distal segment is identified and serially sectioned until patency and normal-appearing mucosa is defined. Care should be taken to maximize tubal length. Bleeding points in the muscularis and serosa should be controlled with fine-needle-tip or bipolar cautery.

With adequate definition of the tubal segments and patency assured, a suture of 4-0 polyglactin should be placed through the mesosalpinx to draw the segments into proximity and relieve tension at the site of anastomosis. Anastomosis should then be accomplished with microscopic guidance. Initially, the mucosa is reapproximated with 4 to 5 sutures with care taken not to violate the interior of the tube (although no clear-cut information regarding any disadvantage to violation of the lumen exists; depending on circumstances, passage of a stent through the interior may be necessary for adequate anastomosis). Reinforcing stitches are placed in the mesosalpinx as necessary. The serosa is then reapproximated with a similar technique. In circumstances in which a discrepancy of the tubal width (e.g., isthmic–ampullary or cornual–isthmic anastomoses) exists, care should be taken to fit the narrower proximal segment into the wider distal segment. Chromotubation may be performed to ensure patency or a No. 1 suture may be placed through the two segments to be anastomosed and the anastomosis performed around it. Ease of removal at the conclusion of the procedure ensures patency.

Depending on the type of anastomosis performed, placement of the sutures in the mucosal segments may vary (Figures 14-4 and 14-5). A marked discrepancy in the luminal diameters may make it necessary to fishmouth the narrower segment and fit this segment into the broader distal segment. Alternatively, when luminal discrepancy exists, the opening in the wider (usually distal) segment may be limited to a diameter to match the narrower lumen. A blunt probe may be helpful passing the probe gently from the distal-most segment into the proximal segment and incising over the probe.

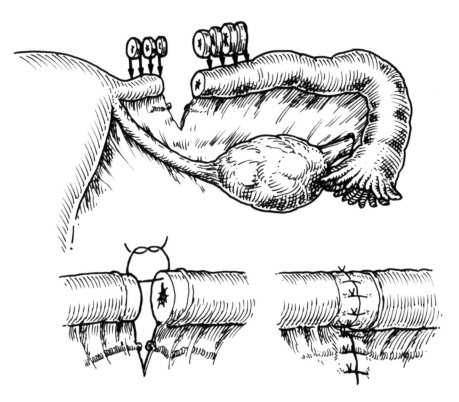

Figure 14-4   Isthmic–isthmic anastomosis. In isthmic–isthmic anastomosis, the tube is serially sectioned both proximally and distally to determine both distal and proximal patency to preserve as much of the tubal length as possible. Closure is performed in two layers using fine suture (bottom).

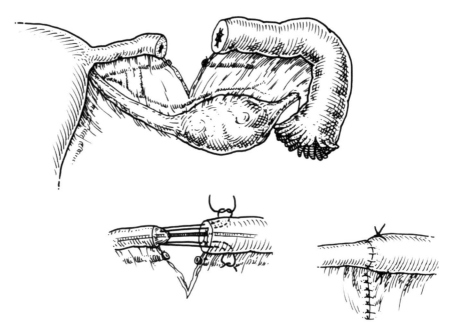

Figure 14-5   Isthmic–ampullary anastomosis. Isthmic–ampullary anastomosis is performed after defining the patency of the proximal and distal tubal segments. In place is a stent that may be used in lieu of a transcervical or
transfimbrial catheter system to ensure tubal patency at the conclusion
of the procedure (bottom).

The size of the opening can then be tailored to more closely match the narrower proximal segment (a frequent situation in isthmic–ampullary anastomoses). When only one tube is operable, removal of the remaining tubal
segments of the inoperable side should be considered. Ectopic pregnancies
have been described in these tubal remnants after unilateral anastomosis.[54]

Laparoscopic Anastomosis

Tubal anastomosis is a procedure that is transitioning from a microsurgical
to an endoscopic technique. Various endoscopic techniques are available
with excellent outcomes. Laparoscopic repair has become a viable and less
invasive option to microsurgery.[33,55–59] The proximal and distal segments to
be anastomosed should be opened using a laser or fine micro-scissors. After
patency is established, the ends may be anastomosed by a variety of techniques. Laparoscopic techniques vary from a standard two-layer closure
incorporating 4 to 5 sutures on each layer to one or two sutures placed at the
12 o'clock position.[60] In a two stitch repair, the first stitch approximates the
mesosalpinx and the second the tubal muscularis. In occasional circumstances, a third may be necessary. In a single suture tubal anastomosis, the
suture is placed at the 12 o'clock position on the antimesenteric borders of

the tube.[61] Outcomes from these two procedures are comparable. With these techniques patency may be achieved 95% of the time and pregnancy rates within 6 months to 4 years were 60%. An adjunct to laparoscopic anastomosis is the hysteroscopic passage of a stent through the cornua and across the anastomotic site. The stent provides a guide for drawing the tubal segments together and facilitates suture placement. Cost analyses of tubal anastomoses by laparoscopy or laparotomy indicate that laparoscopy costs $8610, and laparotomy $13,480. Of particular note. After laparoscopy, patients spent more time in the recovery room but avoided hospitalization after laparotomy. Time in the operating room was similar for these two groups of patients. Several series suggest that microsurgical anastomosis may be done with 24-hour (or less) hospitalization. The advent of endoscopic reversals may make 24-hour hospitalization even more feasible.

However, the laparoscopic skill required to perform these procedures may preclude them from widespread use in the general practice population.[62] Robotic assistance may improve outcomes as described in preliminary trials. Other options have been tried. Fibrin gluing is an alternative to conventional microsurgical suturing technique, particularly when luminal matches are nearly identical. When wider and discrepant lumens are considered, the risk of fistula formation and incomplete anastomosis preclude its use. If surgery will yield less than ideal results, consideration should be given to IVF except in unusual circumstances.

Other Conditions

Microsurgical anastomosis remains the best surgical technique for SIN if intervention is elected.[63,64] However, transcervical tubal catheterization may also be used for the diagnosis and treatment of proximal and isthmic tubal obstruction associated with SIN. In this setting and when proximal tubal obstruction is present, 70 to 80% of patients achieved tubal patency with pregnancy rates ranging from 25 to 30%.[65,66] Of particular note, 5% of these pregnancies were ectopic in keeping with the concept that perhaps SIN does identify patients at risk for ectopic pregnancies.

Postoperative Surveillance

If a pregnancy has not been achieved in 6 to 12 months (depending on the patient's age and type of tubal anastomosis), an HSG or referral for IVF is indicated. Tubal patency is present in 60 to 85% of cases after anastomoses. However, HSG has not been sensitive in detecting pelvic adhesive disease in these patients.[67] Selective salpingography and tubal cannulation are other options for further evaluating the tubal patency and in removing adhesions present within the tubal lumen after anastomosis.[68–70] In one study, cannulation was not successful in any patient who had evidence of tubal strictures or fistulous tract formation. In those with stenosis only, the cannulation succeeded in establishing patency in 13 of 15 tubes. Three patients became pregnant in a time interval ranging from 1 to 16 months after the procedure. Transcervical recannulation may be carefully considered as an alternative to IVF when obstruction is demonstrated. If a pregnancy has not been achieved after cannulation, the patient should be referred for IVF and any further evaluation avoided. These options are for patients who prefer to avoid IVF. If IVF is an option, referral is indicated if no pregnancy is achieved in 6 to 12 months after anastomosis without further evaluation.

Evaluation Prior to ART

For most patients with isthmic tubal obstruction, regardless of etiology, IVF is appropriate as first-line management. For patients who request microsurgery or operative laparoscopy and fail to conceive after 6 to 12 months postoperatively, referral for IVF is indicated.[70] Evaluation of endometrial cavity is indicated prior to IVF. Otherwise, no further evaluation is needed.

Outcomes Analysis

Various interrelated factors, such as the type of anastomosis, the type of tubal ligation repaired, the length of tube at the conclusion of the anastomosis, and the age of the patient, influence the success of tubal anastomosis. The overall rates of term delivery, abortion, and ectopic pregnancy are on average 50% (range, 37 to 79%), 10%, and 5%, respectively. The most reversible procedure is use of the Falope ring, Hulka clip, or Pomeroy resection. After reversal, conception occurs in approximately 7 months.[71–73] Optimal circumstances for pregnancy exist when the total tubal length is 6 cm or more (75% compared with 42% if tubal length is shorter than 6 cm).[74] Decisions to proceed with surgery must be carefully weighed against IVF success rates factoring the patient's age and personal preferences.[75]

The most successful tubal anastomoses are isthmic–isthmic and cornual–isthmic, with pregnancy rates of 75 and 71% within 1 year, respectively. Success in these circumstances is probably related to the technical ease of anastomosing tubal segments of nearly equal size, to the greater length of tube present after anastomoses involving these segments of tube and intact ampullary segments. There is an inverse relationship between the length of the tube and the interval between the surgery and conception. When tubal length exceeds 6 cm, most pregnancies occur within the first five menstrual cycles. If the tubal length is less than 4 cm, the interval between surgery and conception is approximately 20 months. Anastomosis is not recommended for cornual–ampullary repair.

Age also influences outcome. Optimal conditions include age of less than 31 years, and success decreases progressively with advancing age. Encouraging results have been described in older age groups but IVF should be the first option. Extreme care is required in patient selection when age is greater than

30 years. In one series in which women aged 40 to 45 years underwent micro-surgical anastomosis, an intrauterine pregnancy rate of 45% and an ectopic pregnancy rate of 4% were reported. Twenty-six percent of first pregnancies ended in spontaneous first-trimester abortion, and the live birth rate was 44%. The mean duration between reversal and first pregnancy was 5.5 months.[32] Laparoscopic anastomosis in several series has had success rates similar to microsurgical anastomosis.[76–79] In the largest study, 54 patients underwent this procedure with a 78% intrauterine pregnancy rate.[56] There was one ectopic pregnancy. This technique is applicable regardless of the technique of tubal ligation or type of anastomosis required.

Summary and Recommendations

Microsurgery and operative laparoscopy has markedly improved outcomes for surgical repair of the isthmic segment of the tube. Understanding of the contribution of SIN in infertility and ectopic pregnancy remains poor, but clinical data correlate these clinical events with SIN. On the basis of the literature available, the following recommendations may be made.

- Microsurgery and operative laparoscopy are the primary options for patients considering reversal of tubal ligation when adequate tubal segments are suggested by review of the operative report. Surgery should not be considered for patients who have had a distal or partial salpingectomy including the fimbria or an outright fimbriectomy (Kroener procedure).
- Operative and histology reports should be reviewed, when possible, to determine the extent and type of sterilization performed and to ensure that adequate tubal segments are available for anastomosis.
- IVF should be considered as the primary management for patients who have tubes whose final length cannot be reconstructed to more than 4 cm or patients with previous fimbriectomy sterilization and any patient older than 35 years or failed surgical reversal.
- Microsurgery or operative laparoscopy should be considered for the repair of congenital isthmic absence or to anastomose segments of tube after a segmental resection in the management of an isthmic ectopic pregnancy.
- The presence of SIN does not immediately mandate surgery but should be considered in the overall clinical picture. Surgery for the excision of SIN and tubocornual anastomosis is an option depending on clinical setting.

References

1. Christian SL. A new method of anastomosing the ovarian tube or vas deferens. JAMA 1913;61:2157–2159.

2. Siegler AM. Tubal plastic surgery: the past, the present, and the future. Obstet Gynecol Surv 1960;15:680–688.

3.   Hellman LM. The use of polyethylene in human tubal plastic operations. Fertil Steril 1951;2:498–504.

4.   Aldridge AH. Temporary surgical sterilization with a subsequent pregnancy. Am J Obstet Gynecol 1934;27:741–745.

5.   Urman B, Gomel V, McCumb P, Lee N. Midtubal occlusion: etiology, management, outcome. Fertil Steril 1992;57:747–750.

6.   Schwartz DB, Wingo PA, Antarsh L, Smith JC. Female sterilizations in the United States, 1987. Fam Plann Perspect 1989;21:209–212.

7.   Wilcox LS, Chu SY, Eaker ED, et al. Risk factors for regret after tubal sterilization: 5 years of follow-up in a prospective study. Fertil Steril 1991;55:927–933.

8.   Wilcox LS, Chu SY, Peterson HB. Characteristics of women who considered or obtained tubal reanastomosis: results from a prospective study of tubal sterilization. Obstet Gynecol 1990;75:661–665.

9.   Trussell J, Guilbert E, Hedley A. Sterilization failure, sterilization reversal, and pregnancy after sterilization reversal in Quebec. Obstet Gynecol 2003;101:677–684.

10.   Hardy E, Bahamondes L, Osis MJ, et al. Risk factors for tubal sterilization regret, detectable before surgery. Contraception 1996;54:159–162.

11.   Langer M, Hick P, Nemeskeri N, et al. Psychological sequelae of surgical reversal or of IVF after tubal ligation. Int J Fertil Menopausal Stud 1993;38:44–49.

12.   Chi IC, Jones DB. Incidence, risk factors, and prevention of poststerilization regret in women: an updated international review from an epidemiological perspective. Obstet Gynecol Surv 1994;49:722–732.

13.   Winston RM. Why 103 women asked for reversal of sterilisation. Br Med J 1977;ii:305–307.

14.   Leader A, Galan N, George R, Taylor PJ. A comparison of definable traits in women requesting reversal of sterilization and women satisfied with sterilization. Am J Obstet Gynecol 1983;145:198–202.

15.   Petta CA, Bahamondes L, Hidalgo M, et al. Follow-up of women seeking sterilization reversal: a Brazilian experience. Adv Contracept 1995;11:157–163.

16.   Brooks J, Taylor PJ, Freedman B, Pattison HA. The fate of women requesting reversal of tubal sterilization. Fertil Steril 1987;47:876–878.

17.   Goldberg JM, Friedman CI. Noncanalization of the fallopian tube. A case report. J Reprod Med 1995;40:317–318.

18.   Szlachter N, Weiss G. Distal tubal pregnancy in a patient with a bicornuate uterus and segmental absence of the fallopian tube. Fertil Steril 1979;32:602–603.

19.   Kurcz JA, Sharp MS. Congenital absence of one ovary associated with contralateral tubal pregnancy. Am J Obstet Gynecol 1948;55:1065–1067.

20.   Wheeler JE. Diseases of the fallopian tube. In: Kurman RJ, ed. Blaustein's pathology of the female genital tract, 3rd edn. New York: Springer Verlag, 1987.

21.   Chiari H. Zur pathologischen anatomie des eileiterlatarrhs. Ztschr Heilk 1887;8:457.

22.   Kontopoulos VG, Wang CF, Siegler AM. The impact of salpingitis isthmica nodosa on infertility. Infertility 1978;1:137–153.

23. Benjamin CL, Beaver DC. Pathogenesis of salpingitis isthmica nodosa. Am J Clin Pathol 1951;21:212–222.

24. Jenkins CS, Williams SR, Schmidt GE. Salpingitis isthmica nodosa: a review of the literature, discussion of clinical significance and consideration of patient management. Fertil Steril 1993;60:599–607.

25. Freakley G, Norman WJ, Ennis JT, Davis ER. Diverticulosis of the Fallopian tubes. Clin Radiol 1974;25:535–542.

26. Majmudar B, Henderson PH 3rd, Semple E. Salpingitis isthmica nodosa: a high-risk factor for tubal pregnancy. Obstet Gynecol 1983;62:73–78.

27. Honore LH. Salpingitis isthmica nodosa in female infertility and ectopic tubal pregnancy. Fertil Steril 1978;29:164–168.

28. Creasy JL, Clark RL, Cuttino JT, Groff TR. Salpingitis isthmica nodosa. Radiologic and clinical correlates. Radiology 1985;154:597–600.

29. Homm RJ, Holtz G, Garvin AJ. Isthmic ectopic pregnancy and salpingitis isthmica nodosa. Fertil Steril 1987;48:756–760.

30. McComb PF, Rowe TC. Salpingitis isthmica nodosa: evidence it is a progressive disease. Fertil Steril 1989;51:542–545.

31. Neuhaus W, Bolte A. Prognostic factors for preoperative consultation of women desiring sterilization: findings of a retrospective analysis. J Psychosom Obstet Gynaecol 1995;16:45–50.

32. Trimbos-Kemper TC. Reversal of sterilization in women over 40 years of age: a multicenter survey in the Netherlands. Fertil Steril 1990;53:575–577.

33. van Noord-Zaadstra BM, Looman CW, Alsbach H, et al. Delayed childbearing: effect of age on fecundity and outcome of pregnancy. BMJ 1991;302:1361–1365.

34. Novy MJ. Reversal of Kroener fimbriectomy sterilization. Am J Obstet Gynecol 1980;137:198–206.

35. Rouzi AA, McComb PF. A new selection criterion for fimbriectomy reversal. Fertil Steril 1995;64:185–186.

36. Opsahl MS, Klein TA. The role of laparoscopy in the evaluation of candidates for sterilization reversal. Fertil Steril 1987;48:546–549.

37. Taylor PJ, Leader A. Reversal of female sterilization: how reliable is the previous operative report? J Reprod Med 1982;27:246–248.

38. Groff TR, Edelstein JA, Schenke RS. Hysterosalpingography in a preoperative evaluation of tubal anastomosis candidates. Fertil Steril 1990;53:417–420.

39. Karasick S, Ehrlich S. The value of hysterosalpingography before reversal of sterilization procedure involving the fallopian tubes. Am J Roentgenol 1989;153:1247–1248.

40. Yankskas BC, Kerner TC, Cuttino JT, Clark RL. Post-ligation dilatation of the fallopian tube. Invest Radiol 1992;27:578–582.

41. Gurgan T, Urman B, Yarali H, et al. Salpingoscopic findings in women with occlusive and nonocclusive salpingitis isthmica nodosa. Fertil Steril 1994;61:461–463.

42.   American Society of Reproductive Medicine. Classification of adnexal adhesions, distal tubal occlusion, tubal occlusion secondary to tubal ligation, tubal pregnancies, Müllerian abnormalities, and intrauterine adhesions. Fertil Steril 1988;49:944–955.

43.   Rouzi AA, Mackinnon M, McComb PF. Predictors of success of reversal of sterilization. Fertil Steril 1995;64:29–36.

44.   Grunert GM, Drake TS, Takaki NK. Microsurgical reanastomosis of the fallopian tube for reversal of sterilization. Obstet Gynecol 1981;58:148–151.

45.   Siegler AM, Hulka J, Peretz A. Reversibility of female sterilization. Fertil Steril 1985;43:499–510.

46.   Watson A, Vandekerckhove P, Lilord R. Techniques for pelvic surgery in subfertility. Cochrane Database Syst Rev 2003:CD000221.

47.   Seiler JC. Factors influencing outcome of microsurgical tubal ligation reversals. Am J Obstet Gynecol 1983;146:292–298.

48.   Henderson SR. The reversibility of female sterilization with the use of microsurgery: a report on 102 patients with more than one year of follow up. Am J Obstet Gynecol 1984;149:57–65.

49.   Vasquez G, Winston RM, Boeckx W, Brosens I. Tubal lesions subsequent to sterilization and their relation to fertility after attempts at reversal. Am J Obstet Gynecol 1980;138:86–92.

50.   Awartani K, McComb PF. Microsurgical resection of nonocclusive salpingitis isthmica nodosa is beneficial. Fertil Steril 2003;79:1199–1203.

51.   Daniel RK. Microsurgery: through the looking glass. N Engl J Med 1979;300:1251–1257.

52.   Kim SN, Shin CJ, Kim JG, et al. Microsurgical reversal of tubal sterilization. Fertil Steril 1997;68:865–870.

53.   Edozien LC, Anastassopulos D, Mander AM. Reversal of sterilisation by the railroad technique. Br J Obstet Gynaecol 1997;104:92–95.

54.   Armstrong A, Neihardt AB, Alvery R, Sahara F, Segars J. The role of fallopian tube anastomosis: a survey of current reproductive endocrinology fellows and practitioners. Fertil Steril 2004;82:495–497.

55.   Glock JL, Kim AH, Hulka JF, et al. Reproductive outcome after tubal reversal in women 40 years of age or older. Fertil Steril 1996;66:863–865.

56.   Yoon TK, Sung HR, Cha SH. Fertility outcome after laparoscopic microsurgical tubal anastomosis. Fertil Steril 1997;67:18–22.

57.   Tsin DA, Mahmood D. Laparoscopic and hysteroscopic approach for tubal anastomosis. J Laparoendosc Surg 1993;3:63–66.

58.   Sitko D, Commenges-Ducos M, Roland P. IVF following impossible or failed surgical reversal of tubal sterilization. Human Reprod 2001;16:683–685.

59.   Kao LW, Giles HR. Laser-assisted tubal anastomosis. J Reprod Med 1995;40:585–589.

60.   Yoon TK, Sung HR, Kang HG, et al. Laparoscopic tubal anastomosis: fertility outcome in 202 cases. Fertil Steril 1999;72:1121–1126.

61.   Dubuisson JB, Swolin K. Laparoscopic tubal anastomosis (the one stitch technique): preliminary results. Hum Reprod 1995;10:2044–2046.

62. Barjot PJ, Marie G, Von Theobald P. Laparoscopic tubal anastomosis and reversal of sterilization. Hum Reprod 1999;14:1222–1225.

63. Awartani K, McComb PF. Microsurgical resection of nonocclusive salpingitis isthmica nodosa is beneficial. Fertil Steril 2003;79:1199–1203.

64. Gurgan T, Urman B, Yarali H, et al. Salpingoscopic findings in women with occlusive and nonocclusive salpingitis isthmica nodosa. Fertil Steril 1994;61:461–463.

65. Thurmond AS, Burry KA, Novy MJ. Salpingitis isthmica nodosa: results of transcervical fluoroscopic catheter recanalization. Fertil Steril 1995;63:715–722.

66. Silva PD, Schaper AM, Meisch JK, Schauberger CW. Outpatient microsurgical reversal of tubal sterilization by combined approach of laparoscopy and minilaparotomy. Fertil Steril 1991;55:696–699.

67. Young GP, Ott DJ, Chen MY, et al. Postoperative hysterosalpingography. Radiographic appearances and clinical results following tubal surgery. J Reprod Med 1993;38:924–928.

68. Lang EK, Dunaway HH. Transcervical recanalization of strictures in the postoperative fallopian tube. Radiology 1994;191:507–512.

69. Dunphy BC, Greene C. Failed reversal of sterilization: transcervical transostial recannulation of occluded fallopian tube. Am J Obstet Gynecol 1994;171:274–275.

70. Thurmond AS, Brandt KR, Gorrill MJ. Tubal obstruction after ligation reversal surgery: results of catheter recanalization. Radiology 1999;210:747–750.

71. Zhang YJ, Fan HM, Huang XM, Zhang JH. Microsurgical recanalization of fallopian tubes after tubosterilization and its related factors. Report of 278 cases. Chin Med J (Engl) 1993;106:433–436.

72. Rachagan SP, Jaafar Y. Fertility following reversal of female sterilization. Med J Malaysia 1993;48:225–228.

73. Dubuisson JB, Chapron C, Nos C, et al. Sterilization reversal: fertility results. Hum Reprod 1995;10:1145–1151.

74. Prabha S, Burnett Lunan C, Hill R. Experience of reversal of sterilisation at Glasgow Royal Infirmary. J Fam Plann Reprod Health Care 2003;29:32–33.

75. Yossry M, Aboulghar M, D'Angelo A, Gillett W. In vitro fertilisation versus tubal reanastomosis (sterilisation reversal) for subfertility after tubal sterilisation. Cochrane Database Syst Rev 2003.

76. Istre O, Olsboe F, Trolle B. Laparoscopic tubal anastomosis: reversal of sterilization. Acta Obstet Gynecol Scand 1993;72:680–681.

77. Lee CL, Lai YM, Huang HY, Soong YK. Laparoscopic rescue after tubal anastomosis failure. Hum Reprod 1995;10:1806–1809.

78. Katz E, Donesky BW. Laparoscopic tubal anastomosis. A pilot study. J Reprod Med 1994;39:497–498.

79. Daniell JF, McTavish G. Combined laparoscopy and minilaparotomy for outpatient reversal of tubal sterilization. South Med J 1995;88:914–916.

15 *Endometriosis and Ovarian Endometriomas*

If one can be reasonably sure the ovaries can be stripped completely of endometrial growth . . . conservatism will yield a gratifying result.
— *L. R. Wharton, 1929*

Endometriosis

Clinical descriptions of endometriosis first appeared in 1696. These were isolated cases of interest but clearly of unknown importance. Its clinical significance was reported at the turn of the twentieth century. In 1899, Russell described in a case report an ovarian cyst that contained uterine glands and interconnective tissue suggestive of an endometrioma.[1] Clinical interest continued as cases of cysts and peritoneal implants containing "uterine-type tissue" were described.[2] Despite an increasing body of information, the condition remained poorly understood. The subject became the focus of a review in 1908 when Cullen published *Adenomyoma of the Uterus*, which summarized the understanding of endometriosis of the time.[3] This publication raised the level of awareness and brought the issue into the foreground of clinical care. Several hypotheses regarding the etiology of endometriosis were proposed. The most prominent was described in 1921 by Sampson[4] and is now known as the classic *reflux menstruation* theory. This theory is one of the more commonly cited of several for the development of endometriosis.

In spite of poor understanding regarding etiology, several treatment modalities were described with variable success. Hysterectomy and oophorectomy became the mainstays of therapy based on a suggestion that endometriosis was dependent on ovarian hormones.[5] In 1929, Wharton suggested that radical surgery could be avoided. He described conservative surgery involving excision of only the "endometrial growth" in a series of four patients.[6] Shortly thereafter, a description of "excision of ovarian adenomas" lent further support to the conservative, organ-sparing approach.[7,8] Conservative surgical therapy with preservation of the ovaries heralded a new era of conservative therapy for endometriosis. Conservative therapies evolved rapidly through the 1940s and 1950s and led to the dictum that only minimal surgery be the treatment of choice for anyone of reproductive age.

Though surgery remained the primary treatment modality, interest in drug therapy evolved in parallel to understanding the hormonal underpinnings of the disease. Medical management with testosterone was initially proposed in the 1930s. A series in 1943 by Hirst described androgens for "endometriosis externa".[9] This therapy was limited because of masculinizing side effects. Later reports described high-dose estrogens to induce regression. Continuous combination oral contraceptives emerged as a conservative, safe option in the late 1960s and 1970s.[10] On the basis of the potential influence of androgens on regression of endometriosis, an attenuated androgen, danazol, was used with moderate success,[11] although widespread use was limited because of serious side effects. Danazol was supplanted with the advent of gonadotropin-releasing hormone (GnRH) analogs, now considered a mainstay of medical therapy.

Classic options range from aggressive surgical management with ablation or removal of all visible endometriotic lesions, to a combination of medical and surgical therapies designed to minimize the endometriotic lesions with GnRH analogs and surgical excision, to a conservative combination of assisted reproductive technologies with either observation or laparoscopic drainage of an endometrioma. This chapter discusses etiologies of endometriosis, its influence on reproduction, and approaches for the surgical and medical management in conjunction with ART to maximize reproductive potential. The relationship of pelvic pain and endometriosis is complex and beyond the scope of this chapter. That topic is not included in the discussion.

Etiology

In spite of the clinical significance of, and the intense interest by physicians, public, and lay press in endometriosis, the exact etiology of endometriosis is still unknown.[12] Understanding of the causes of endometriosis and its relationship to infertility has evolved significantly over the past 5 years, but controversy still abounds. The focus of the controversy is on the processes influencing the development of endometriotic implants in locations both near and far from the endometrium. Three important questions are pertinent: from where does the endometrial tissue arise? What contributes to its progression? How does it exert its clinical impact?

Contemporary proposals suggest three possible sources of the tissue that contribute to the development of endometriosis: the endometrium, peritoneal mesothelium via cell rests or coelomic metaplasia, and reactive metaplasia. The endometrium has been suggested as the most likely origin for several reasons, especially the well-known mechanisms for its dissemination (i.e., retrograde menstruation and possible venous transmission). Retrograde menstruation occurs in 75% of women and could provide a population of endometrial cells within the peritoneal cavity. In addition, endometrial cells retain viability in culture and in regions outside the uterine cavity. In this scenario, angiogenesis in the region of the endometrial cell population is enhanced by an estrogen-mediated increase in vascular endothelial growth factor (VEGF).[13,14] Normal clearance of these cells is inhibited by macrophage inhibitory factor. Both processes permit the perpetuation of endometrial implants within the peritoneal cavity.

The two other proposed origins, coelomic and reactive metaplasia, are hypothetically attractive but largely unproved. These two theories maintain that decreased responsiveness in cell-mediated immunity permits implantation and growth of the ectopic endometrium or, alternatively, the presence of endometrium in locations other than the uterus may provoke humoral or cell-mediated autoimmune mechanisms. Alterations in immune response figure largely into these theories, both as fostering the growth of the implants and as a cause of infertility.

A variety of cell and humoral mechanisms may permit the progression of endometriosis. These theories maintain that decreased responsiveness in cell-mediated immunity may permit implantation and growth of the ectopic endometrium. Cell-mediated immune responses in normal physiology typically contribute to the elimination of foreign antigens and cells. There is also an intrinsic ability of the immune systems to recognize and eliminate altered autologous cells. Effective methods of policing ectopic endometrial cells may be altered and enable implantation and perpetuation of the implants. This hypothesis holds that such reduction in cellular immunity could lead to a susceptibility to endometrial implantation in ectopic sites. Functional changes in cells of the immune system, including monocytes, natural killer cells, cytotoxic T lymphocytes, and B lymphocytes, occur in association with endometriosis.[15,16] These changes include a decreased surveillance, recognition, and destruction of endometrial cells and enhanced likelihood of implantation and progression.

The development of endometriosis may also be secondary to altered maturation and function of peritoneal macrophages.[17] Associated granulocyte-macrophage colony-stimulating factors are present in both endometrial and endometriotic epithelial cells and may explain the influence by endometriosis on peritoneal macrophage activity. Although leukocyte subpopulations are in peritoneal fluid and in endometrial tissue of women with and without endometriosis, the leukocyte profiles are different between these two groups. Significant elevations in the total number of leukocytes, macrophages, lymphocytes, and natural killer cells are present in patients with endometriosis. These disturbances in cellular immunity potentially could lead to a progression of endometriosis in the peritoneal cavity.[18,19]

Alterations in the cytotoxic activity of natural killer cells and activation of T-cells in the peritoneal cavity of women with endometriosis may also be instrumental in disease progression. Decreased natural killer cell cytotoxicity in the peritoneal fluid of women with endometriosis may be due to a functional defect in cells with concomitant reduction in activated T-cells. In advanced stages of endometriosis, natural killer cell activity is impaired. This impairment persists in the postoperative state in spite of cytoreductive surgery. This reduction in natural killer cell activity and changes in macrophage clearance may contribute to an impairment in the normal mechanisms for clearing ectopic endometrium.[20] Though decreased natural killer cell activity is unlikely to be a primary etiologic factor in the development of endometriosis, this decreased surveillance may influence the establishment and development of the lesions and implants characteristic of endometriosis. These data further suggest the possibility that alterations in the hormonal milieu may influence the regression of endometriosis based on potential improvement in immunocompetence with changing hormonal environment. Peripheral blood monocytes from patients with endometriosis secrete several different cytokines that may be involved in both the pathogenesis and symptomatology of endometriosis. Interleukin-8, a macrophage-derived angiogenic factor, is present in the peritoneal fluid of women with endometriosis, and may contribute to the pathogenesis of endometriosis by promoting the neovascularization of ectopic endometrial implants.[21] Local secretion of chemotactic factors could contribute to the attraction of macrophages into the peritoneal cavity of women with endometriosis. The increase in macrophages and local cytokines may contribute to the growth and inflammation of these implants.

Clinical Impact: Endometriosis and Infertility

Exactly how endometriosis causes infertility is unclear. A variety of hypotheses have been proposed (Table 15-1). None has been proven *conclusively* that endometriosis is a cause of infertility or is a symptom of a systemic problem that is adversely influencing reproduction. Multiple factors associated with or caused by endometriosis may impact fertility. The patient populations with endometriosis-related infertility are a heterogeneous group. True mechanical factors such as tubal damage and adhesions secondary to inflammation may be instrumental in moderate and severe cases. Diminished oocyte quality and ovarian reserve may also be implicated in these settings. There may also be distinct subpopulations of patients whose infertility is caused by more subtle systemic problems such as autoimmunity, changes in prostaglandin metabolism, the influence of growth factors on endometrial development and maturation and a genetic or familial predisposition. There is emerging evidence that endometriosis-associated infertility may be related to functional changes within the endometrium. These alterations may contribute to both the development of endometriosis at ectopic sites and implantation failure.

Autoimmune mechanisms have been hypothesized as one possible etiology of infertility associated with endometriosis.[26,27] These theories maintain that the presence of ectopic endometrium may provoke a local and systemic humoral or cell-mediated autoimmune response that is responsible for the infertility associated with endometriosis. Several lines of evidence demonstrate markedly altered immune mechanisms in patients with endometriosis.

Table 15-1.
Possible Factors in Endometriosis-Associated Infertility

- **Mechanical**
  - o Alteration in tubal motility caused by adhesions, prostaglandins, or both
  - o Pelvic adhesions resulting in ovum entrapments
  - o Tubal obstruction secondary to adhesions or endometriotic lesions

- **Peritoneal**
  - o Direct toxic effects of prostaglandins
  - o Macrophage activation and local immune response

- **Immunologic**
  - o Alterations of cell-mediated immunity
  - o Heightened systemic immune response (antiendometrial antibodies)

- **Ovulatory**
  - o Abnormal follicular development
  - o Luteal-phase defects
  - o Luteinized unruptured follicle syndrome

- **Endometrial receptivity**
  - o Abnormal gene expression in histologically normal endometrium
  - o Abnormalities of implantation
  - o Possible increase in early spontaneous first-trimester loss

---

Complement levels, both C3 and C4, are present in higher concentrations in both serum and peritoneal fluid of patients with endometriosis than in controls.[24] Similarly, the level of activity of peritoneal macrophages in both sperm phagocytosis and the synthesis of androgens in the peritoneal fluid are increased in patients with endometriosis compared with activity and synthesis in controls.[25]

Autoimmune etiologies gain further credence with the demonstration of endometrial autoantibodies in the serum, endometrial implants, and peritoneal fluid of patients with endometriosis. These circulating antiendometrial antibodies could interfere, theoretically, with ovum pickup and implantation.[26,27] Any fertility-enhancing effect associated with hormonal therapy, such as danazol or GnRH analogs, may possibly achieve its result not so much by inducing a regression of the endometrial implants as by altering immune responsiveness. Endometriosis is also associated with autoantibody production against endometrium-related antigens.[28]

An enhanced amount of prostaglandin release by peritoneal macrophages in endometriosis could explain several aspects of endometriosis-associated infertility. Prostaglandins may also be etiologic in the development of endometriosis and associated symptoms of pain and infertility. Increases in PGF_{2a} and PGE_2 and the prostaglandin metabolites of thromboxane B_2 (TXB_2) and 6-ketoprostacyclin $F_{1\alpha}$ are increased in the peritoneal fluid in patients with endometriosis. However, subsequent studies could find only an increase in 6-ketoprostacyclin $F_{1\alpha}$,[29] but the results of these studies were confounded because peritoneal fluid was sampled at varying times in the menstrual cycle, a factor known to influence the concentration of the prostaglandins.[30] Differences in both the amount and activity of peritoneal macrophages may result in increased prostaglandin release, thereby affecting uterine and tubal contractility and, ultimately, fertility.

The maintenance of endometrial implants is dependent on continued secretion of ovarian steroids and a variety of growth factors. A possible role for the insulin-like growth factor system as a mediator for the proliferative effect of estradiol on the implants has been demonstrated.[31,32] The actions of fibrogenic growth factors provide a role in stromal proliferation and response to progesterone and also in the repair and regeneration of endometrium following menstruation.[33] The expression of epidermal growth factor and fibrogenic growth factors is similar in both endometrium and endometriotic implants.[34] Vascular endothelial growth factor, an estrogen sensitive factor is expressed by peritoneal macrophages in the setting of endometriosis.[35]

A familial tendency for endometriosis has long been suspected. Extended case reports and retrospective reviews describe such an association. In a study of 123 families with histologically proven endometriosis, 6% of the sisters and 8% of the mothers of patients with endometriosis were affected, in contrast to only 1% of affected patients' husbands' families.[36,37] Concordance for endometriosis has been described in monozygotic twins. Three genetic possibilities are suggested by these findings: polygenic or multifactorial inheritance, a single mutant autosomal dominant or autosomal recessive gene, or a single mutant gene occurring in a small subset of patients with endometriosis. The polygenic multifactorial inheritance pattern is supported by the absence of any HLA linkage for endometriosis. An international endogene collaboration has been established to assemble both clinical data and DNA for linkage in association with studies on endometriosis. Genome-wide linkage analysis using sib pair analysis has identified several regions of exclusion but no specific linkages have yet been recorded. Early studies suggest chromosomal alterations involving trisomy 11, monosomy 16, and monosomy 17 in late stage endometriosis. A loss of only the p53 tumor suppressor gene rather than loss of chromosome 17 seems to be a pivotal event.

Molecular Basis for Endometriosis-Associated Infertility

Infertility associated with endometriosis may in part be due to a failure of implantation.[17] The endometrium is receptive to implantation during a temporally defined window. Genes currently known to be aberrantly expressed during the window of implantation and at other times of the cycle in women with versus without endometriosis include the following: aromatase, integrins $\alpha(v)\beta(3)$, hepatocyte growth factor, 17β-hydroxy steroid dehydrogenase, HoxA-10, HoxA-11, leukemia inhibitory factor, matrix metalloproteinase 7 and 11. Implantation failure may be secondary to altered environment within the endometrium.

Two complimentary aspects of the endometrium may now be evaluated using two techniques: *structure* with biopsy and histology and *function* with microarray techniques. Endometriosis-associated infertility may have as a core issue changes in functional aspects of the endometrium. Evaluation of the endometrium may provide a clinical tool for identifying this dysfunction through a search for altered expression of genes.[38,39] The traditional standard for evaluating the endometrium has been the endometrial biopsy performed in the late luteal phase. Considerable attention has historically been placed on endometrial histology to assess the structural competence (sometimes referred to as *adequacy*) of the luteal phase. Increasing attention has been focused on assessing the functional aspects of the endometrium, particularly in women with endometriosis. This search focuses on histologically normal but functionally abnormal endometrial environments at the time of implantation.

A number of molecules may be dysregulated in the endometrium of women with endometriosis and detectable by genetic analysis of an endometrial biopsy. Genome-wide analyses using microarray technologies may be used to assess this dysfunction. Using this technique, it is now possible to investigate large-scale gene expression in the endometrium. As noted above, endometrial biopsies have traditionally been used for the histologic evaluating or dating of the endometrium. In the classic sense, any discrepancy between the chronologic timing of the menstrual cycle and the histologic appearance of the endometrial biopsy would suggest what was commonly referred to as a *luteal phase defect*. Microarray technologies go beyond standard histologic evaluations. Recent studies suggest that in patients with endometriosis, the endometrium may be histologically normal but functionally abnormal during the window of implantation. Several genes or gene products may be aberrantly expressed in the endometrium during this window or at other times during the cycle in women with endometriosis. This aberrant gene expression may find its clinical expression in either failure of implantation or contribute to the establishment and growth of endometriotic cells in areas other than within the endometrial cavity. Thus compromised fertility in patients with endometriosis may be related to abnormalities in the endometrium or aberrant gene expression during the time of implantation. Microarray technology to assess endometrial gene expression in endometrial stroma cells may provide insight regarding the etiology of infertility in these patients and be targeted in specific therapy for these abnormalities.

Dysfunctional, nonreceptive endometrium is emerging as a cause for endometriosis-associated infertility. The receptivity of the endometrium may be assessed using a variety of biomarkers. Candidate biomarkers include progesterone-induced proteins such as insulin-like growth factor binding protein and glycodelin, and endometrial integrins. Together these proteins account for a majority of the total endometrial proteins expressed in the mid- to late secretory phase and both have been suggested as useful for the study of endometrial growth, development and function. Glycodelin A is a specific product of the secretory endometrium. This endometrial protein may play an important role in implantation. Using microarrayed oligonucleotides this protein is reduced in mid-secretory eutopic endometrium in patients with endometriosis compared wiht normal subjects. This finding suggests a possible role of diminished glycodelin A within the eutopic endometrium in patients with endometriosis-associated infertility as a reason for implantation failure.

Several immune-related gene products are also increased in endometriotic implants compared with normal endometrium. These encode immunoglobulins and compliment proteins that are important components to normal endometrium. In laboratory studies the proto-oncogene c-erb-B2 is overexpressed in endometriotic implants. The c-myc proto-oncogene is also expressed in the ectopic endometrium in patients with endometriosis. The upshot of these evolving genomic technologies is focusing on the molecular aspects of reproduction to compliment the traditional hormonal and surgical management techniques that have long been the mainstay of endometriosis therapies. It is possible that inhibitors of overexpressed oncogenes might be of benefit in the treatment of endometriosis.

Integrins are another endometrial component altered in endometriosis. Integrins are heterodimeric transmembrane cell adhesion receptors composed of an α and β subunit. Integrins are the major receptors by which cells attach to the extracellular matrix and mediate cell-to-cell adhesion. As a result of integrin binding, intracellular signals are transduced to enhance regulation of cell phenotype. Integrins are the best characterized immunohistochemical markers of uterine receptivity. An increasing interest in integrins in the reproductive tract regarding both fertilization and implantation has emerged as data accumulate regarding the impact of endometrial function on these outcomes. Integrins serve as receptors for ECM ligands and act as modulators of cellular function. Three integrins are expressed by the endometrium in a cycle specific pattern coincidental to the window of implantation: $\alpha(1)\beta(1)$, $\alpha(4)\beta(1)$ and $\alpha(v)\beta(3)$ are co-expressed on glandular epithelium only during cycle days 20–24 corresponding to the putative window of implantation. Alterations in these integrins may be involved in the pathogenesis of endometriosis and the development of ectopic endometrial implants. Alterations in integrins within the eutopic endometrium in patients with endometriosis-associated infertility may also be a component to implantation failure in these patients. In this latter circumstance, $\alpha(v)\beta$ integrin and its extracellular matrix ligand osteopontin may regulate endometrial receptivity. Dependent on ovarian steroid secretion, $\alpha(v)\beta$ integrin expression may be stimulated by epidermal growth factor while osteopontin is stimulated by progesterone. In patients with endometriosis, $\alpha(v)\beta3$ expression is reduced during the implantation window. Osteopontin appears to be unaffected. These findings suggest that the etiology of infertility in patients with endometriosis may be related to dysfunctional eutopic endometrium resulting in reduced cycle fecundity.

This understanding is a fundamental change in thinking regarding endometriosis. In this circumstance, the paradigm has shifted from an endometrial assessment that focuses on structure, i.e. the dating of a secretory endometrium, to one that focuses on function, i.e. factors apart from the histology. While an in-phase secretory endometrium has been considered the gold standard for evaluating endometrial adequacy, endometrial abnormalities may not be in fact reflected by altered histology. Subtle endometrial deficiencies leading to implantation failure may exist. These deficiencies are not detected using standard endometrial histology. These defects reflect changes in the functional aspects of the endometrium in spite of normal structure, i.e., in-phase secretory endometrium. Two endometrial defects have been described. Type 1 defect reflects a lack of endometrial expression of integrins associated with the histologic delay (the classic luteal phase deficiency) and the Type 2 defect reflects changes where the endometrium is histologically normal (i.e., no histologic delay noted, no luteal phase defect) but associated with the absence of expression of important markers of uterine receptivity. This latter defect is found largely in women with minimal or mild endometriosis and in women with hydrosalpinges.

Other Causes of Endometriosis-Associated Infertility

Other factors may also be instrumental and altered with endometriosis. Nitric oxide is a potential contributor to endometriosis-associated infertility.[40] High levels of nitric oxide will adversely affect sperm motility, implantation, and tubal function. Peritoneal macrophages in patients with endometriosis-associated infertility express higher levels of nitric oxide synthase, have higher levels of nitric oxide enzyme activity, and produce more nitric oxide in response to immune stimulation. A hypothetical treatment for endometriosis-associated infertility may be reducing or blocking nitric oxide production or effects respectively in the peritoneal fluid. Matrix metalloproteinases (MMP) are a family of endopeptidases that are instrumental in the degradation and turnover of extracellular matrix proteins. Their action is regulated by tissue inhibitors. There is an altered equilibrium between MMP-9 in the peritoneal fluid and the tissue inhibitors of women with endometriosis suggesting that endopeptidases and their tissue inhibitors may be instrumental in the pathogenesis of endometriosis.[41]

Endometriosis-related infertility may also involve the follicle, with alterations relating to follicle maturation and oocyte and embryo quality. Concentrations of interleukin-6 are diminished in the serum of patients with endometriosis and vascular endothelial growth factor (VEGF) is present in lower concentrations in the follicular fluid of patients with endometriosis. These findings suggest that alterations within the follicular dynamics may impair fertility.[42–45]

Ovarian endometriomas represent one of the more severe forms of endometriosis. The endometriomas may be isolated findings without any other evidence of pelvic or abdominal endometriosis or they may be part of a progressive process of evolving endometriosis associated with a variety of lesions, as noted above.[46] Any of the peritoneal lesions characteristic of endometriosis may be found on the ovary. Ovarian endometriomas may be associated with extensive pelvic adhesive disease and induce sufficient tissue reaction to compromise tubal function and structure. Any approach to the surgical excision of ovarian endometriomas must also provide the possibility of an extensive adhesiolysis and tubal repair.

Clinical Correlates

The exact prevalence of endometriosis is dependent on the population studied. The prevalence among reproductive age women ranges from 10 to 50% depending on clinical complaints and methods of detection. When laparoscopy is used as a diagnostic tool a higher incidence is detected secondary to the sensitivity of the evaluation and selection of symptomatic patients undergoing the tests. Consequently, asymptomatic and unevaluated cases are not identified, which leads to a falsely lowered incidence. A prevalence of 5% is described in a fertile population undergoing tubal ligation,[26] suggesting this as the true incidence in the general fertile population. As long as the diagnosis of endometriosis requires an operative procedure, the prevalence estimates will be biased by the types of women selected for evaluation. Age at diagnosis ranges from 10 to 83 years, with a median age of 29 years. The high frequency of endometriosis calls into question whether a process diagnosed with such frequency is a pathologic process. Subpopulations of patients have a higher predeliction. The prevalence of the disease is not surprisingly higher in patients with infertility (30.5%) and chronic pelvic pain (45%).

Endometriosis continues to be one of the most common reasons for hospitalization in patients 15 to 44 years old.[47] In a pre- and adolescent population aged 10 to 19 years examined for cyclic pelvic and abdominal pain, a prevalence rate as high as 55% was described.[48] Costs for treatment range from approximately $600 million for inpatient care to $3 billion if costs for managing pelvic pain secondary to endometriosis are included.[49] The most common clinical presentations of endometriosis are infertility and pelvic pain. The relationship between infertility and endometriosis is well-described, ranging from 30 to 50%.[50] In advanced stages, this infertility may be secondary to distortions in pelvic anatomy. In minimal and mild cases of endometriosis the causes are unclear, with monthly fecundity rates of these women less than those of the general population. The second-most-common clinical manifestation is chronic pelvic pain, ranging from 20% to 80%.[51] The frequency of these complaints in association with endometriosis varies according to the age group studied. In general, the presentation of both infertility and chronic pelvic pain is clustered at age extremes: pelvic pain is more frequent in adolescent years and infertility more frequent in ages 38 to 42 years.

Autoimmune diseases are part of the clinical picture of endometriosis. The immune system appears to be altered in infertility patients with endometriosis as noted above.[52] A systemic autoimmune mechanism may be instrumental in both the etiology of endometriosis and the infertility associated with endometriosis. These abnormalities may be manifested clinically by features of autoimmune disease. A strong correlation is noted between the presence of lupus anticoagulant and antinuclear antibody with both IgM and IgG autoantibodies.[53] These observations suggest that endometriosis is associated with abnormal activation of polyclonal B lymphocytes, a classic characteristic of autoimmune disease. Further support for this theory is suggested by the demonstration that immunoglobulin levels, particularly IgG, are elevated in patients with endometriosis and more so in lupus anticoagulant-positive patients than in lupus anticoagulant-negative patients.[54] Antiendometrial antibodies in the serum and peritoneal fluid of infertile patients with endometriosis have also been demonstrated.[55,56] These data suggest that part of the clinical profile for patients with endometriosis may be an autoimmune phenomenon with management implications attendant to autoimmune diseases. The presence of endometriosis, regardless of clinical complaint, should thus prompt consideration of the need for further evaluation to rule out associated autoimmune disease by history or testing.

Classification Systems

Because of the relationship between endometriosis and infertility, various classification systems have been devised to determine influence of endometriosis on the incidence of infertility and the most effective therapies on a stage-by-stage assessment of the disease. The first classification designed to predict outcome, preposed in 1973,[57] was based on an anatomic description of the amount of pelvic involvement and intended to predict the likelihood of achieving pregnancy after a specific intervention. A numeric classification was described in a 1978 system based on a cumulative score that calculated the degree of peritoneal, ovarian, and tubal involvement of the endometriotic implants.[58] However, even after revision in 1985, the numeric system did not prove to be a reliable predictor of pregnancy.[59] Given these shortcomings, reliance on any classification system to predict outcome is open to question. The insensitivity of these classifications may be due to the multifactorial and heterogeneous nature of endometriosis, the failure to diagnose the true extent of the disease by visualization alone or account for factors contributing to implantation failure. These factors may influence fertility far beyond the anatomic distortion that current classification schemes attempt to quantify. This method for describing the location, morphology, and extent of endometriosis continues to be a means of communicating between clinicians, but is of limited value in predicting outcome.

Diagnostic Studies

Imaging techniques are useful in detecting adnexal masses suggestive of endometriosis. They are of no value in detecting minimal or mild disease. Ovarian abnormalities are frequently detected as part of a routine clinical examination by bimanual examination or by transvaginal or transabdominal ultrasound scans. Transvaginal ultrasound imaging (TVS) to screen ovaries as part of routine medical care has led to the diagnosis of cystic adnexal masses with increasing frequency and to the need for conservative approaches in the management. Image characteristics lend insight into the diagnosis. Most cystic adnexal masses are benign. These masses must be carefully characterized and followed with serial examinations to rule out the presence of a neoplasm.[60] Management depends in part on the appearance of the mass on the ultrasound scan. In certain circumstances, magnetic resonance imaging (MRI) with fat saturation may further refine the diagnosis, especially in circumstances in which a dermoid is suspected.

Transvaginal Ultrasound Imaging

On TVS, cystic enlargements of the ovary have a variety of appearances. The most likely diagnosis is suggested by the echo patterns and size on imaging. Functional ovarian cysts may have no internal echoes, a smooth wall, and enhanced through transmission. These masses may contain low-level echoes representing blood, fat, or cellular debris. In a predominantly cystic mass, low-level echoes may also arise from proteinaceous or mucinous material suggestive of a complex differential diagnosis. Endometriomas have varying sonographic appearances ranging from anechoic to strongly echogenic and from a loculated complex to septated cystic structures, depending on the amount and viscosity of the internal cystic architecture (Figures 15-1 and 15-2).[61,62] The borders may be irregular. Hemorrhagic cysts and dermoids frequently are part of the differential diagnosis and have similar appearances. In one series, ultrasound as a screening tool had a sensitivity of only 11% in detecting endometriomas when all symptomatic patients were included and not just patients with a suspected pelvic mass or endometrioma.[63] The suspicion of an endometrioma may be raised when the characteristics described above are consistently demonstrated by serial examinations. In questionable circumstances, color Doppler sonography may be helpful.[64] Ultimately, questionable cases require advanced diagnostic studies.

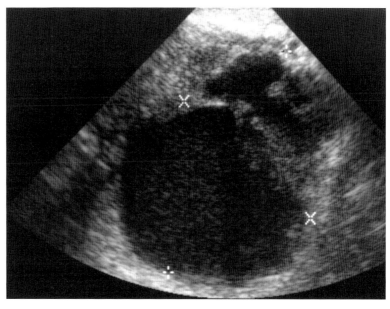

Figure 15-1   Transvaginal ultrasound image of ovarian endometrioma demonstrating mixed echogenicity.

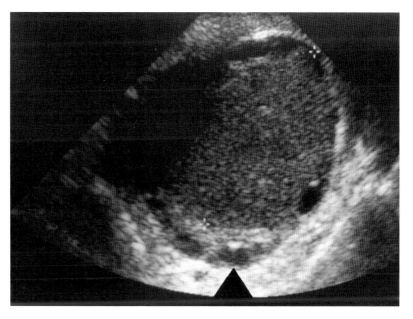

Figure 15-2   Transvaginal ultrasound image of diffuse echo pattern characteristic of endometriomas surrounded by follicles.

Magnetic Resonance Imaging

Endometriomas have a classic appearance on MRI because of the signal characteristics of blood (Figure 15-3).[65,66] Since hemoglobin contains iron, which affects the signal behavior of a lesion, hemorrhage is easily identified with MRI. Endometriomas are imaged as multiple cystic lesions with signal characteristics of hemorrhage. Hemorrhagic cysts, bowel, mesenteric fat, and other hemorrhagic lesions such as cystadenoma and neoplasms may mimic the appearance of a single endometrioma.[67] The sensitivity of MRI for the diagnosis of endometriomas ranges from 64 to 71% and the specificity as 60 to 82%.[68] The low sensitivity is caused by the inability of MRI to identify small lesions in serosal implants. Solitary lesions contribute to both false-positive and false-negative diagnoses. Large endometriomas may be diagnosed when the lesion is larger than 1 cm in diameter and hyperintense on T1- and T2-weighted images. Fat saturation MRI may be required to differentiate the hemorrhage in an endometrioma from the oil and sebaceous content of a dermoid (Figure 15-4).[69,70] Use of this modality for saturation in addition to conventional images is suggested in the assessment of any questionable ovarian mass. MRI may also be useful in assessing response to ovarian suppressive therapy and in planning surgical intervention based on cyst reduction.[71,72]

Serum Markers

No laboratory tests are reliable in the diagnosis of endometriosis. Serum markers are of no value in predicting minimal or mild disease but may be a

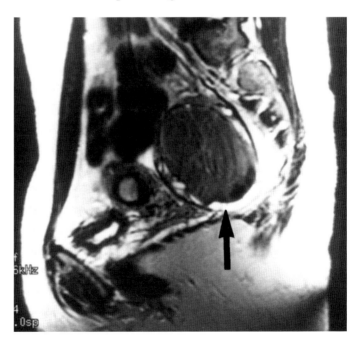

Figure 15-3   MRI demonstrating characteristic appearance of an endometrioma (arrow). Note follicles on the periphery of the endometrioma.

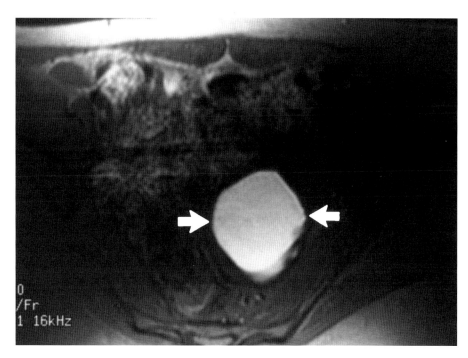

Figure 15-4   Fat saturation of MRI consistent with an endometrioma (arrows). MRI can differentiate the fatty debris of cystic dermoids from blood-containing endometriomas.

useful adjunct in severe endometriosis. Testing for endometriosis with serum markers has consistently given conflicting results regarding sensitivity and specificity. Serum CA-125 determinations have a relatively low sensitivity and are not recommended for general screening of infertility populations. Serum CA-19-9, a high-molecular-weight glycoprotein is also elevated and correlates with severity of endometriosis. It is no more sensitive or specific than CA-125. Depending on the signs and symptoms suggestive of endometriosis, these tests may be helpful in select circumstances. They are not designed to replace clinical assessment or laparoscopy when visual or histologic confirmation of endometriosis is essential. When used in conjunction with TVS, they may provide further insight to the nature of an ovarian abnormality.[73] Additional serum markers such as leptin, CD-10 and soluble intercellular adhesions molecule-I have had preliminary evaluation but are of uncertain clinical utility.

Diagnostic Laparoscopy

Although the imaging techniques of TVS and MRI in conjunction with serum markers are sensitive and specific for large endometriomas, direct visualization is essential for minimal to mild endometriosis.[74] The variable appearance of endometriosis has led to the recommendation that peritoneal biopsy of any suspicious lesion may increase the frequency of diagnosis and improve management.[75] Despite the increased ability to detect pigmented and nonpigmented endometriotic lesions, 13% of patients with normal-appearing peritoneum will have histologic evidence of endometriosis.[76] Microscopic endometriosis has been discovered by random biopsies of normal-appearing peritoneum by visual examination in 25% of patients.

The variable appearances of endometriosis may be the result of an age-related evolution in the appearance of endometriosis. Clear lesions progress to red or vascular and then to dark brown or black powder-burn lesions characteristic of older, long-standing endometriosis. The appearance of the lesions at laparoscopy suggests that endometriosis is a progressive disease; hence, the recommendation that peritoneal biopsy and histologic evaluation by directed biopsy at a suspicious lesion or by random biopsies may enhance diagnostic accuracy.

Pelvic endometriosis is classically divided into bulky lesions displacing ovarian substance (ovarian endometriomas) and as lesions that disort the peritoneum as isolated or coalesced black puckered spots (so-called powder burns). To accommodate this spectrum there has been a gradual movement away from classic visual criteria (an absolute requirement of a "powder burn" lesion for diagnosis) to a broader visual spectrum of peritoneal changes suggestive of endometriosis and a more liberal use of laparoscopic-directed biopsy to confirm suspected cases. Two aspects regarding visual diagnosis of endometriosis at laparoscopy are noteworthy.

The first is the gross appearance of the lesions.[59] Appearances of the gross peritoneal lesions suggestive of endometriosis can be variable. The morphology of the peritoneal and ovarian implants may be categorized as red (red, red-pink, and clear lesions), white (white, yellow-brown, and peritoneal defects), and black (black and blue lesions). The assessment of the morphologic appearance of these lesions recognizes that endometriosis may assume a variety of appearances rather than the classic "powder burn". A high index of suspicion and familiarity with the broad spectrum of appearances is essential.

The second is on the depth of infiltration of the endometriotic lesions.[77] Two different lesions with varying clinical implications were described and labeled "superficial" and "deep". Superficial endometriosis is located only on the surface of the peritoneum and has the classic irregularities of brownish discoloration and variable size. Deep endometriosis is found by biopsy and histologic examination and is associated with pelvic pain. It is more frequently associated with increasing age, further suggesting that endometriosis is a progressive disease. The depth of infiltration of deep endometriosis requires biopsy to fully differentiate the depth. Deep endometriosis is defined as pelvic endometriosis infiltrating deeper than 5 mm; very deep is greater than 10 mm.

Categorization is further refined by type or form. Three forms of deep endometriosis, classified as types 1, 2, and 3, are clinically significant. Type 1 lesions are conical, infiltrative lesions. These lesions line the largest surface area of the peritoneal cavity. Type 2 lesions are present when the pelvic anatomy is grossly disturbed with peritoneal retraction, scarring, and adhesions over the lesion. In the most common form, the adhesions associated with type 2 are present over the uterosacrals and the pouch of Douglas and cover the entire lesion. Type 3 lesions are defined as deep lesions with their largest area under the peritoneal surface in a pelvis with an otherwise intact anatomy. The significance of depth of infiltration and type may be related to clinical presentation. A correlation may exist between superficial and deep endometriosis and infertility and chronic pelvic pain. Superficial lesions may be active disease associated with infertility. The deeper endometrial implants may be associated with pelvic pain. These correlations fit with clinical findings and await comparative data for confirmation.

Variations in appearance, morphology, and depth of infiltration of endometriosis add to the technical difficulties of the diagnosis and management of this disease. Skill in identification of the different forms of endometriosis as much as skill in surgical technique to assure adequate precise excision is a prerequisite for effective surgical management. The varying appearance and clinical presentation of endometriosis suggests that two separate conditions may exist: minimal or mild endometriosis and moderate or severe endometriosis.[78] Each condition may be clinically and pathologically separate. Minimal or mild endometriosis may have no relationship to infertility, may be equally shared by both normal and infertile populations, and may be considered an almost incidental finding. Moderate or severe endometriosis may be associated with infertility secondary to anatomic distortion. This differentiation has important implications for fertility therapies. Patients with mild endometriosis and infertility may be managed expectantly, but patients with moderate or severe endometriosis require more aggressive management with medical, surgical, or combination therapy.

Management

Management of endometriosis is complex and requires individualization of therapy. Not all patients who have endometriosis require therapy. For patients who do require treatment, the therapy must be tailored to the symptoms associated with the endometriosis (pain or infertility). Options include medical or surgical management, a combination of both therapies, or in some patients, immediate referral for IVF. In select patients with pelvic pain and documented endometriosis, medical management alone is a viable option as definitive therapy after any other medical or social factors are excluded.

Because of its dynamic nature endometriosis will progress in 60% of untreated women.[78] In treated patients, the degree of progression varies according to the treatment used. Thirty-three and twenty-two percent of patients with medical and surgical treatment respectively, will progress to more advanced states.[79] Progression may be related to the depth and extent of the endometriosis. In these patients, medical management may offer a temporary relief of pain, arrest progression, and provide an opportunity for normal immunologic mechanisms to induce a regression of the disease. However, management of patients with large endometriomas, especially in the setting of infertility, requires a more aggressive approach with surgery or immediate referral for IVF.

Medical Management

Medical protocols for endometriosis are complex and require careful patient selection. The indications for medical management are primarily in the long-term control of pain or as a prelude or integral part of ART. Suppression of ovarian function, the mainstay of medical management is one option for pain management. There is no ideal medical protocol for the management for endometriosis. Medical management consists of GnRH analogs to induce hypoestrogenism and/or continuous combination and/or cyclic oral contraceptives to eliminate cyclic ovarian function. The goal is to reduce or eliminate any stimulation of endometriotic implants by ovarian steroids and improve symptoms.[80] They have been shown to reduce pelvic pain in select cases and may be useful preoperatively to enhance the ease of operation and removal of an endometrioma.[81] Medical protocols of continuous oral contraceptives, progestins, and GnRH analogs are appropriate first-line management for patients with chronic pelvic pain.[82] These agents may be used in conjunction with other fertility therapies but have a questionable role as sole management for fertility secondary to endometriosis. Prolonged suppression (viz, 2 months) may enhance fertility when used as part of the suppression protocol prior to IVF.[83–85] Care is required in balancing pain control and fertility plans in patients over 35 years old. A prolonged course of ovarian suppression may not be an appropriate investment of time in patients of advanced reproductive age.

Surgical Management

The surgical approach to endometriosis has evolved from exploratory laparotomy as a standard to operative laparoscopy as the contemporary paradigm.[86,87] Most patients, even those with extensive endometriosis or endometriomas, may be managed laparoscopically. Severe pelvic adhesive disease, large endometriomas, and severely distorted and immobile pelvic anatomy may require laparotomy in extreme cases. However, a significant reduction in hospital days and costs may result from laparoscopy as compared with laparotomy (72 days versus 258 days, respectively, and $223,600 versus $424,500, respectively, for 120 patients equally divided in each group).[88] Good clinical judgment is essential, both preoperatively in planning the surgery and intraoperatively.

Endometriomas are managed laparoscopically by a combination of incision, drainage and fulguration with low-power, continuous laser or cautery.[89] Simple drainage of the endometrioma with irrigation may be optimal in select cases when IVF is planned, though recurrence rates range from 50 to 75%.[90] Incision and drainage, irrigation, removal of the cyst wall, and coagulation of the ovarian bed (if necessary) may be required to minimize risk of recurrence. In some patients with extensive, severe pelvic adhesions and in whom adequate visualization is impossible, consideration should be given to either laparotomy and excision of the endometrioma for pain management or postponement of further surgery and immediate referral for IVF depending on age of patient and indications for surgery.

Laparoscopy is an option in two circumstances: normal evaluation and images suggestive of endometriosis. When the infertility evaluation is normal including history, clinical examination, hysterosalpingography, and transvaginal ultrasonography, risk of extensive endometriosis is low but finite. Laparoscopy in the setting of normal imaging studies and negative history is a controversial issue. In this setting, if endometriosis is present, it is probably at a minimal or mild degree. It is unclear whether this degree of endometriosis contributes to infertility (see below). The management of minimal and mild endometriosis for fertility enhancement is open to question. Fulguration of minimal or mild endometrial implants is appropriate if laparoscopy is performed as part of the evaluation for pain or infertility.[91,92] Formerly an integral "next step" in the infertility evaluation, the high likelihood of a negative exam in this setting has reduced its role.

Surgical therapy is appropriate for moderate to severe endometriosis for any patient with pelvic pain and infertility or a desire for future children. Surgery is undertaken to excise the endometrioma and preserve the maximum amount of normal ovarian architecture, fulgurate any endometrial implants, lyse adhesions, and restore pelvic anatomy to normal. As a sole approach for fertility enhancement, the decision to proceed with surgery turns in part on the age of the patient, previous surgeries, size of the endometrioma, and the role and timing of IVF. In select cases, drainage of the endometrioma and preservation of ovarian architecture and proceeding directly to IVF in the immediate postoperative period may be appropriate.[91,92] The degree of fertility enhancement by excising endometriomas is a matter of debate. Two large collaborative studies yielded differing results. In one, no change in fecundity between treated and untreated patients was observed. However, in a second study, a doubling of fecundity was observed after excision.[94] The discrepancy may be a reflection of the diversity of causes of endometriosis-related infertility.

Patient Selection

The treatment of endometriosis includes precise assessment of extent regarding type, location, and depth of infiltration and an accurate assessment of goals (pain control versus fertility). Ablation of deep or retroperitoneal endometriosis, correction of abnormal pelvic anatomy with adhesiolysis, excision of ovarian endometriomas, and reconstruction of tubal abnormalities are important considerations in making the assessment. Care is required in selecting patients to be managed surgically versus IVF for management of infertility.

Surgical management of ovarian endometriomas may be planned according to the size on preoperative ultrasound imaging.[95,96] Endometriomas of less than 5 mm may be coagulated with cautery or laser. Histologically, these structures have glands and stroma penetrating for 1–2 mm. The infiltration into ovarian stroma of smaller lesions can be variable; hence, vaporization should include 2 to 4 mm of normal-appearing stroma. For endometriomas ranging from 5 mm to 2 cm, an assessment of the cyst wall, depth of penetration, and ease of dissection should be made, and a decision made regarding coagulation and excision versus drainage and referral for IVF. Most endometriomas regardless of size are manageable laparoscopically by cyst drainage, excision of cyst wall and ablation of any endometriosis of the ovarian bed.[97] When endometriomas exceed 5 cm, difficult dissection and inadequate excision as well as prolonged laparoscopic surgery and an increased chance of recurrence are concerns. In excising the cyst wall, the operative mandate is to preserve as much normal ovarian architecture as possible, maintain ovarian reserve and reduce the likelihood of recurrence.

Operative Technique

The ovarian capsule overlying the endometrioma is incised with needle-tip cautery or laser. The cyst may then be drained and irrigated. Two sets of graspers will facilitate cyst-wall enucleation. One set is used to grasp the normal ovarian tissue, a second to grasp the cyst wall. Through a 5-mm puncture, a set of operating scissors is used to dissect a cleavage plane between normal ovarian stroma and cyst wall. Gentle traction and countertraction are exerted with the grasping forceps. A search is made for an adequate plane between the cyst wall and ovarian tissue. A plane of dissection is developed carefully and slowly along the margin of the endometrioma wall and the normal ovary.

The cyst wall may be peeled out by using a corkscrew motion or by gentle traction on the cyst wall and countertraction on the ovary. The cyst wall may be friable and easily fragmented when removal is attempted. Blunt and sharp dissection of the cyst from the ovarian capsule may be needed. Alternatively, the cyst can be shelled out intact with traction and countertraction. In this case, when the cyst is removed from the ovary, it is drained intra-abdominally into a pouch and then removed through the laparoscope. After the cyst is removed, the ovary may be left open. The base of the endometrioma should be irrigated generously and a search made for any residual traces of endometriosis within the depths of the ovary. These areas should be carefully ablated with cautery or laser vaporization. The goal in this ablation is twofold: reduce recurrence risk and maintain ovarian reserve. The edges of the ovary may be left unsutured.[95,98,99] Application of a barrier to the operative site will reduce the likelihood of recurrence. If the risk of extensive damage to ovarian architecture exists, drainage and referral to IVF may be the best option.

Recurrent Endometriomas

Considerable care is required in the surgical management of severe endometriosis in patients who have undergone one procedure for excision of an ovarian endometrioma. The decision to reoperate on recurrent endometriomas must be weighed against the likelihood of success with in vitro fertilization.[100–102] In patients who have recurrent endometriomas, surgery should be deferred. The patient is best treated with in vitro fertilization. There is the risk of compromised ovarian function and a negative impact on IVF outcomes after multiple surgeries for ovarian endometriomas.

Evaluation Prior to ART

The evaluation prior to ART depends on the extent of endometriosis, prior treatment, and age (Table 15-2). These patients do not require further laparoscopic evaluation prior to ART. In patients with minimal to mild endometriosis, a Cochrane database review described an improvement in pregnancy rates with laparoscopic ablation. In any patient with ovarian endometriomas the two most important aspects in management are the patient's age and history of previous surgery. In patients who are 38 years or older, consideration should be given to proceeding with assisted reproductive technologies prior to any surgery and immediate referral for IVF. Cyst drainage and immediate IVF are options, with suggestion in several reports of improved pregnancy rates with IVF after drainage. This should be balanced against the patient's pain pattern. In vitro fertilization should also be considered in patients with a history of at least one ovarian cystectomy for endometriomas. In this circumstance, careful review of the operative report and assessment of damage of normal ovarian stroma should be made. Assessment of ovarian reserve is particularly important in this group of patients because of potential compromise to ovarian reserve after extensive ovarian surgery. Diminished ovarian response and decreased implantation

---

Table 15-2.
Evaluation Prior to ART: Endometrioma

- Avoidance of multiple ovarian surgeries for recurrent endometriomas
  Ovarian reserve assessment of particular importance if prior ovarian surgery

- Identification of the location of endometriomas within the ovary and verification that follicular sites are within access to a retrieving needle

- Possible role of long-term (3-months) ovarian suppression with GnRH analogs depending on age

- Possible role for autoimmune and endometrial receptivity evaluation

and pregnancy rates with in vitro fertilization may occur after surgery for recurrent ovarian endometriomas particularly in patients who are older than 35 years of age.[102] Patients with severe endometriosis and of advanced reproductive age with a previous ovarian cystectomy for ovarian endometriomas are best referred for in vitro fertilization, postponing surgery until after IVF. In patients with severe endometriosis and undergoing in vitro fertilization, a prolonged suppression with GnRH analogs prior to stimulation may improve pregnancy rates. The possible mechanisms of this are probably related to changes in functional aspect of the endometrium. The data regarding outcome after a second ovarian cystectomy are variable. A second operation should be carefully weighed against the impact this may have on ovarian reserve and outcome of in vitro fertilization.

Outcomes Analysis

Since the underlying mechanisms contributing to infertility associated with endometriosis are not clearly understood, most therapies are empiric. Since endometriosis is a heterogeneous disorder, it is not unexpected that prescribed therapies may be beneficial for some but not for others. The ultimate measure of efficacy in endometriosis therapy, for patients presenting with infertility, is a clinical pregnancy and live birth, and for patients with pain, the relief of chronic pelvic pain. Early studies assessing the effectiveness of medical and surgical management of endometriosis and infertility were anecdotal and observational clinical studies without proper randomization or controls. The pregnancy rates in the literature were very broad. Quality of the data is further compromised by variable follow-up intervals, varying definitions of success rates, and a variety of staging classifications as an example. In a review of literature evaluating laser and electrocautery for endometriosis, stage for stage, the range in pregnancy rates quoted is 10 to 100%.[107] Although providing descriptive information, previous data provide little guidance for counseling patients and making operative decisions about which type of therapy (no treatment, medical, surgical, or referral for in vitro fertilization) is the most appropriate management for a patient.

Despite these limitations, the literature provides some useful insights into outcomes to guide decision-making treatments.[108–113] For patients with minimal and mild disease, in comparisons of no treatment, laparoscopy, or laparotomy, similar pregnancy rates of 67, 68, and 74%, respectively, are reported for 3-year estimated, cumulative life-table pregnancy rates. After laparoscopic resection and ablation of mild to minimal endometriosis (stages I and II), the fecundity rate is 4.7% as compared with 2.4% for patients who only underwent the diagnostic procedure for endometriosis. Two meta-analyses of surgery and medical management found no benefit of surgical or medical therapy whereas two large-scale studies support surgical ablation of minimal and mild disease to improve fertility rates. However, the Cochrane review noted above suggests a benefit.

Management of moderate and severe endometriosis by laparoscopy or laparotomy yield similar results. For patients with moderate and severe disease, operative laparoscopy and laparotomy resulted in rates of 62 and 44%, respectively, for 3-year estimated, cumulative life-table pregnancy rates. For patients with endometriomas, operative laparoscopy and laparotomy yielded rates of 52 and 46%, respectively, for 3-year estimated, cumulative life-table pregnancy rates. Stage by stage comparisons were also similar. Cumulative pregnancy rates at 1, 2, and 3 years were 39, 46, and 51% for stage I; 31, 47, and 58% for stage II; 30, 41, and 54% for stage III; and 25, 47, and 47% for stage IV.[114] Thus, surgical management, stage-for-stage, appears to offer similar success rates, regardless of whether laparoscopy or laparotomy was used.

Though clearly appropriate as first-line medical management for pelvic pain, hormonal therapy for fertility enhancement for minimal and mild disease is appropriate only in unique clinical circumstances.[115] Medical management with GnRH agonists may play a role in combination with surgery or for pain management after laparoscopy. Medical management in the postoperative period for fertility, however, was not shown to be clearly beneficial in well-designed studies. The role of these medications as either sole management or postoperative management may not enhance fertility rates. There is increasing evidence that patients with severe endometriosis (stage IV) and those aged 38 years or more are best treated by in vitro fertilization as an initial approach for their infertility. Controversy exists whether pregnancy rates are enhanced by drainage or reduced by excision. Further data are required. Careful individualization of therapy is essential.

While several studies of assisted reproduction suggest decreased pregnancy rates among women with endometriosis, meta-analysis suggested similar pregnancy rates in women with endometriosis and tubal factor infertility. The general trend in the literature is that there is no difference in pregnancy rates on a stage-by-stage comparison of endometriosis and other indications for IVF.[116] Overall, a 38% pregnancy rate per cycle, 41% rate per retrieval, and 43% rate per transfer may be expected. In a stage-by-stage comparison, pregnancy rates of 39, 48, 45, and 40% for minimal, mild, moderate, and severe endometriosis, respectively, have been described.

Summary and Recommendations

The clinical aspects and management of endometriosis have changed considerably in the recent past. Better definitions of the various forms of endometriosis have enabled a more precise diagnosis. Emerging cohesive explanations for the etiology of the disease and the associated infertility have improved treatment plans. Endometriosis is associated with subfertility in its mild forms and infertility in its severe forms. DNA microarray technology has provided expanded insight into the etiology of endometriosis-associated infertility.[117] A scrutiny of the literature on medical and surgical management of endometriosis for pelvic pain and infertility has brought into better focus which therapies are most appropriate on a stage-by-stage basis. Despite this evolution in understanding, questions remain regarding the optimal management of patients with endometriosis-associated infertility. On the basis of recent literature including prospective, randomized studies, meta-analyses, and reviews, the following recommendations may be made for infertility management:

- For minimal and mild endometriosis, no hormonal management has been shown to be of benefit. No treatment or laparoscopic vaporization with cautery or laser may have a beneficial effect on pregnancy rates, but properly controlled trials are needed.
- For moderate and severe endometriosis, surgery is one option. There is no clear-cut advantage of laparoscopy to laparotomy. Laparoscopy has a distinct economic advantage, with substantial savings. Adjunctive therapy with a GnRH analog may facilitate surgery in select circumstances.
- Infertility associated with endometriosis may be due to adverse changes in endometrial growth factors.
- Controversy exists whether drainage or excision of an ovarian endometrioma prior to IVF enhances fertility rates.
- Patients with endometriosis may have a maturational delay and fail to express $\alpha(v)\beta(3)$ integrin during the window of implantation. Subsets of infertile women with endometriosis may be identified on the basis of biochemical marker proteins in the endometrium. On the basis of failed expression, there are some women with minimal or mild disease who have a dysfunctional endometrium compared with women without this disorder.
- There is no clear-cut role for postoperative ovarian suppression in patients who have had adequate surgical treatment. A possible role does exist, however, in patients who have had inadequately excised endometriomas or extensive peritoneal endometriosis not amenable to vaporization. The exact enhancement of fertility, however, is unclear.
- In patients who have failed to achieve a pregnancy after surgical management, IVF offers pregnancy rates similar to rates in a control population without any appreciable decrease in pregnancy rates on a stage-by-stage basis.
- Second surgeries for excision of ovarian endometriomas to enhance fertility should be avoided because of the possibility of compromising ovarian response to stimulation during IVF.
- Prolonged suppression (2 to 3 months) with GnRH analogs prior to ovarian stimulation may improve outcomes with IVF.
- Gives the diverse profiles of endometriosis, what may emerge as a therapeutic paradigm is a two-step process of profiling the cause(s) of endometriosis-related infertility for a given patient through a series of studies including evaluation of endometrial function and tailoring a therapeutic plan that meets this unique profile.

References

1. Russell WW. Aberrant portions of the mullerian tract found in an ovary: ovarian cysts of mullerian origin. Bull Johns Hopkins Hosp 1899;10:8–12.

2. Pick W. Ueber neubildungen am genitale. Arch Gynecol 1905;76:251.

3. Cullen TS. Adenomyoma of the uterus. Philadelphia: WB Saunders, 1908.

4. Sampson JA. Perforating hemorrhagic (chocolate) cysts of the ovary. Their importance and especially their relation to pelvic adenomas of endometrial type ("adenomyoma" of the uterus, rectovaginal septum, sigmoid). Arch Surg 1921;3:245–248.

5. Sampson JA. Heterotopic or misplaced endometrial tissue. Am J Obstet Gynecol 1925;10:649–653.

6. Wharton LR. Conservative surgical treatment of pelvic endometriosis. South Med J 1929;22:267–271.

7. Meigs JV. Endometrial hematomas of the ovary. Boston Med Surg J 1922;187:1.

8. Holmes SR. Endometriosis. Am J Obstet Gynecol 1942;43:255–262.

9. Hirst JC. Conservative treatment and therapeutic tests for endometriosis by androgens. Am J Obstet Gynecol 1947;53:483–488.

10. Karnaky KJ. The use of stilbestrol for endometriosis. Preliminary report. South Med J 1948;41:1109–1111.

11. Lauersen NH, Wilson KH, Birnbaum S. Danazol: an antigonadotropic agent in the treatment of pelvic endometriosis. Am J Obstet Gynecol 1975;123:742–747.

12. Schmidt CL. Endometriosis: a reappraisal of pathogenesis and treatment. Fertil Steril 1985;44:157–173.

13. Shifren JL, Tseng JF, Zaloudek CJ, et al. Ovarian steroid regulation of vascular endothelial growth factor in the human endometrium: implications for angiogenesis during the menstrual cycle and in the pathogenesis of endometriosis. J Clin Endocrinol Metab 1996;81:3112–3118.

14. Yamashita Y, Ueda M, Takehara M, et al. Influence of severe endometriosis on gene expression of vascular endothelial growth factor and interleukin-6 in granulosa cells from patients undergoing controlled ovarian hyperstimulation for in vitro fertilization-embryo transfer. Fertil Steril 2002;78:865–871.

15. Halme J, Becker S, Hammond MG, Raj S. Pelvic macrophages in normal and infertile women: the role of patent tubes. Am J Obstet Gynecol 1982;142:890–895.

16. Halme J, Becker S, Wing R. Accentuated cyclic activation of peritoneal macrophages in patients with endometriosis. Am J Obstet Gynecol 1984;148:85–90.

17. Mahutte NG, Arici A. New advances in the understanding of endometriosis related infertility. J Reprod Immunol 2002;55:73–83.

18. Steele RW, Dmowski WP, Marmer DJ. Immunologic aspects of human endometriosis. Am J Reprod Immunol 1984;66:33–36.

19. Gomez-Torres MJ, Acien P, Campos A, Velasco I. Embryotoxicity of peritoneal fluid in women with endometriosis. Its relation with cytokines and lymphocyte populations. Hum Reprod 2002;17:777–781.

20.   Kats R, Metz CN, Akoum A. Macrophage migration inhibitory factor is markedly expressed in active and early-stage endometriotic lesions. J Clin Endocrinol Metab 2002;87:883–899.

21.   Ryan IP, Tseng JF, Schriock ED, et al. Interleukin-8 concentrations are elevated in peritoneal fluid of women with endometriosis. Fertil Steril 1995;63:929–932.

22.   Gleicher N, Pratt D, Dudkiewicz A. What do we really know about autoantibody abnormalities and reproductive failure: a critical review. Autoimmunity 1993;16:115–140.

23.   Hill JA. Immunology and endometriosis. Fertil Steril 1992;58:262–264.

24.   Isaacson KB, Coutifaris C, Garcia CR, Lyttle CR. Production and secretion of complement component 3 by endometriotic tissue. J Clin Endocrinol Metab 1989;69:1003–1009.

25.   Muscato JJ, Haney AF, Weinberg JB. Sperm phagocytosis by human peritoneal macrophages: a possible cause of infertility in endometriosis. Am J Obstet Gynecol 1982;144:503–510.

26.   Mathur S, Garza DE, Smith LF. Endometrial autoantigens eliciting immunoglobulin (Ig)G, IgA, and IgM responses in endometriosis. Fertil Steril 1990;54:56–63.

27.   Wild RA, Satyaswaroop PG, Shivers AC. Epithelial localization of antiendometrial antibodies associated with endometriosis. Am J Reprod Immunol Microbiol 1987;13:62–65.

28.   Hatayama H, Imai K, Kanzaki H, et al. Detection of antiendometrial antibodies in patients with endometriosis by cell ELISA. Am J Reprod Immunol 1996;35:118–122.

29.   Ylikorkala O, Koskimies A, Laatkainen T, et al. Peritoneal fluid prostaglandins in endometriosis, tubal disorders, and unexplained infertility. Obstet Gynecol 1984;63:616–620.

30.   Badawy SZ, Marshall L, Cuenca V. Peritoneal fluid prostaglandins in various stages of the menstrual cycle: role in infertile patients with endometriosis. Int J Fertil 1985;30:48–53.

31.   De Leon FD, Vijayakumar R, Brown M, et al. Peritoneal fluid volume, estrogen, progesterone, prostaglandin, and epidermal growth factor concentration in patients with and without endometriosis. Obstet Gynecol 1986;68:189–194.

32.   Giudice LC, Dsupin BA, Gargosky SE, et al. The insulin-like growth factor system in human peritoneal fluid: its effects on endometrial stromal cells and its potential relevance to endometriosis. J Clin Endocrinol Metab 1994;79:1284–1293.

33.   Di Blasio AM, Centinaio G, Carniti C, et al. Basic fibroblast growth factor messenger ribonucleic acid levels in eutopic and ectopic human endometrial stromal cells as assessed by competitive polymerase chain reaction amplification. Mol Cell Endocrinol 1995;115:169–175.

34.   Shifren JL, Tseng JF, Zaloudek CJ, et al. Ovarian steroid regulation of vascular endothelial growth factor in the human endometrium: implications for angiogenesis during the menstrual cycle and in the pathogenesis of endometriosis. J Clin Endocrinol Metab 1996;81:3112–3118.

35.   Vercellini P, Frontino G, Piertropaolo G, et al. Deep endometriosis: definition, pathogenesis and clinical management. J Am Assoc Gynecol Laparosc 2004;11:153–161.

36.   Simpson JL, Elias S, Malinak LR, Buttram VC Jr. Heritable aspects of endometriosis. I. Genetic studies. Am J Obstet Gynecol 1980;137:327–331.

37.   Simpson JL, Malinak LR, Elias S, et al. HLA associations in endometriosis. Am J Obstet Gynecol 1984;148:395–397.

38.   Taylor RN. The future of endometriosis research genomics and proteomics. Gynecol Obstet Invest 2004;57:47–49.

39.   Daftary GS, Taylor HS. Emx2 gene expression in the female reproductive tract and dbe expression in the endometrium of patients with endometriosis. J Clin Endocrinol Metab 2004;89:2390–2396.

40.   Osborn BH, Haney AF, Misukonis MA, Weinberg JB. Inducible nitric oxide synthase expression by peritoneal macrophages in endometriosis-associated infertility. Fertil Steril 2002;77:46–51.

41.   Szamatowicz J, Laudanski P, Tomaszewska I. Matrix metalloproteinase-9 and tissue inhibitor of matrix metalloproteinase-1: a possible role in the pathogenesis of endometriosis. Hum Reprod 2002;17:284–288.

42.   Toya M, Saito H, Ohta N, et al. Moderate and severe endometriosis is associated with alterations in the cell cycle of granulosa cells in patients undergoing in vitro fertilization and embryo transfer. Fertil Steril 2000;73:344–350.

43.   Lyons RA, Djahanbakhch O, Saridogan E, et al. Peritoneal fluid, endometriosis, and ciliary beat frequency in the human fallopian tube. Lancet 2002;360:1221–1222.

44.   Diaz I, Navarro J, Blasco L, et al. Impact of stage III-IV endometriosis on recipients of sibling oocytes: matched case-control study. Fertil Steril 2000;74:31–34.

45.   Hull MG, Williams JA, Ray B, et al. The contribution of subtle oocyte or sperm dysfunction affecting fertilization in endometriosis-associated or unexplained infertility: a controlled comparison with tubal infertility and use of donor spermatozoa. Hum Reprod 1998;13:1825–1830.

46.   Gruppo italiano per lo studio dell'endometriosi. Prevalence and anatomical distribution of endometriosis in women with selected gynaecological conditions: results from a multicentric Italian study. Hum Reprod 1994;9:1158–1162.

47.   Mathias SD, Kuppermann M, Liberman RF, et al. Chronic pelvic pain: prevalence, health-related quality of life, and economic correlates. Obstet Gynecol 1996;87:321–327.

48.   Wheeler JM. Epidemiology of endometriosis-associated infertility. J Reprod Med 1989;34:41–46.

49.   Zhao SZ, Wong JM, Davis MB, et al. The cost of inpatient treatment: an analysis based on the Health-care Cost and Utilization Project Nationwide Inpatient Sample. Am J Manag Care 1998;4:1127–1134.

50.   Redwine DB. The distribution of endometriosis in the pelvis by age groups and fertility. Fertil Steril 1987;47:173–175.

51.   Garcia CR, David SS. Pelvic endometriosis: infertility and pelvic pain. Am J Obstet Gynecol 1977;129:740–747.

52.   Gleicher N, el-Roeiy A, Confino E, Friberg J. Is endometriosis an autoimmune disease? Obstet Gynecol 1987;70:115–122.

53.   Meek SC, Hodge DD, Musich JR. Autoimmunity in infertile patients with endometriosis. Am J Obstet Gynecol 1988;158:1365–1373.

54.   Dmowski P, Braun DP. Immunology of endometriosis. Best Prac Res Clin Obstet Gynecol 2004; 18:245–263.

55.   Goari I, Ishikawa M, Onose R, et al. Antiendometrial autoantibodies are generated in patients with endometriosis. Am J Reprod Immunol 1993;29:116–123.

56.   Fernandez-Shaw S, Hicks BR, Yudkin PL, et al. Anti-endometrial and anti-endothelial auto-antibodies in women with endometriosis. Hum Reprod 1993;8:310–315.

57.   Acosta AA, Buttram VC Jr, Besch PK, et al. A proposed classification of pelvic endometriosis. Obstet Gynecol 1973;42:19–25.

58.   American Society of Reproductive Medicine. Classification of endometriosis. Fertil Steril 1979;32:633–638.

59.   Schenken RS, Guzick DS. Revised endometriosis classification: 1996. Fertil Steril 1997;67:815–816.

60.   Prys-Davies I. The adnexal mass: benign or malignant? Evaluation of a risk of malignancy index. Br J Obstet Gynaecol 1993;100:927–931.

61.   Bazot M, Darai E, Hourani R, et al. Deep pelvic endometriosis: MR imaging for diagnosis and prediction of extension of disease. Radiology 2004;232:379–389.

62.   Sugimura K, Okizuka H, Imaoka I, et al. Pelvic endometriosis: detection and diagnosis with chemical shift MR imaging. Radiology 1993;188:435–438.

63.   Guerriero S, Mais V, Ajossa S, et al. The role of endovaginal ultrasound in differentiating endometriomas from other ovarian cysts. Clin Exp Obstet Gynecol 1995;22:20–22.

64.   Fleischer AC, Cullinan JA, Jones HW 3rd, et al. Serial assessment of adnexal masses with transvaginal color Doppler sonography. Ultrasound Med Biol 1995;21:435–441.

65.   Ishijima H, Ishizaka H, Inoue T. Distinguishing between cystic teratomas and endometriomas of the ovary using chemical shift gradient echo magnetic resonance imaging. Australas Radiol 1996;40:22–25.

66.   Takahashi K, Ikada S, Okada M, et al. Magnetic resonance relaxation time in evaluating the cyst fluid characteristics of endometrioma. Hum Reprod 1996;11:857–860.

67.   Takahashi K, Okada M, Okada S, et al. Studies on the detection of small endometrial implants by magnetic resonance imaging using a fat saturation technique. Gynecol Obstet Invest 1996;41:203–206.

68.   Tanaka YO, Itai Y, Anno I, et al. MR staging of pelvic endometriosis: role of fat-suppression T1-weighted images. Radiat Med 1996;14:111–116.

69.   Ascher SM, Agrawal R, Bis KG, et al. Endometriosis: appearance and detection with conventional and contrast-enhanced fat-suppressed spin-echo techniques. J Magn Reson Imaging 1995;5:251–257.

70.   Thickman D, Gussman D. Magnetic resonance imaging of benign adnexal conditions. Magn Reson Imaging Clin N Am 1994;2:275–289.

71.   Sugimura K, Okizuka H, Kaji Y, et al. MRI in predicting the response of ovarian endometriomas to hormone therapy. J Comput Assist Tomogr 1996;20:145–150.

72.   Takahashi K, Okada S, Okada M, et al. Prognostic application of magnetic resonance imaging in patients with endometriomas treated with gonadotrophin-releasing hormone analogue. Hum Reprod 1996;11:1083–1085.

73.   Guerriero S, Mais V, Ajossa S, et al. Transvaginal ultrasonography combined with CA-125 plasma levels in the diagnosis of endometrioma. Fertil Steril 1996;65:293–298.

74.   Cook AS, Rock JA. The role of laparoscopy in the treatment of endometriosis. Fertil Steril 1991;55:663–680.

75.   Davies JA. Endometriosis: a scientific and clinical challenge. Br J Obstet Gynaecol 1994;101:267–268.

76.   Murphy AA, Green WR, Bobbie D, et al. Unsuspected endometriosis documented by scanning electron microscopy in visually normal peritoneum. Fertil Steril 1986;46:522–524.

77.   Koninckx PR, Martin DC. Deep endometriosis: a consequence of infiltration or retraction or possibly adenomyosis externa. Fertil Steril 1992;58:924–928.

78.   Redwine DB. Age-related evolution in color and appearance of endometriosis. Fertil Steril 1987;48:1062–1063.

79.   Candiani GB, Vercellini P, Fedele L. Laparoscopic ovarian puncture for correct staging of endometriosis. Fertil Steril 1990;53:984–987.

80.   Donnez J, Nisolle M, Gillerot S, et al. Ovarian endometrial cysts: the role of gonadotropin-releasing hormone agonist and/or drainage. Fertil Steril 1994;62:63–66.

81.   Fedele L, Bianchi S, Bocciolone L, et al. Pain symptoms associated with endometriosis. Obstet Gynecol 1992;79:767–769.

82.   Olive DL, Pritts EA. Treatment of endometriosis. N Engl J Med 2001;345:266–275.

83.   Surrey ES, Silverberg KM, Surrey MW, Schoolcraft WB. Effect of prolonged gonadotropin-releasing hormone agonist therapy on the outcome of in vitro fertilization-embryo transfer in patients with endometriosis. Fertil Steril 2002;78:699–704.

84.   Dicker D, Goldman JA, Levy T, Feldberg D, Ashkenazi J. The impact of long-term gonadotropin-releasing hormone analogue treatment on preclinical abortions in patients with severe endometriosis undergoing in vitro fertilization-embryo transfer. Fertil Steril 1992;57:597–600.

85.   Marcus SF, Edwards RG. High rates of pregnancy after long-term down-regulation of women with severe endometriosis. Am J Obstet Gynecol 1994;171:812–817.

86.   Gant NF. Infertility and endometriosis: comparison of pregnancy outcomes with laparotomy versus laparoscopy techniques. Am J Obstet Gynecol 1992;166:1072–1081.

87.   Adamson GD, Hurd SJ, Pasta DJ, Rodriguez BD. Laparoscopic endometriosis treatment: is it better? Fertil Steril 1993;59:35–44.

88.   Luciano AA, Lowney J, Jacobs SL. Endoscopic treatment of endometriosis-associated infertility. Therapeutic, economic and social benefits. J Reprod Med 1992;37:573–576.

89.   Fayez JA, Vogel MF. Comparison of different treatment methods of endometriomas by laparoscopy. Obstet Gynecol 1991;78:660–665.

90.   Candiani GB, Vercellini P, Fedele L, et al. Conservative surgical treatment for severe endometriosis in infertile women: are we making progress? Obstet Gynecol Surv 1991;46:490–498.

91.   Wong BC, Gillman NC, Oehninger S, et al. Results of in vitro fertilization in patients with endometriomas: surgical removal beneficial? Am J Obstet Gynecol 2004;191:597–606.

92. Meden-Vrtovec H, Tomazevic T, Verdenik I. Infertility treatment by in vitro fertilization in patients with minimal or mild endometriosis. Clin Exp Obstet Gynecol 2000;27:191–193.

93. Tinkanen H, Kujansuu E. In vitro fertilization in patients with ovarian endometriomas. Acta Obstet Gynecol Scand 2000;79:119–122.

94. Barnhart K, Dunsmoor-Su R, Coutifaris C. Effect of endometriosis on in vitro fertilization. Fertil Steril 2002;77:1148–1155.

95. Mage G, Canis M, Manhes H, et al. Laparoscopic management of adnexal cystic masses. J Gynecol Surg 1990;6:71–79.

96. Suganama N, Wakahara Y, Ishida D, et al. Pretreatment for ovarian endometrial cyst before in vitro fertilization. Gynecol Obstet Invest 2002;54:36–40.

97. Marconi G, Vilela M, Quintana R, Sueldo C. Laparoscopic ovarian cystectomy of endometriomas does not affect the ovarian response to gonadotropin stimulation. Fertil Steril 2002;78;876–878.

98. Daniell JF, Kurtz BR, Gurley LD. Laser laparoscopic management of large endometriomas. Fertil Steril 1991;55:692–695.

99. Canis M, Mage G, Wattiez A, et al. Second-look laparoscopy after laparoscopic cystectomy of large ovarian endometriomas. Fertil Steril 1992;58:617–619.

100. Donnez J, Wyns C, Nisolle N. Does ovarian surgery for endometriomas impair ovarian response to gonadotropin? Fertil Steril 2001;76:662–665.

101. Pagidas K, Falcone T, Hemmings R, Miron P. Comparison of reoperation for moderate (stage III) and severe (stage IV) endometriosis-related infertility with in vitro fertilization-embryo transfer. Fertil Steril 1996;65:791–795.

102. Aboulghar MA, Mansour RT, Serour GI, et al. The outcome of in vitro fertilization in advanced endometriosis with previous surgery: a case-controlled study. Am J Obstet Gynecol 2003;188:371–375.

103. Shulman A, Marom H, Oelsner G, et al. The effect of adnexal surgery on the ovarian response to stimulation in in vitro fertilization. Eur J Obstet Gynecol Reprod Biol 2002;103:158–162.

104. Canis M, Pouly JL, Tamburro S, et al. Ovarian response during IVF-embryo transfer cycles after laparoscopic ovarian cystectomy for endometriotic cysts of >3 cm in diameter. Hum Reprod 2001;16:2583–2586.

105. Geber S, Ferreira DP, Spyer Prates LF, et al. Effects of previous ovarian surgery for endometriosis on the outcome of assisted reproduction treatment. Reprod Biomed Online 2002;5:162–166.

106. Busacca M, Fedele L, Bianchi S, et al. Surgical treatment of recurrent endometriosis: laparotomy versus laparoscopy. Hum Reprod 1998;13:2271–2274.

107. Garcia-Velasco JA, Mahutte NG, Corona J, et al. Removal of endometriomas before IVF does not improve fertility outcomes. Fertil Steril 2004;81:1194–1197.

108. Hughes EG, Fedorkow DM, Collins JA. A quantitative overview of controlled trials in endometriosis-associated infertility. Fertil Steril 1993;59:963–970.

109. Vercellini P, Chapron C, De Giorgi O, et al. Coagulation or excision of ovarian endometriomas? Am J Obstet Gynecol 2003;188:606–610.

110. Adamson GD, Pasta DJ. Surgical treatment of endometriosis-associated infertility: meta-analysis compared with survival analysis. Am J Obstet Gynecol 1994;171:1488–1504.

111. Napolitano C, Marziani R, Mossa B, et al. Management of stage III and IV endometriosis: a 10–year experience. Eur J Obstet Gynecol Reprod Biol 1994;53:199–204.

112. Olivennes F, Feldberg D, Liu HC, et al. Endometriosis: a stage by stage analysis–the role of in vitro fertilization. Fertil Steril 1995;64:392–398.

113. Guzick DS, Silliman NP, Adamson GD, et al. Prediction of pregnancy in infertile women based on the American Society for Reproductive Medicine's revised classification of endometriosis. Fertil Steril 1997;67:822–829.

114. American Society for Reproductive Medicine. Revised American Society for Reproductive Medicine classification of endometriosis: 1996. Fertil Steril 1997;67:817–821.

115. Waller KG, Shaw RW. Gonadotropin-releasing hormone analogues for the treatment of endometriosis: long-term follow-up. Fertil Steril 1993;59:511–515.

116. Geber S, Paraschos T, Atkinson G, et al. Results of IVF in patients with endometriosis: the severity of the disease does not affect outcome, or the incidence of miscarriage. Human Reprod 1995;10:1507–1511.

117. Eyster KM, Boles AL, Brannian JD, Hansen KA. DNA microarray analysis of gene expression markers of endometriosis. Fertil Steril 2002;77:38–42.

16 *Polycystic Ovary Syndrome*

The treatment of amenorrhea and sterility in this group of patients was at first conservative using endocrine preparations. Eventually, the treatment became surgical.
— *Irvin F. Stein and Michael L. Leventhal 1938*

Recognition of abnormal ovarian structure occurred well before any understanding of ovarian function. Polycystic ovaries (polycystic ovary syndrome, PCOS) were described as early as the nineteenth century. Gross sclerocystic changes in the ovary were described by Chereau in 1845. An association of ovarian morphology and menstrual function emerged and with it, proposals for treatment. Surgical management with ovarian resection became a standard of care in the late 1890s in Europe by Gusserow and Sweifel. In the American literature, Finley described a "cystic degeneration of the ovary" in 1904.[1] Though the etiology of this degeneration was unclear, he proposed that partial wedge resection was appropriate management for restoration of menses. The general thinking at the turn of the century was that the polycystic appearance of the ovaries and its impact on menstruation, ovulation, and reproduction was anatomic in origin and required surgical management.

In 1921, Achard and Thiers described what is now recognized as insulin resistance and hyperandrogenism. Ovulation disturbances were increasingly thought at this time to have an endocrine basis. This hypothesis was furthered in 1930 by Witchi, who proposed two local regulators necessary for gonadal development and ovulation labeled *cortenine* and *medullarine*.[2] In 1935, Stein and Leventhal in a report of seven patients described a syndrome of amenorrhea, infertility, and hirsutism.[3] They later expanded this series to 100 patients and included the entity of obesity as part of the syndrome. Ovulation induction with a variety of medications, was tried with variable success. Surgical management remained the mainstay and Stein and Leventhal, after failed attempts at ovulation induction with hormonal therapy, suggested that the best way to achieve normalization of ovarian function was through surgery.[4]

PCOS has evolved from an anatomic abnormality into a complex endocrine process with changes in ovarian morphology secondary to systemic endocrine and metabolic abnormalities and alterations in the ovarian microenvironment. Debates over causation have focused on adrenal, pituitary, and ovarian origins. PCOS was recognized as a heterogeneous abnormality with a variety of endocrine changes that resulted in the commonalities of anovulation and hirsutism and an ovary containing multiple follicles. Consequently, the name "Stein-Leventhal syndrome" has fallen into disuse and PCOS or polyfollicular ovaries has been adopted as a general term for this diverse spectrum of clinical abnormalities.

Management remained surgical until the 1950s when pituitary gonadotropin preparations became available, such as *Gestyl*.[6,7] With the development of antiestrogens and urinary gonadotropin preparations, ovulation induction reverted to medical management as first-line care and surgery was largely abandoned. In 1964, it was recognized that the ovaries were important sources of androgens and it was suspected that polycystic ovaries were a result of failure to ovulate and the syndrome secondary to androgen secretion by both the adrenal glands and ovaries.[8] This appreciation marked a transition in understanding. In 1976 when Kahn described a syndrome of extreme insulin resistance, diabetes, and virilization the suggestion was made that insulin could be involved in the etiology of PCOS.

The complexity and diversity of ovarian function is better understood today. Though an integrated theory to completely explain all the diverse metabolic reproductive and cosmetic aspects of PCOS is lacking, the pathophysiology is in better focus. Contemporary concepts of PCOS include interactions between insulin, insulin-like growth factors (IGF), and binding proteins, luteinizing hormone (LH), and follicle-stimulating hormone (FSH) and the interaction of these hormones on the pituitary, ovary, and endometrium. The metabolic implications of the alterations include adverse changes in lipid and glucose metabolism in addition to problems of anovulation, infertility, and hirsutism.[9,10] Increasingly, the terms *metabolic syndrome*, *syndrome x* and PCOS are used together, focusing on the broad metabolic aspects of PCOS. Treatment is increasingly focused on maintenance of well-being, management of metabolic complications, primarily insulin resistance and dyslipidemias, and when indicated, ovulation induction. Long-term deleterious sequelae involving abnormal glycemic control and cholesterol metabolism are part of this syndrome. As the most prevalent cause of anovulatory infertility, further elucidation and treatment regarding its basic pathogenesis focusing on insulin resistance will result in more effective therapies. Medical management has expanded to include insulin-sensitizing agents in addition to the more conventional hormonal therapies. Ironically, contemporary therapies have come full circle; they now include the surgical option of ovarian diathermy, a variation on wedge resection. Surgically induced ovulation has been described by a variety of terms including ovarian drilling, ovarian electrocautery, ovarian punch biopsy, and ovarian diathermy. This chapter describes the endocrine and metabolic aspects of PCOS, diagnostic techniques, and the management both medically and surgically. The objective of this chapter is to review the basis of polycystic ovary syndrome and the various methods of management, both medical and surgical, of this entity.

Etiology

The etiology of PCOS remained enigmatic until recent studies focused on the role of local regulators in ovarian function and on cross-reactivity of several hormones, primarily insulin-like growth factors and binding proteins with ovarian receptors (Figure 16-1). Though several questions remain unanswered and a unifying explanation to account for the diversity of PCOS is lacking, significant insight has been gained. What has evolved is an understanding of the complex interaction and cross reaction of hormones within a common ovarian pathway.[11,12] These abnormalities are modulated by insulin, insulin-like growth factors, and luteinizing hormone, which are responsible for a cascade of events leading eventually to anovulation, alterations in glycemic control and cholesterol metabolism, and possibly obesity.[13]

The common pathway is in part through an association of PCOS, obesity, and insulin resistance (Figure 16-2). This association is manifested as the classic type A syndrome of acanthosis nigricans, severe insulin resistance, and ovarian hyperandrogenism. The initial clinical description of this syndrome was published in 1975; the genetic alterations described in 1988.[14,15] Patient profiles range from patients who have normal glycemic control with increased insulin secretion (insulin resistance) to patients who have type II diabetes and hypercholesterolemia. The etiology may be an intrinsic defect in target cells (numerous receptor mutations have been described) and secondary factors such as obesity affecting target cells and altering response. The increased insulin secretion as part of the syndrome of insulin resistance results in a marked stimulation of ovarian androgen production, acting through the insulin-like growth factor family of receptors.

An understanding of the relationship between insulin, the ovary, and PCOS is based on clarification of the local ovarian environment and local regulators. Insulin-like growth factors (IGF) function as co-gonadotropins in the

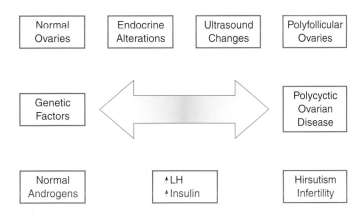

Figure 16-1   Spectrum of changes in the clinical syndrome of PCOS.

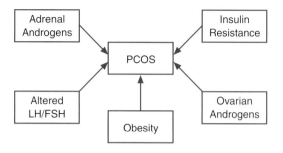

Figure 16-2   Etiologies of PCOS.

microenvironment of the ovary, facilitating steroidogenesis and folliculo-genesis, and regulating granulosa and thecal cell activity. Insulin-like growth factor binding proteins 1 to 5 are expressed in the ovary and act primarily to regulate IGF action. In PCOS, insulin-like growth factor I (IGF-I) and follicle stimulating hormone (FSH) levels are normal. High levels of insulin-like growth factor binding proteins (IGF BP) are present in these follicles and modulate IGF action, resulting in an arrested stage of folliculogenesis.[16] These follicles have a higher androgen to estradiol content and the follicular growth is usually arrested at the antral stage. This arrest gives the ovaries an appearance of multicystic, small, 8- to 12-mm follicles on TVS imaging.

Insulin resistance may be the underlying and cardinal metabolic defect that leads to the clinical expression of PCOS. Insulin resistance in PCOS may result in insulin acting on surrogate receptors, such as the family of IGF receptors, and increasing androgen production. Although the precise roles of the insulin-like growth factor system in the pathogenesis of PCOS and associated states of hyperandrogenism require more precise definition, clear trends are emerging. The so-called insulin resistance syndrome (IR syndrome or metabolic syndrome) also has associated with it a higher likelihood of developing type II diabetes mellitus, accelerated atherosclerosis, hypertension, and increased incidences of colon cancer. The most prominent manifestation because of its impact on menstrual cyclicity is polycystic ovary syndrome.[17,18] This association can be independent of body weight.

Ovarian androgen production may also be driven by insulin. Insulin appears to be a general augmenter of androgen production in conjunction with luteinizing hormone. Hyperinsulinism enhances the expression of hyperandrogenemia by increasing the availability of androgens within the ovary itself. The increased androgen production by ovarian stroma is driven both by insulin via insulin-like growth factors and increased LH secretion. Pituitary LH hypersecretion in synergism with insulin further leads to increased ovarian androgen production and further contributes to an androgen-rich microenvironment. The end result is characteristic morphologic changes in ovarian follicles most notable on transvaginal ultrasound examination.

Altered gonadotropin-releasing hormone secretion secondary to insulin also contributes to the development of PCOS. Hyperinsulinism may drive the pituitary gonadotrophs to hypersecrete LH. An increased pulse frequency and amplitude of LH is an integral part of the pathophysiology of the syndrome. Thecal androgen production is augmented by increased LH secretion. There are also altered dynamics of FSH secretion. Inadequate concentrations and inappropriate pulsatility of FSH ultimately lead to anovulation and limited estradiol secretion by the granulosa cells. Both the absolute concentrations and proper pulsatility of FSH fail to result in maturation of a follicle and ovulation.

There is no consensus regarding the genetics of PCOS. Studies of family clusters in relatives of affected probands show a high incidence of affected relatives.[19] A dominant mode of inheritance rather than a recessive one may be involved. Multiple genetic causes of hyperandrogenism and chronic anovulation (two key elements to PCOS) have been identified, but consistent abnormalities and a unifying cause for PCOS have not. Both quantitative linkage analysis and candidate gene approaches are areas being pursued in polycystic ovary syndrome. These studies may reveal that polycystic ovary syndrome is composed of a variety of subtypes influenced by one or more dominant gene causes. Microarray analysis suggests that a stable molecular phenotype of PCOS theca cells may be part of the pathophysiology of the syndrome. These genes may be specifically responsible for the excess ovarian androgen production.[20] Various genes have been suggested as candidates for polycystic ovary syndrome.

Clinical Correlates

PCOS has evolved into a multifaceted and variably expressed endocrine disorder manifested by an abnormal gonadotropin, estrogen and androgen milieu leading to hypothalamic dysfunction, hyperandrogenism, and associated adrenal function, hyperinsulinemia, and LH hypersecretion (Figure 16-3). PCOS has a varied and heterogeneous clinical expression. Clinical endocrine and metabolic abnormalities include the classic triad of obesity, anovulation, and infertility. In addition, a broader spectrum of clinical abnormalities – insulin resistance and glucose intolerance, acanthosis nigricans, sleep apnea, excessive cardiovascular disease, and increased first-trimester loss – has been associated with PCOS (Figure 16-4).[21] This spectrum brings significant implications for the long-term management and health surveillance for these patients.[22–31] Prevalence estimates are race dependent and range from 4 to 5% for white and 3 to 4% for African-American women. These prevalence figures translate to approximately 3 to 4 million women of reproductive age in the United States with PCOS.

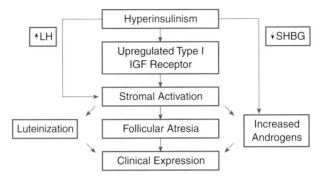

Figure 16-3   Schematic of role of insulin and cascade of endocrine events.

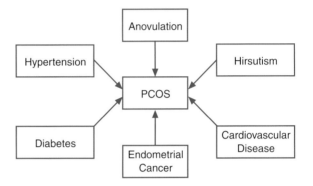

Figure 16-4   Spectrum of clinical conditions associated with PCOS.

Obesity

There is a strong association of obesity with PCOS and with the increasing incidences of obesity and PCOS in Western society. The incidence of obesity remained relatively stable from 1960 to 1980 according to the Obesity Prevalence Data of the National Center for Health Statistics.[32] There has been a gradual and progressive increase over the past 5 to 10 years of obesity in Western countries and particularly the United States.[34] It is now estimated that 60% of people in Western countries are overweight with 40% obese. The affluence of Western society, activity patterns, and dietary preferences contribute in part to the increased incidence. Obesity is now considered one of the most common nutritional diseases in the United States and a major contributor to morbidity and mortality.[35] Sixty-five percent of patients with a body mass index of 27 will have at least one comorbid condition. The most sinister of these comorbid conditions is diabetes. Premenopausal patients who are obese also have a two times higher incidence of colon cancer. The trend in obesity is particularly disturbing among children, who now represent the largest at-risk population for the development of diabetes. Children aged 2 to 11 and 12 to 19 years have an incidence of 10 and 15% obesity, respectively.[36] The various therapies for obesity including medical and surgical management, and lifestyle alterations have been largely ineffective.[36–38] These trends in obesity run counter to an increasing awareness of the benefits of dietary restriction and exercise on overall well-being. The intersection of obesity and polycystic ovary syndrome derives in large part through the high incidence of insulin resistance in patients who are overweight and obese.

In addition to the impact of insulin resistance and hyperandrogenism, obesity and alterations in lipid metabolism place these patients at risk for long-term morbidity. Obesity is associated with an increased incidence of hirsutism, elevated testosterone concentration, and increased rates of infertility and anovulation. Serum concentrations of free fatty acids are markedly increased in these patients and are closely associated with lower insulin sensitivity and lower glucose intolerance in these patients. These patients also have an increased risk of premature subclinical atherosclerosis.[22] Significant increases in the intima to media thickness have been found in cases of PCOS when compared with controls, suggesting substantial build-up of plaque within the carotid system.[23] In these patients, there were significant differences in insulin, total cholesterol, low-density lipoprotein, cholesterol, and body mass index.

Body Weight, Body Composition, and PCOS

Over 85% of women with PCOS are obese. This figure compares with an overall 40 to 50% incidence of obesity in the general population. Among obese PCOS patients, the most unfavorable endocrine profile can be observed in those patients with upper body/truncal obesity. An increased waist-to-hip ratio is associated with androgenicity, increased basal and post-glucose load blood insulin levels, and diminished insulin sensitivity. In women with abdominal visceral obesity such as those in PCOS, androgen production rates are elevated. Moreover, obesity is associated with decreased sex hormone binding globulin levels, increased androgens, and a relative hyperestrogenic state due to extra-gonadal conversion of gonadal androgens by fat tissue. The degree of insulin resistance also seems amplified in obese patients with PCOS. There is a correlation between circulating levels of leptin, a product of the adipocyte, and adiposity or body mass index in PCOS patients. Leptin may regulate the adipose tissue endocrine compartment apart from insulin. Obese patients with PCOS represent a subgroup with more pronounced endocrine disturbances and more profound ovarian dysfunction. For ovulation induction, these obese patients require higher doses of either clomiphene or gonadotropins compared with their lean counterparts. An increased body mass index was, in part, the only differentiating factor between responders and nonresponders to clomiphene citrate.

The metabolic heterogeneity of PCOS is reflected by the observation that levels of insulin, lipids, and lipoproteins may or may not be independent from body mass index. Patients may exhibit a variety of hormonal profiles, including severe forms of insulin resistance and hyperandrogenism. PCOS may be associated with insulin resistance as well as defective insulin secretion in up to 50% of all patients. These abnormalities, together with obesity itself, explain the substantially increased prevalence of glucose intolerance in PCOS.[24] Insulin resistance seems to be related to excessive serine phosphorylation of the insulin receptor due to an extrinsic factor controlling insulin receptor signaling. This phosphorylation also appears to modulate the activity of a key regulatory enzyme of androgen biosynthesis, $P450_{c17}$.

Diagnosis

Clinical Evaluation

No consensus exists regarding diagnostic criteria for PCOS. For clinical purposes, a simple classification of anovulatory infertility and hyperandrogenism was initially proposed and modified by both the World Health Organization and the European Society for Human Reproduction and Embryology. According to these classifications, patients fit into three categories. Patients presenting with low levels of gonadotropins and negligible endogenous estrogen levels constitute Group I (hypothalamic pituitary origin of anovulation). Patients with low estrogen concentrations but gonadotropin levels that are elevated suggesting an ovarian origin of the anovulation constitute Group III (i.e., premature ovarian failure). Women in both of these categories usually present with amenorrhea rather than oligomenorrhea due to low or absent estrogen exposure. The majority of patients with anovulation such as PCOS present with low serum FSH and estradiol levels within the low to normal range and are classified as Group II. PCOS is characterized by chronic hyperandrogenic anovulation and is one of the most common abnormalities in reproductive age women and a major cause of infertility. Most cross-sectional studies find associations between various clinical features such as hirsutism, anovulation, and hyperandrogenism. The criteria of elevated androgens (total and free testosterone, DHEA-S, DHEA, androstenedione) with normal serum concentrations of FSH and elevated LH (ratio of greater than 2:1) and a polycystic ovary morphology on transvaginal ultrasound examination are frequently used to define PCOS.[40,41]

Though various criteria and classifications have been debated, a clinically useful tool is essential for the day-to-day practice. The clinical criteria for the diagnosis of PCOS (amenorrhea, hirsutism, and obesity) are by contemporary standards inadequate. This definition grossly underestimates the prevalence of the disease and risks inadequate therapy and surveillance. Clinical and biochemical heterogeneity is very common in these patients. If one were to adhere strictly to the original diagnostic criteria a large number of cases would go undetected.[41] Ultrasonography is one technique for diagnosis.

Ultrasound screening of ovaries in women of reproductive age and assessment of ovarian morphology provide one of the more sensitive means of detecting PCOS.[42] Ovaries are described as polycystic or polyfollicular if there are 10 or more cysts or follicles 2 to 8 mm in diameter arranged around a dense hyperechoic stroma occupying more than 25% of ovarian volume or scattered throughout an increased amount of stroma (Figure 16-5). Enlarged polycystic ovaries are strongly associated with hyperandrogenemia, high LH values, and clinically irregular cycles in the absence of any overt evidence of hyperandrogenism such as hirsutism or acne. These changes may be noted during the postmenarchal period and appear to persist throughout the reproductive years. However, more than 20% of women with regular menstrual cycles have ovaries that fit the description of polycystic upon transvaginal ultrasonographic examination. In these patients, normal-appearing ovaries during the postmenarchal period may evolve and assume a polycystic ovarian appearance with an increase in volume later on during the reproductive life. The diagnosis of PCOS on ultrasound is strongly associated with exaggerated ovarian androgen and estrogen responses to provocative testing with GnRH.[43,44]

The appearance of the ovaries on ultrasound does not predict the severity of the syndrome. In select circumstances where the ovaries are clearly polycystic in appearance and no endocrine abnormalities are noted, serial follow-up examination and monitoring may be necessary. There may be a time lapse between the morphologic ovarian changes and actual endocrine expression.[45] Limitations in this diagnostic study do exist. Ultrasound diagnosis of PCOS

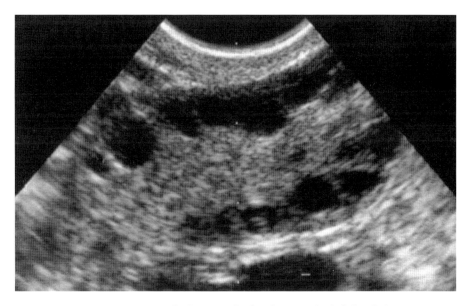

Figure 16-5   Transvaginal ultrasound of polycystic (polyfollicular) ovary. Note multiple small follicles at periphery and central hyperechoic stroma.

may be limited by its inability to display either ovary in 15% of patients. Sensitivity of 91% and specificity of 100% was described in one series.[46] With ultrasound diagnosis, polycystic ovaries may be found in 20% of women with amenorrhea, 87% of women with oligomenorrhea, 92% of women with hirsutism, and 22% of normal volunteers.[47] Ultrasound endocrinopathies are seen in 20 to 40% of "normal" women.[45] The diagnosis of PCOS with MRI has not been shown to be more effective than the less-expensive ultrasound.[48,49]

A combination of findings is frequently the most useful approach to diagnose PCOS that includes ultrasonographic, hormonal, and clinical parameters. Any patient with oligo-ovulation or anovulation who has at least three of the following criteria is likely to fit the syndrome: polycystic ovaries by ultrasonography, hirsutism, and hyperandrogenism. The hyperandrogenism is determined biochemically by evaluating total and serum free testosterone levels, androstenedione concentrations, and sex hormone binding globulin concentrations.

Management

Weight Loss

The first method of management for anovulation, associated with obesity, should be a weight loss protocol. Weight loss is associated with significant improvements in menstruation abnormalities, ovulation, and fertility. The management of obesity is increasingly recognized as a cognitive issue. Part of managing polycystic ovary syndrome associated with obesity should be in counseling the patients regarding the association of obesity and anovulation. When appropriate, consultation with weight reduction clinics may provide a drug-free option for patients interested in ovulation induction. These programs are frequently effective, but difficult, in part because of motivational issues and in part because of the relatively slow process associated with weight loss and restoration of ovulation. Though weight loss may be, in part, related to motivation, it is increasingly apparent that there are specific hormones related to weight loss that may provide an opportunity for drug therapy in the future.[50]

There is a complex interaction between obesity, ovulation and hormones relating to calorific intake. Three hormones figure heavily into weight control. The significance of these hormones in the management of polycystic ovary syndrome may be, in part, as portals for manipulation for weight loss. Leptin is a hormone produced and released by the adipocytes in a pulsatile manner.[51] It acts at the level of the hypothalamus to inhibit food intake and increase energy expenditure. Studies in animal models suggested that it is instrumental in weight loss and normalization of insulin–glucose interactions.[52] Leptin and body mass index are important predictors of ovarian response during ovulation induction. The second hormone is ghrelin. This hormone is produced by the stomach. It increases with food intake and participates in an adaptive response to weight loss. It is noted to rise during dieting and may act in a "feed me" fashion. Appetite may stimulate its production and it is noted to rise sharply before and decrease after every meal. Of particular note is the suppression of this hormone associated with gastric bypass surgery possibly contributing to the weight-reducing effect of that procedure.[53] The third hormone is resistin. Resistin is an adipocyte-derived peptide and has a possible role as an antagonist to insulin. It is elevated in obesity.[54] This hormone is of particular interest to polycystic ovary syndrome, in part because of its relation to insulin resistance and in part because it is down-regulated with treatment using metformin.[55,56] In spite of an increasing understanding of obesity, satiety, and their relationship to hormones, there are as yet no effective anti-obesity agents. Medical management of obesity has been side tracked because of ineffective protocols and the recent association with fen-phen with valvular heart disease. Long-term success is also open to question. Medical management of weight loss is frequently associated with a weight loss of 10–15% followed by a plateau and gradual gain.[57] However, with understanding of the hormonal basis of hunger and satiety, effective antagonists to block or agonists to mimic these urges are now possible.

Weight loss should be discussed with all patients who are presenting for ovulation induction with polycystic ovary syndrome associated with obesity. In addition to this, for patients who are morbidly obese, consultation with appropriate maternal–fetal medical specialists prior to conception is also be recommended. For those patients who elect not to undertake a weight loss protocol, medical ovulation induction is the next option.

Medical Management

Anti-estrogens are the first method of ovulation induction for patients with polycystic ovary syndrome (Figure 16-6). These medications have the advantage of ease of use, but because of the complex issues surrounding anovulation in PCOS, are not the most effective options. The anti-estrogens are first-line management for anovulation secondary to PCOS. Clomiphene may be used at doses ranging from 50 mg to 150–200 mg for 5 days per cycle. Tamoxifen is a second option at doses of 25 mg for 5 to 7 days per cycle. A cardinal principle in their use is a rigid definition of success and a firm plan for monitoring response. The patient should have ultrasound assessment of follicular activity and endometrial thickness periodically through a cycle. If follicular dominance is not established in a reasonable period of observation, the dose should be increased and the monitoring repeated. Success has a two-part definition: consistent and predictable ovulation and pregnancy. If no ovulation has occurred after increasing doses to the maximum limit, clomiphene should be discontinued. If ovulation has occurred over 3 to 6 cycles and no pregnancy has occurred, consideration should be given to gonadotropins of IVF.

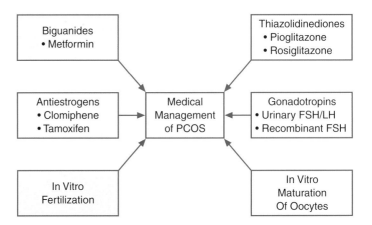

Figure 16-6   Options for medical management of PCOS.

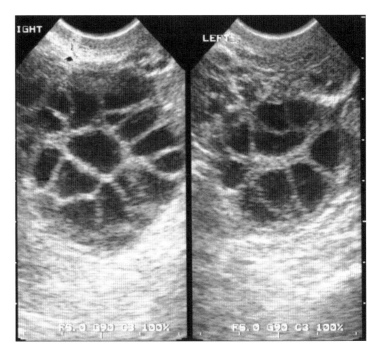

Figure 16-7   Transvaginal ultrasound image of right and left ovary showing multiple follicular development characteristic of ovarian hyperstimulation syndrome in PCOS.

In patients who do not ovulate with anti-estrogens, the next two options are ovulation induction with gonadotropins and in vitro fertilization. Ovulation induction using gonadotropins is a more effective method for patients who do not respond to clomiphene. It has a higher likelihood of successful ovulation and pregnancy. It is also associated with a higher incidence of ovarian

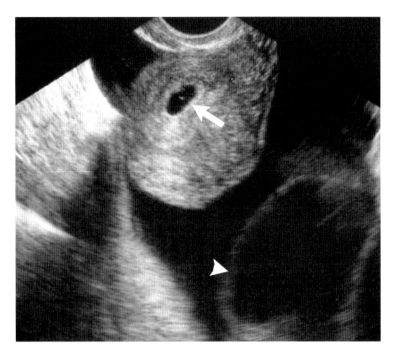

Figure 16-8   Transvaginal ultrasound image of ascites, ovarian cysts (arrow-head) and intrauterine gestation (arrow) in ovarian hyperstimulation syndrome.

hyperstimulation syndrome and multiple pregnancies (Figures 16-7 and 16-8). Management with gonadotropins is a complex and intricate process. There are both urinary and recombinant products available. Similar outcomes have been described for each, although the recombinant FSH preparations appear to fit more precisely with the pathophysiology of the process. The dosing of the medications should be based in part on the patient's weight. The starting dose should be as low as possible to avoid the possibility of multiple follicles developing and a high risk of multiples and ovarian hyper-stimulation syndrome. Monitoring with ultrasound and serum estradiol concentrations are standard. However, extreme care is required in interpreting these data. This information is intended to guide decision-making regarding dose of medication and the decision and timing of HCG administration. Studies however question the accuracy of this dual monitoring approach in predicting high order multiples. Hence, an individualized approach is necessary. When one, two or three follicles have reached maturity with diameters of 18–22 mm, HCG may be given. An essential part of counseling any patient for ovulation induction with gonadotropins is the possibility of multiple pregnancies, ovarian hyperstimulation syndrome, and the possibility that the cycle will either be canceled or converted to a cycle of in vitro fertilization. Only after the above options have been exhausted is it appropriate to consider surgical techniques for ovulation induction in polycystic ovary syndrome.

Insulin-sensitizing agents offer another alternative for medical management of PCOS. The mainstay for medical management of polycystic ovary syndrome with insulin-sensitizing agents is with metformin.[58,59] Given the role of hyperinsulinism and the pathophysiology of polycystic ovary syndrome, insulin-sensitizing agents have found a role in the management of this syndrome. Metformin is the insulin-sensitizing agent studied in the most detail and in the largest groups of women. It is a second-generation biguanide introduced in the United States in 1995. Metformin lowers serum glucose levels and, consequently, serum insulin levels. Peripheral insulin resistance is decreased by the drug's ability to activate glucose transporters in both muscle and hepatic cells.[60] Most published studies have shown an increase in menstrual cyclicity, spontaneous ovulation, and fertility rates in polycystic ovary syndrome at doses ranging from 1000 to 2000 mg of metformin daily.[61,62] The quality of the evidence supporting the use of metformin in these circumstances is extremely varied.[63] Case reports, case series, uncontrolled studies and randomized, placebo-controlled trials have all suggested a role for metformin. Androgen profiles appear to normalize and an improvement in both total and free serum testosterone levels were noted with metformin. In addition, sex hormone binding globulin levels have been noted to increase.

Though metformin is first line management rosiglitazone and pioglitazone are alternatives for patients who cannot tolerate metformin. These agents enhance insulin action without directly stimulating insulin secretion. These drugs demonstrated improvements in blood pressure, androgen parameters, and lipid profiles. There are, however, no long-term studies that clearly demonstrate enhanced effectiveness of these agents over metformin. Rosiglitazone and pioglitazone drugs are category C and have been demonstrated to retard fetal development. D-*chiro*-inositol is a phosphoglycan mediator of insulin action and is decreased in patients with insulin resistance. There is a suggestion that this compound may be effective in managing anovulation secondary to polycystic ovary syndrome. Insulin-sensitizing agents may be used in conjunction with either clomiphene citrate, gonadotropins, or ovarian drilling.

Evaluation Prior to ART

Patients who fail to conceive through conservative options may consider in vitro fertilization. The decision to proceed with IVF may be reached after failure to achieve ovulation with gonadotropins, failure to achieve a pregnancy after 3 to 6 ovulatory cycles, cancellations due to excessive stimulation and higher than acceptable rate of multiples. There are no set criteria for reaching this decision. A combination of factors including previous responses to either anti-estrogens or gonadotropins, degree of risk a couple may be willing to face regarding multiples and ovarian hyperstimulation syndrome (OHSS), and likelihood of success may weigh considerably into the decision. Options for protocols address the issues of insulin resistance, oocyte quality, the tendency toward ovarian hyperstimulation syndrome, and variable endometrial receptivity (Table 16-1). Ultimately, simpler,

Table 16-1.
Evaluation Prior to ART: Polycystic Ovary Syndrome
• Weight loss is essential
• Possible role of insulin-sensitizing agents
• Assessment of endometrium: endometrial thickness, echogenic pattern, and receptivity
• Assessment of ovaries: basal antral follicle count and ovarian size in three dimensions
• Careful calculation of gonadotropin dosage based on BMI and prior responses (if available)
• Possible role of long-term (1 month) GnRH suppression prior to ovarian stimulation
• Assessment of ovarian reserve (if possible) in patients who have undergone previous ovarian diathermy and are ovulatory
• Counseling regarding ovarian hyperstimulation syndrome
• Cancellation of cycle or conversion to IVF in patients undergoing ovulation induction if stimulation is excessive and risk of multiples is high

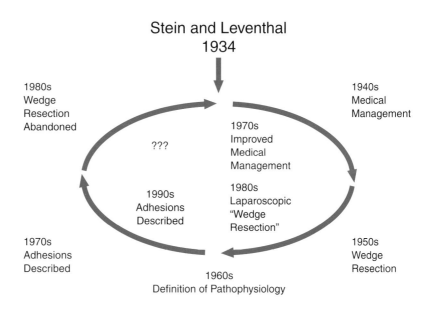

Figure 16-9   Summary of surgical and medical management of anovulation of polycystic ovary disease from the initial description by Stein and Leventhal in 1934 to contemporary methods of ovarian electrocautery.

less-expensive protocols may supplant current practice for IVF in PCOS. The options of in vitro maturation of oocytes may provide one avenue to minimize ovarian stimulation and reduce the risk of full-blown OHSS and the complexity of the stimulation protocols. In those patients who do not conceive with IVF, refuse to accept the risks and expenses of IVF or have ethical or religious objections, surgical ovulation induction may be considered.

Surgical Management

Therapies for PCOS have evolved considerably since Stein and Leventhal's initial description of wedge resection (Figure 16-9). Selection of optimal therapy now requires careful consideration of a variety of parameters and options. Medical management remains the mainstay of therapy. Ovulation is induced with clomiphene or gonadotropins to achieve reproductive potential.[64-66] IVF is the next most aggressive option. IVF may be considered as first-line therapy depending on age.

Only after exhaustion of these regimens should any consideration be given to surgical therapy (Table 16-2). Potential advantages of surgical induction of ovulation include possible normalization of ovulatory cycles from a single

---

Table 16-2.
Surgical Ovulation Induction

- **Indications**

  Clomiphene-resistant patients undergoing diagnostic laparoscopy
  Poor response to any ovulation-inducing agent, whether clomiphene citrate or gonadotropins

- **Techniques**

  Laser
  Cautery
  Multiple punch biopsies

- **Clinical Advantages**

  Improved endocrine profiles
  Spontaneous ovulation
  Reduction in gonadotropin doses for ovulation induction
  Improvement in pregnancy rates
  Reduction in multiple pregnancy rates and first-trimester loss rates and incidence of ovarian hyperstimulation syndrome

- **Clinical Disadvantages**

  Adhesion formation
  Compromise to ovarian function
  Influence on age of menopause onset unclear

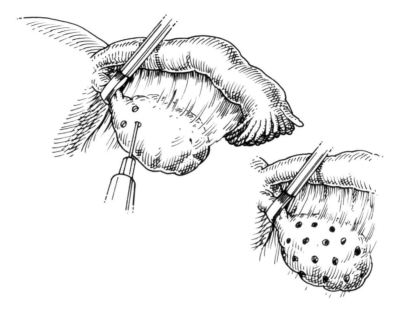

Figure 16-10   Ovarian electrocautery. The ovary is gently grasped at the ovarian–uterine ligament. Grasping in this region permits rotating the ovary on its axis for access to all surfaces. With needle-tip cautery, several burns are placed throughout the ovarian surface. In lieu of needle-tip cautery, a laser fiber may be used.

treatment, no risk of ovarian hyperstimulation or multiple gestation, and the possibility of a higher live-birth rate because of a lower incidence of miscarriage[67–71]. Disadvantages include adhesion formation and premature menopause caused by postoperative ovarian atrophy has been reported (Table 16-2).[72] Data from uncontrolled studies suggest that surgical techniques for ovulation induction may have a role in PCOS in patients who do not respond to maximal doses of clomiphene and who are unable or unwilling to undergo gonadotropin therapy.[67,68] The exact mechanism by which laparoscopic procedures induce ovulation, however, remains unclear.[69]

Operative Technique

A standard laparoscopic approach is utilized. Using grasping forceps, the uterine ovarian pedicle is identified and gently grasped. This procedure enables the ovary to be rotated on its axis so that both lateral and medial aspects of the ovary can be visualized (Figure 16-10). With needle-tip cautery and low wattage, isolated cauterization is then undertaken for approximately 1 to 2 mm in depth and 5 to 6 mm in width. The number of cauterization points may depend on the size of the ovary, but 8 to 12 points per ovary should be undertaken, with the cauterization sites spaced approximately 2 to 3 mm apart. Duration of cauterization should be 4 to 6 seconds at each point

	Table 16-3.		
	Outcomes After Surgical Treatment of PCOS		
Technique	**Ovulation‡** **Rate %**	**Conception‡** **Rate %**	**Periadnexal Adhesion‡** **Formation %**
Cautery	81% (74, 86)	55% (47, 63)	36% (27, 46)
Nd:YAG laser	70% (57, 81)	46% (33, 59)	35% (24, 48)
CO_2/KTB laser	71% (60, 80)	56% (45, 67)	20% (5, 49)

‡ Percentages and 95% confidence interval
References 67–83

at 300 to 400 watts. This procedure is performed on anterior, posterior, and lateral aspects of the ovary and bilaterally for even distribution. A KTP or CO_2 laser may be used if preferred by the surgeon.

Outcomes Analysis for Surgical Management

Normalization of endocrine profiles in PCOS has been reported after ovarian electrocautery.[73–78] A significant decrease in androstenediol, dihydrotestosterone, androstenedione, and testosterone levels occurs. Estradiol concentrations are increased. No change has been described in serum concentrations of sex hormone binding globulin, prolactin dehydroepiandrosterone (DHEA), DHEA sulfate, 17-hydroxyprogesterone, and FSH. Markedly reduced basal serum LH concentration and normalization of menstrual cyclicity occurs in approximately 50% of patients after laparoscopic ovarian electrocautery. Significantly higher rates of ovulation and pregnancy have been reported in some series after these techniques when compared with gonadotropin-stimulated cycles (Table 16-3). In those patients who fail to conceive after ovarian electrocautery, there is also a significant reduction in the amount of mediation and duration for ovulation induction with gonadotropins. A favorable profile for conception includes a shorter duration of infertility (less than 3 years), treatment with diathermy (rather than laser), higher preoperative LH levels (greater than 10 mIU/mL), younger age, and ultrasonographic evidence of PCOS. In one study, the success rate in women with infertility of less than 3 years duration treated with diathermy and in whom preoperative LH was more than 10 reached 79%.

Age is an important consideration, especially for patients considering IVF as an alternative. In one study of the effects of ovarian surgery on ovarian function and menopause, the age of onset of menopause in patients who underwent ovarian surgery at an age of less than 30 years was found to be significantly younger than a control group. For women who had undergone bilateral wedge biopsy and ovarian drilling greater than 35 years there is no suggestion of changes in age of menopause.[79,80]

Several series have described these techniques using needle-tip cautery or laser surgical management of PCOS and for ovulation induction.[81] Current studies are of variable quality. Pregnancies after surgical induction of ovulation have been reported in 56 to 94% of treated patients (Table 16-3). In a Cochrane review, no difference in cumulative pregnancy rates could be demonstrated between ovarian drilling and ovulation induction. However, multiple pregnancy ranges were significantly reduced after ovarian drilling.[82,83] In a series of 252 women with PCOS treated with ovarian laparoscopic electrocautery, ovulation was induced in 92% and resulted in an 84% pregnancy rate. In another study, the cumulative pregnancy rate 12 months after laparoscopic ovarian drilling for anovulatory infertility, clomiphene-resistant polycystic ovary syndrome was 50%. Clomiphene citrate in patients who become pregnant after ovarian electrocautery increased the pregnancy rate to an overall rate of 89%. Most pregnancies occur within six ovulatory cycles. Failure to conceive within this time frame warrants further investigation, including either second-look laparoscopy and lysis of adhesions or more probably referral for IVF. The response rate to ovarian electrocautery is influenced by body weight; ovulation rates of 97% in slim patients decrease to 70% in moderately obese patients. The limiting factor of these techniques is postoperative adhesions. Occurrence of adhesions varies from 0 to 100% (Table 16-3). Ovarian electrocautery may be considered as surgical management for patients with PCOS, especially patients undergoing laparoscopy for other reasons, or for whom IVF or ART are not options.[81] Careful, detailed counseling is essential. This approach is not first-line management and patient selection is critical.

Summary and Recommendations

Patients with PCOS who fail to ovulate using clomiphene citrate or gonadotropins are candidates for ovarian electrocautery. This procedure is an alternative to IVF in select cases. Patients should be carefully counseled regarding the complications of the procedure, including adhesion formation, a potential compromise to ovarian function, and the possibility of complete loss of ovarian function. Success rates for this procedure should be compared to IVF including details of costs and rate of multiples. The advantages of the procedure are marked improvement in the endocrine milieu, a reduction in the amount of medication required for those patients who do not resume ovulation spontaneously, and a reduction in the complications of multiple gestation and ovarian hyperstimulation in those patients who do require gonadotropin therapy. The following recommendations may be made.

- Consideration should be given to surgical induction of ovulation in any patient with PCOS who is clomiphene citrate-resistant or has hyperstimulation on gonadotropins or for whom IVF is not an option.
- Postoperative adhesion formation may occur in 30 to 100% of patients

undergoing this procedure. Early second-look laparoscopy or the use of a barrier may reduce the incidence of adhesion formation and its potential impact on fertility.
- In those patients who do not achieve a pregnancy, consideration should be given to IVF.

References

1. Findley P. Cystic degeneration of the ovary: an anatomic and clinical study of 180 cases. Am J Obstet Dis Women Child 1904;49:762–765.

2. Mahesh VB, Greenblatt RB. Steroid secretions of the normal and polycystic ovary. Recent Prog Horm Res 1964;20:341–394.

3. Stein IF. Amenorrhea associated with bilateral polycystic ovaries. Am J Obstet Gynecol 1935; 29:181–186.

4. Stein RF, Cohen MR. Results of bilateral ovarian wedge resection in 47 cases of sterility. Am J Obstet Gynecol 1949;58:267–274.

5. Meaker SR. Ovarian resection for the relief of sterility. Fertil Steril 1950;1:293.

6. Gemzeli CA, Diczfalusy E, Tillinger KC. Clinical effect of human pituitary follicle-stimulating hormone. J Clin Endocrinol 1958;18:1333.

7. Lunenfeld B, Lunenfeld E. Gonadotropic preparation – lessons learned. Fertil Steril 1997;67:812–814.

8. Yen SS, Vela P, Rankin J. Inappropriate secretion of follicle-stimulating hormone and luteinizing hormone in polycystic ovarian disease. J Clin Endocrinol Metab 1970;30:435–442.

9. Legro RS. The genetics of polycystic ovary syndrome. Am J Med 1995;98:9S–16S.

10. Nestler JE, Jakubowicz DJ, de Vargas AF, et al. Insulin stimulates testosterone biosynthesis by human thecal cells from women with polycystic ovary syndrome by activating its own receptor and using inositolglycan mediators as the signal transduction system. J Clin Endocrinol Metab 1998; 83:2001–2005.

11. Adashi EY, Resnick CE, Hernandez ER, et al. Insulin-like growth factor I as an intraovarian regulator: basic and clinical implications. Ann N Y Acad Sci 1991;626:161–168.

12. Adashi EY. Growth factors and ovarian function: the IgF-I paradigm. Horm Res 1994;42:44–48.

13. Barbieri RL, Smith S, Ryan KJ. The role of hyperinsulinemia in the pathogenesis of ovarian hyperandrogenism. Fertil Steril 1988;50:197–212.

14. Moloer DE, Flier JS. Detection of an alteration in the insulin-receptor gene in a patient with insulin resistance acanthosis nigricans, and the polycystic ovary syndrome (type A insulin resistance). N Engl J Med 1988;319:1526–1529.

15. Adashi EY. Intraovarian regulation: the IgF-I example. Reprod Fertil Dev 1992;4:497–504.

16. Giudice LC. The insulin-like growth factor system in normal and abnormal human ovarian follicle development. Am J Med 1995;98;48S–54S.

17. Morin-Papunen LC, Vauhkonen I, Koivunen RM, et al. Insulin sensitivity, insulin secretion, and meta-
     bolic and hormonal parameters in healthy women and women with polycystic ovarian syndrome.
     Hum Reprod 2000;15:1266–1274.

18. Fruehwald-Schultes B, Oltmanns KM, Toschek B, et al. Short-term treatment with metformin
     decreases serum leptin concentration without affecting body weight and body fat content in normal-
     weight healthy men. Metabolism 2002;51:531–536.

19. Rajkhowa M, Bicknell J, Jones M, Clayton RN. Insulin sensitivity in women with polycystic ovary syn-
     drome: relationship to hyperandrogenemia. Fertil Steril 1994;61:605–612.

20. Wood JR, Nelson VL, Ho C, et al. The molecular phenotype of polycystic ovary syndrome (PCOS)
     theca cells and new candidate PCOS genes defined by microarray analysis. J Biol Chem
     2003;278:26380–26390.

21. Meirow D, Yossepowitch O, Rosler A, et al. Insulin resistant and non-resistant polycystic ovary syn-
     drome represent two clinical and endocrinological subgroups. Hum Reprod 1995;10:1951–1956.

22. Guzick DS, Talbott EO, Sutton-Tyrrell K, et al. Carotid atherosclerosis in women with polycystic ovary
     syndrome: initial results from a case-control study. Am J Obstet Gynecol 1996;174:1224–1229.

23. Talbott E, Guzick D, Clerici A, et al. Coronary heart disease risk factors in women with polycystic
     ovary syndrome. Arterioscler Thromb Vasc Biol 1995;15:821–826.

24. Legro RS, Kunselman AR, Dodson WC, Dunaif A. Prevalence and predictors of risk for type 2 diabetes
     mellitus and impaired glucose tolerance in polycystic ovary syndrome: a prospective, controlled study
     in 254 affected women. J Clin Endocrinol Metab 1999;84:165–169.

25. Birdsall MA, Farquhar CM, White HD. Association between polycystic ovaries and extent of coronary
     artery disease in women having cardiac catheterization. Ann Intern Med 1997;126:32–35.

26. Holte J, Bergh T, Berne C, Lithell H. Serum lipoprotein profile in women with the polycystic ovary
     syndrome: relation to anthropometric, endocrine and metabolic variables. Clin Endocrinol
     1994;41:463–471.

27. Singh KB, Mahajan DK, Wortsman J. Effect of obesity on the clinical and hormonal characteristics of
     the polycystic ovary syndrome. J Reprod Med 1994;39:805–808.

28. Wild RA. Obesity, lipids, cardiovascular risk, and androgen excess. Am J Med 1995;98:27S–32S.

29. Talbott E, Guzick D, Clerici A, et al. Coronary heart disease risk factors in women with polycystic
     ovary syndrome. Arterioscler Thromb Vasc Biol 1995;15:821–826.

30. Balen AH, Conway GS, Kaltsas G, et al. Polycystic ovary syndrome: the spectrum of the disorder in
     1741 patients. Hum Reprod 1995;10:2107–2111.

31. Haas DA, Carr BR, Attia GR. Effects of metformin on body mass index, menstrual cyclicity, and ovula-
     tion induction in women with polycystic ovary syndrome. Fertil Steril 2003;79:469–481.

32. Pi-Sunyer FX, Laferrere B, Aronne LJ, Bray GA. Therapeutic controversy: Obesity – a modern-day epi-
     demic. J Clin Endocrinol Metab 1999;84:3–12.

33. Brunner EJ, Wunsch H, Marmot MG. What is an optimal diet? Relationship of macronutrient intake to
     obesity, glucose tolerance, lipoprotein cholesterol levels and the metabolic syndrome in the Whitehall
     II study. Int J Obes Relat Metab Disord 2001;25:45–53.

34. Manson JE, Bassuk SS. Obesity in the United States: a fresh look at its high toll. JAMA 2003;289:229–230.

35. Bray GA. Obesity: a time bomb to be defused. Lancet 1998;352:160–161.

36. Howard BV, Wylie-Rosett J. Sugar and cardiovascular disease: A statement for healthcare professionals from the Committee on Nutrition of the Council on Nutrition, Physical Activity, and Metabolism of the American Heart Association. Circulation 2002;106:523–527.

37. Subar AF, Krebs-Smith SM, Cook A, Kahle LL. Dietary sources of nutrients among US adults, 1989 to 1991. J Am Diet Assoc 1998;98:537–547.

38. U.S. Preventive Services Task Force. Behavioral counseling in primary care to promote physical activity: recommendation and rationale. Ann Intern Med 2002;137:205–207.

39. Homburg R. What is polycystic ovarian syndrome? A proposal for a consensus on the definition and diagnosis of polycystic ovarian syndrome. Hum Reprod 2002;17:2495–2499.

40. The ESHRE Capri Workshop Group. Anovulatory infertility. Hum Reprod 1995;10:1549–1553.

41. van der Westhuizen S, van der Spuy ZM. Ovarian morphology as a predictor of hormonal values in polycystic ovary syndrome. Ultrasound Obstet Gynecol 1996;7:335–341.

42. Farquhar CM, Birdsall M, Manning P, et al. Prevalence of polycystic ovaries on ultrasound scanning in a population of randomly selected women. Aust NZ J Obstet Gynaecol 1994;34:67–72.

43. Suikkari AM, MacLachlan V, Montalto J, et al. Ultrasonographic appearance of polycystic ovaries is associated with exaggerated ovarian androgen and oestradiol responses to gonadotropin-releasing hormone agonist in women undergoing assisted reproduction treatment. Hum Reprod 1995;10;513–519.

44. Filicori M, Flamigni C, Campaniello E, et al. The abnormal response of polycystic ovarian disease patients to exogenous pulsatile gonadotropin-releasing hormone: characterization and management. J Clin Endocrinol Metab 1989;69:825–831.

45. Gulekli B, Turhan NO, Senoz S, et al. Endocrinological, ultrasonographic and clinical findings in adolescent and adult polycystic ovary patients: a comparative study. Gynecol Endocrinol 1993;7:273–277.

46. Fox R, Hull M. Ultrasound diagnosis of polycystic ovaries. Ann N Y Acad Sci 1993;687:217–223.

47. Botsis D, Kassanos D, Pyrgiotis E, Zourlas PA. Sonographic incidence of polycystic ovaries in a gynecological population. Ultrasound Obstet Gynecol 1995;6:182–185.

48. Maubon A, Courtieu C, Vivens F, et al. Magnetic resonance imaging of normal and polycystic ovaries. Preliminary results. Ann N Y Acad Sci 1993;687:224–229.

49. Kimura I, Togashi K, Kawakami S, et al. Polycystic ovaries: implications of diagnosis with MR imaging. Radiology 1996;201:549–552.

50. Bray GA. Pharmacological treatment of obesity. In: Bray GA, Bouchard C, James WPT, eds. Handbook of Obesity. New York: Marcel Dekker, Inc. 2001;953–975.

51. Janeckova R. The role of leptin in human physiology and pathophysiology. Physiol Res 2001;50:443–459.

52. Shintani M, Ikegami H, Fujisawa T, et al. Leptin gene polymorphism is associated with hypertension independent of obesity. J Clin Endocrinol Metab 2002;87:2909–2912.

53. Cummings DE, Weigle DS, Frayo RS, et al. Plasma ghrelin levels after diet-induced weight loss or gastric bypass surgery. N Engl J Med 2002;346:1623–1630.

54. Janke J, Engeli S, Gorzelniak K, et al. Resistin gene expression in human adipocytes is not related to insulin resistance. Obes Res 2002;10:1–5.

55. Steppan CM, Lazar MA. Resistin and obesity-associated insulin resistance. Trends Endocrinol Metab 2002;13:18–23.

56. Shuldiner AR, Yang R, Gong DW. Resistin, obesity and insulin resistance – the emerging role of the adipocyte as an endocrine organ. N Engl J Med 2001;345:1345–1346.

57. Sims EA. Are there persons who are obese, but metabolically healthy? Metabolism 2001;50:1499–1504.

58. Heard MJ, Pierce A, Carson SA, Buster JE. Pregnancies following use of metformin for ovulation induction in patients with polycystic ovary syndrome. Fertil Steril 2002;77:669–673.

59. Van Gaal L, Scheen AJ. Are all glitazones the same? Diabetes Metab Res Rev 2002;18:S1–S4.

60. Moghetti P, Castello R, Negri C, et al. Metformin effects on clinical features, endocrine and metabolic profiles, and insulin sensitivity in polycystic ovary syndrome: a randomized, double-blind, placebo-controlled 6-month trial, followed by open, long-term clinical evaluation. J Clin Endocrinol Metab 2000;85:139–146.

61. Nestler JE, Stovall D, Akhter N, et al. Strategies for the use of insulin-sensitizing drugs to treat infertility in women with polycystic ovary syndrome. Fertil Steril 2002;77:209–215.

62. Norman RJ, Kidson WJ, Cuneo RC, Zacharin MR. Metformin and intervention in polycystic ovary syndrome. Endocrine Society of Australia, the Australian Diabetes Society and the Australian Paediatric Endocrine Group. Med J Aust 2001;174:580–583.

63. Lord JM, Flight IH, Norman RJ. Insulin-sensitising drugs (metformin, troglitazone, rosiglitazone, pioglitazone, D-chiro-inositol) for polycystic ovary syndrome. Cochrane Database Syst Rev 2003;(3):CD003053.

64. Dunaif A, Scott D, Finegood D, et al. The insulin-sensitizing agent troglitazone improves metabolic and reproductive abnormalities in the polycystic ovary syndrome. J Clin Endocrinol Metab 1996;81:3299–3306.

65. Acbay O, Gundogdu S. Can metformin reduce insulin resistance in polycystic ovary syndrome? Fertil Steril 1996;65:946–949.

66. Velazquez EM, Mendoza S, Hamer T, et al. Metformin therapy in polycystic ovary syndrome reduces hyperinsulinemia, insulin resistance, hyperandrogenemia, and systolic blood pressure, while facilitating normal menses and pregnancy. Metabolism 1994;43:647–654.

67. Farhi J, Soule S, Jacobs HS. Effect of laparoscopic ovarian electrocautery on ovarian response and outcome of treatment with gonadotropins in clomiphene citrate-resistant patients with polycystic ovary syndrome. Fertil Steril 1995;64:930–935.

68. Kriplani A, Manchanda R, Agarwal N, Nayar B. Laparoscopic ovarian drilling in clomiphene citrate-resistant women with polycystic ovary syndrome. J Am Assoc Gynecol Laparosc 2001;8:511–518.

69. Li TC, Saravelos H, Chow MS, et al. Factors affecting the outcome of laparoscopic ovarian drilling for polycystic ovarian syndrome in women with anovulatory infertility. Br J Obstet Gynaecol 1998;105:338–344.

70. Campo S, Felli A, Lamanna MA, et al. Endocrine changes and clinical outcome after laparoscopic ovarian resection in women with polycystic ovaries. Hum Reprod 1993;8:359–363.

71. Gurgan T, Yarali H, Urman B. Laparoscopic treatment of polycystic ovarian disease. Hum Reprod 1994;9:573–577.

72. Naether OG, Fischer R. Adhesion formation after laparoscopic electrocoagulation of the ovarian surface in polycystic ovary patients. Fertil Steril 1993;60:95–98.

73. Naether OG, Fischer R, Weise HC, et al. Laparoscopic electrocoagulation of the ovarian surface in infertile patients with polycystic ovarian disease. Fertil Steril 1993;60:88–94.

74. Verhelst J, Gerris J, Joostens M, et al. Clinical and endocrine effects of laser vaporization in patients with polycystic ovarian disease. Gynecol Endocrinol 1993;71:49–55.

75. Szilagyi A, Hole R, Keckstein J, Rossmanith WG. Effects of ovarian surgery on the dopaminergic and opioidergic control of gonadotropin and prolactin secretion in women with polycystic ovarian disease. Gynecol Endocrinol 1993;7:159–166.

76. Naether OG, Baukloh V, Fischer R, Kowalczyk T. Long-term follow-up in 206 infertile patients with polycystic ovarian syndrome after laparoscopic electrocautery of the ovarian surface. Hum Reprod 1994;9:2342–2349.

77. Kaaijk EM, Beek JF, van der Veen F. Laparoscopic surgery of chronic hyperandrogenic anovulation. Lasers Surg Med 1995;16:292–302.

78. Johnson NP, Wang K. Is ovarian surgery effective for androgenic symptoms of polycystic ovarian syndrome? J Obstet Gynaecol 2003;23:599–606.

79. Melica F, Chiodi S, Cristoforoni PM, Ravera GB. Reductive surgery and ovarian function in the human – can reductive ovarian surgery in reproductive age negatively influence fertility and age at onset of menopause? Int J Fertil Menopausal Stud 1995;40:79–85.

80. Amer SA, Li TC, Cooke ID. Repeated laparoscopic ovarian diathermy is effective in women with anovulatory infertility due to polycystic ovary syndrome. Fertil Steril 2003;79:1211–1215.

81. Stegmann BJ, Craig HR, Bay RC, et al. Characteristics predictive of response to ovarian diathermy in women with polycystic ovarian syndrome. Am J Obstet Gynecol 2003;188:1171–1173.

82. Farquhar C, Vandekerckhove P, Lilford R. Laparoscopic "drilling" by diathermy or laser for ovulation induction in anovulatory polycystic ovary syndrome. Cochrane Database Syst Rev 2003;3.

83. Farquhar CM, Williamson K, Gudex G, et al. A randomized controlled trial of laparoscopic ovarian diathermy versus gonadotropin therapy for women with clomiphene citrate-resistant polycystic ovary syndrome. Fertil Steril 2002;78:404–411.

84. Buyalos RP, Lee CT. Polycystic ovary syndrome: pathophysiology and outcome with in vitro fertilization. Fertil Steril 1996;65:1–10.

85. Homburg R, Berkowitz D, Levy T, et al. In vitro fertilization and embryo transfer for the treatment of infertility associated with polycystic ovary syndrome. Fertil Steril 1993;60:858–863.

17 *Pelvic Adhesive Disease*

The sequence of formation, lysis and reformation of adhesions last as long as the patient does or the hopeful persistence of the surgeon endures.
— A. E. Hertzler, 1916

Since the advent of abdominal and pelvic surgery, adhesion formation has plagued the surgeon. In one of the earliest reports, Bryant, in 1872, described a case of fatal intestinal obstruction secondary to intra-abdominal and pelvic adhesions after removal of an ovarian tumor.[1] This case introduced into clinical practice the concept of adhesions as a cause of postoperative morbidity and mortality. With this awareness, clinical interest in the process of adhesion formation and prevention began. Early investigations into adhesion prevention were characterized by the kind of trial-and-error that persists even in contemporary practice and clinical investigation. Several trials were undertaken without full knowledge of the pathogenesis or pathology of adhesion formation. Through the late 1800s to the early 1920s, a papain extract was used without success.[2] Both bovine and human amnion were used through the 1930s for prevention of adhesions after extensive abdominal and pelvic surgery,[3–5] a variation on the use of amnion popularized in the plastic surgical repair and reconstruction of traumatic injuries encountered by troops during World War I. Amniotic fluid was then tried. Eli Lily became sufficiently interested that Eli Lily Research Laboratories produced a concentrate of amniotic fluid called Amphitene.[6] Both amnion and amniotic fluid remained in vogue through the 1940s.

In the 1960s, there was a resurgence in clinical research for a method of prevention. The interest broadened as microsurgical techniques became better defined and clinicians sought to identify adjuncts to prevent or retard adhesions. Contemporary management reflects a combination of better understanding of the process of adhesion formation, better tools for intraoperative use, and better methodology for evaluating what works and what does not. This chapter describes the processes of normal peritoneal healing, the changes that occur during surgery or infection that prevent normal healing mechanisms and thus lead to formation of adhesions, and discusses the influence of adhesions on reproduction and their surgical management and intraoperative prevention.

Etiology

Pelvic adhesion formation is a part of peritoneal healing after any trauma. Abdominal and pelvic adhesions are caused by a perturbation in the normal peritoneal healing process of inflammation followed by mesothelial repair and healing, and eventual restoration of normal anatomy.[7,8] An inciting injury is immediately followed by reparative processes that involve an initial inflammatory response characterized by local infiltration of leucocytes, edema, and neovascularization. This process forms the basis for mesothelial repair, peritoneal regeneration, and closure of the defect or injury site. Peritoneal trauma of clinical significance occurs in one of two settings: after any major or minor surgical procedure, and after an infectious process, most typically in gynecology after pelvic inflammatory disease. An understanding of the etiology of adhesion formation requires understanding the normal processes of inflammatory response and peritoneal repair. Perturbations in the process ultimately result in the formation of pelvic adhesions.

Adhesions are typically classified on the basis of formation, i.e., de novo adhesion formation versus reformation, and the character of the adhesions. Classification of adhesions takes into account the type, location, extent, and character of the adhesion. Adhesions are also characterized based on their denseness, ranging from thin, avascular, filmy adhesions that are easily removed using microscissors to those that are thick, dense, and extremely vascular that require a combination of coagulation, excision, and removal. The adhesions may be located in any part of the pelvic or abdominal cavity. They are also classified regarding the degree of organ involvement, expressed as a percentage of surface area ranging from a small area to the entire organ (for example, the degree of adhesion formation on the ovary may involve only 25% or the entire surface area of the ovary).

Any trauma to peritoneal surfaces predisposes to adhesion formation (Table 17-1). The process involved in the formation of adhesions and changes in

Table 17-1. Peritoneal Repair Process
Normal healing: 7 to 10 days after injury
• Mesothelium from primitive mesenchymal cells • Infiltration by macrophages and fibrin complex • Development of basement membrane • Fibrinolysis • Organized mesothelial layer
Adhesion formation: 14 to 21 days after injury
• Prevention of mesothelial cell migration • Absence of mesothelial transformation • Failure of fibrinolytic process • Persistence of fibrin complex • Development of fibrous tissue

anatomic relationships and function involves several events that compromise tissue well-being. Six major contributing factors are trauma, ischemia, presence of foreign bodies, hemorrhage, raw surfaces, and infection. These circumstances may be present in any surgical procedure regardless of techniques used to minimize them. The adhesions formed after surgery are caused by any one or a combination of these factors.[9] Additional causes of peritoneal irritation, such as endometriosis, foreign body reactions, or irradiation, further contribute to the formation of adhesions.

Adhesion Formation as Sequelae to Surgery

As early as 1919, it was suggested that peritoneal healing differed from that of thin-skin healing.[10] A defect made in the peritoneum epithelializes simultaneously, regardless of the size of the defect, not gradually from the borders to within, as is typical of thin-skin healing. Early studies by Clark, in 1958, showed that after destruction and damage of peritoneal mesothelium, repair is accomplished by proliferation of surrounding mesothelial cells from islands of epithelial cells.[11] Mesothelial cells also migrate from the margin of the wound and contribute to the regenerative process. These cells develop from peripheral primitive mesenchymal cells or from subperitoneal fibroblasts. Consequently, large peritoneal wounds re-epithelialize as quickly as do small peritoneal wounds. This aspect of healing is unique to the peritoneum and occurs over an interval of 8 to 10 days.[12]

The process of healing at the dermal level and peritoneal level is different. In both circumstances, a fibrin clot is formed during the inflammatory phase. At this time, the wound site, whether on the peritoneum or the dermal surface, contains neutrophils and macrophages which release growth factors such as vascular endothelial growth factor, transforming growth factor (TGF), and platelet-derived growth factor. Subsequent to this, re-epithelialization and neovascularization occurs, influenced in part by tissue plasminogen activator and matrix metalloproteinases. The healing of the peritoneum takes a different turn at this point. In the peritoneum, inflammation peaks 2 to 3 days after injury. On the second day after injury, epithelialization occurs and is completed within about 12 days. Contraction occurs between the third and the twentieth day of the healing process. Approximately 2 days after injury, peritoneal surfaces are infiltrated with macrophages imbedded within a fibrin complex. Almost immediately, the first signs of peritoneal healing may be noted as mesenchymal cells aggregate at the injury site to initiate the healing process. The process of migration of mesenchymal cells increases during days 3 and 4 after injury, and by day 5, a clearly defined, single-cell layer of mesothelial cells can be noted at the site of the peritoneal injury. At day 6 or 7, a basement membrane is laid beneath the mesothelial cells lining the peritoneum; by day 8, an organized continuous mesothelial layer has formed across the entire injury site. Numerous cytokines such as interleukin-1 and interleukin-2 and growth factors such as transforming growth factor, platelet-derived growth factor-β, and platelet-activating factor are also involved in the normal healing process, though their exact roles in adhesion formation are speculative.[13–15] Adhesions are characterized by greater amounts of TGF-β mRNA and reduced amounts of matrix metallo-proteinase-1 and integrin mRNA than normal peritoneum. When the normal process is interrupted by the presence of ischemia, crush injuries, and blood, occurrences common during the trauma of any surgical procedure, adhesions will form.

Any peritoneal injury has inflammation as the initial response followed by peritoneal regeneration and postinflammatory resolution.[16,17] Trauma to serosal surfaces during a surgical procedure is followed by a release of fibrinogen-rich exudate and deposition of fibrin at the surgical site. Fibrinolysis and resorption of the fibrin matrix is an essential aspect in the resolution of the inflammatory process and is critically dependent on adequate blood supply. The ischemia that occurs during any surgical procedure interferes with the normal fibrinolytic process and causes a reduction in fibrinolysis and the subsequent development of thick and filmy adhesions that may distort anatomy and compromise function.

Adhesion formation occurs during an interval of 10 to 12 days after injury when there is a failure of resorption of the fibrin matrix and a persistence and organization of fibrin at the injury site.[17,18] Early in the process, adhesions have a variety of cell components within the fibrin complex. The complex is gradually replaced with macrophages and fibroblasts. Failure of the normal fibrinolytic process leads to persistence of the fibrin complex with macrophages and prevents the normal mesothelial cell migration. The presence of macrophages and leukocytes in the complex persists to day 5 after injury. At approximately this time, vascularization of the adhesion occurs with migration of the fibroblasts into the injury site. During the next 7 days the cell population within the complex is transformed into one predominantly composed of fibroblasts, which leads to the formation of thick, fibrous bands of tissue without any evidence of the normal mesothelial healing process characteristic of peritoneal injury healing.

Peritoneal adhesions form after any surgical procedure.[19–21] Autopsy data suggest that one-third of cadavers examined have evidence of abdominal and pelvic adhesions without any history significant for adhesion formation.[22] After surgical procedures, adhesion formation may occur in 15 to 100% of patients, depending on the injury being repaired, the surgical technique, and the extent of surgery. Several circumstances may modify the response and influence the degree of adhesion formation. The extent of peritoneal damage and the apposition of damaged surfaces may also be instrumental in the process of adhesion formation. In a murine model, the development of adhesions between serosal surfaces required trauma to *both* contacting peritoneal surfaces.[17] Regardless of the type of injury, when a single peritoneal surface was injured, minimal adhesions were formed. When both surfaces were injured, however, adhesions ranged from 50 to 100%.

Adhesion Formation as a Sequelae to Pelvic Inflammatory Disease

One of the most common clinical scenarios contributing to pelvic adhesive disease is postinflammatory tubal scarring secondary to pelvic inflammatory disease (PID). It is estimated that there are approximately 1,000,000 cases of acute PID per year in the United States, most (approximately 85%) secondary to sexually transmitted diseases.[22] A minority of cases are caused by postoperative infections. These cases have a microbiology different from that of PID. Acute PID is usually polymicrobial and is caused by organisms that ascend from the lower genital tract into the endometrium, migrate to the tubes, and infect the mucosa of the tubes and pelvic peritoneum. The organisms include *Neisseria gonorrhoeae*, *Chlamydia trachomatis*, endogenous aerobic and anaerobic bacteria, and (rarely) genital *Mycoplasma* species. In one series of intra-abdominal cultures, an average of seven different species were cultured from specimens taken directly from the intraperitoneal surfaces.[23] Cultures in 20% of patients with acute PID were positive for *C. trachomatis* and, in approximately 25 to 40% of the patients, for both *N. gonorrhoeae* and *C. trachomatis*. The aerobic and anaerobic species most frequently cultured were *Bacteroides bivius*, *Peptococcus* sp., *Peptostreptococcus* sp., *Gardnerella vaginalis*, *Escherichia coli* and group B streptococci. The roles of ureaplasma and mycoplasma remain unclear, but are demonstrated in anywhere from 2 to 20% of patients having acute PID.[24]

The sequelae of acute PID are significant. Acute PID indirectly contributes to approximately 40 deaths each year, secondary to the effect of PID on tubes and subsequent ectopic pregnancy. Acute PID is also a major cause of infertility secondary to severe tubal damage and pelvic adhesive disease. Before the advent of aggressive antibiotic therapy, approximately 50% of patients who experienced acute PID were infertile. The likelihood of successful surgical repair of adnexal structures damaged by acute PID depends on the extent of the damage and varies from 0 to 50%. The likelihood of becoming infertile after acute PID depends on several factors, such as the number of episodes of PID, the age of onset of PID (the older the patient, the more likely the infertility), and the severity of the infection. Tubal damage and scarring also result in important long-term complications, such as recurrent PID or flare-ups of the disease, chronic pelvic pain, and ectopic pregnancy.[25] Women with one episode of PID are at increased risk for subsequent episodes, presumably because of impaired local defenses.

Infertility caused by tubal occlusion and pelvic adhesions is one of the most serious and costly long-term complications. Infertility from tubal occlusion may develop in 8% of women after a single episode of PID, in 20% after two episodes, and in 40% after three or more episodes.[23] Studies of long-term complications of PID underscore the impact of a silent or atypical disease. As many as 70% of women with infertility secondary to obstructed tubes have serum antibodies to *Chlamydia*, but fewer than 25% of women who are infertile for other reasons have such antibodies.[26,27] Thirty to eighty percent of women with infertility and adnexal scarring had no history of clinically recognizable PID.[28] Presumably, these women had no symptoms or had subtle, mild, or vague symptoms that were not recognized. Similar data link silent disease to ectopic pregnancy. In one study, serologic evidence of a previous chlamydial infection more than doubled the risk of ectopic pregnancy.[29]

Although a clear-cut history of acute PID is related in only 36% of patients (which accounts for the label "silent PID"), careful questioning may suggest symptoms of PID at some point in the past. Of patients without a history of PID but who show laparoscopic evidence of tubal damage and pelvic adhesions, 80% disclose a previous history of lower abdominal pain suggestive of an episode of PID.[30] A history of PID may be an inaccurate predictor of the likelihood of finding significant pelvic adhesive disease. Laparoscopy remains the standard for diagnosis. Recognizing PID has become increasingly difficult because of the variable clinical presentations. Optimal therapy should not only eradicate the infecting organisms, but also preserve reproductive function and prevent the long-term sequelae of both infertility and pelvic pain.

Clinical Correlates

Pelvic adhesions, whether secondary to postoperative healing or to an acute infectious process, have their most significant clinical aspect in infertility and pelvic pain. Pelvic pain is the cause of approximately 3,000,000 annual visits to physicians and results in approximately 300,000 hospital admissions and 150,000 operative procedures per year.[31,32] Data from the Scottish National Health Service Registrar Database revealed that 30 to 50% of all hospitalization readmissions were associated with potential adhesion-associated complications. Approximately 5% are directly related to adhesions. The highest risk category was those patients undergoing gynecologic surgical procedures on the ovaries and tubes. In this survey, 2931 patients were readmitted to the hospital at least once during this interval because of adhesions.[33]

Patients with a history of PID and adhesions are 10 times more likely to be hospitalized for abdominal and pelvic pain, six times more likely to be operated on for endometriosis, and 10 times more likely to be treated for an ectopic pregnancy.[34] The National Hospital Discharge Survey reports the impact of pelvic adhesions on health care costs. The total cost of all hospitalizations for adhesiolysis in the mid-1990s was estimated to be $1.33 billion. The rate of hospitalization reported in the survey for adhesiolysis was relatively constant from 1988 to 1994 at 115.5 per 100,000 persons to 117.3 per 100,000 persons, respectively (this figure in spite of changes in awareness of adhesions and techniques for their prevention). The average hospital stay, however, dropped from 11.2 days to 9.7 days in 1988 to 1994, respectively.[35] The National Hospital Discharge Survey of hospitalizations between 1998 and 2002 described 281,282 hospitalizations for pelvic adhesions and related complications. Of these, 51,100 were related to adhesions solely and 227,882 to cases where adhesions were part of a broader problem. All totaled during this interval, adhesions were directly or indirectly responsible for a cost of $1.18 billion and 948,000 hospital days.[36] In addition to a higher incidence of pelvic pain and ectopic pregnancy, extensive pelvic adhesions may contribute to ovulatory dysfunction and an increased incidence of endometriosis. Infertility secondary to pelvic adhesive disease may result from a restriction in the mobility of the adnexal structures, actual blockage of the distal aspect of the tube, or disruption of the normal tubo-ovarian relationship and ovum pickup.[37]

A major sequelae to pelvic adhesions is pelvic pain. Pelvic pain in this setting may have a multitude of causes. The correlation of pelvic adhesive disease and chronic pelvic pain, however, remains unclear. There is no good correlation between extent of adhesions and degree of patients with pelvic pain found to have adhesions range from 2% to as high as 55% (mean, 40%).[25] Pelvic adhesive disease and endometriosis are the most common findings in women with pelvic pain, but these findings are not consistent, which makes the role of adhesions in pelvic pain controversial. Chronic pelvic pain has multiple contributing factors, including individual differences in pain thresholds and varying social and physical profiles. One theory regarding the etiology of chronic pelvic pain from pelvic adhesive disease is the activation of pain receptors secondary to increased tension on pelvic and abdominal organs. The peritoneum itself is extremely sensitive to irritation. Studies have varied in demonstrating an association of adhesions and pelvic pain. In one study, 38% of patients with pelvic pain had sufficient pelvic adhesive disease to restrict adnexal mobility as compared with 12% for control groups.[38] However, in a subsequent study, no relationship was found regarding the perception of pain and the location and extent of pelvic adhesions in patients with and without pain.[39]

To prove a cause and effect relationship between chronic pelvic pain and pelvic adhesive disease, it is essential to study a significant number of patients with both adhesions and pelvic pain and control for the location, degree, and character of the adhesions and pain and for the familial and social background of the patient. A second approach to study pelvic pain and adhesions would be to demonstrate significant pain relief with lysis of adhesions in patients with a clear-cut cause and effect relationship between pelvic pain and pelvic adhesions. Approximately one-half of patients with and one-third without chronic pelvic pain will have adhesions.[40] Of patients who undergo either laparoscopic or microsurgical adhesiolysis, 75% show an improvement in pain patterns.[41] However, there is a tendency for the pain relief to be of short duration. Long-term follow-up studies are lacking at the present time. Follow-up laparoscopies have failed to correlate the absence of adhesions in patients with adequate pain relief with the recurrence of adhesions in patients who have recurrence of pain.

The second major sequelae of pelvic adhesions is infertility. As with other conditions in reproductive medicine and infertility that require surgical intervention, a standard classification system of pelvic adhesions is helpful but of limited value.[43] Such a system provides a uniform way to describe the extent of the adhesions and outcome after surgery. One classification differentiates between minimal, mild, moderate, and severe pelvic adhesions.[43] A second scoring system defines the prognosis of conception on the basis of the score applied to the adnexa with the *least amount of pathology*, the importance of the fimbriated end of the fallopian tube, and the differentiation between filmy and dense adhesions. This scoring system includes a point system to designate the thickness (filmy or dense) of the adhesions and the degree to which the adhesions encase the ovary and tube. In some clinical circumstances, a descriptive narrative including comments about the character of the adhesions (filmy or dense, vascular or avascular) and extent of pelvic or abdominal involvement may be more appropriate.

Descriptions of degree of adhesions and any scoring system are observer dependent. Interobserver and intraobserver variability in the laparoscopic assessment and scoring of pelvic adhesions is minimal. Agreement has been demonstrated between examiners in estimating the likelihood of a pregnancy after surgery and in recommending IVF when the prognosis was considered poor.[44,45] In one study, however, this scoring system did not appear to predict outcome or influence management decision.[46] The surgeon's fundamental impression of the adhesions within the pelvis was the more powerful predictor. Inspection of the tubes and ovary is critical. There is no correlation between the degree of peritubal adhesions and the mucosal status in patients with a hydrosalpinx. Hence, evaluation of the status of the tube apart from adhesion assessment is essential in considering any patient for an adhesiolysis.[47]

Diagnostic Studies

The definitive diagnosis of pelvic adhesive disease can be made only by direct visualization with either laparoscopy or laparotomy. A combination of factors in the patient's history, physical examination, and radiographic adjuncts such as hysterosalpingography (HSG) may suggest the diagnosis.

A history significant of acute PID or previous abdominal or pelvic surgery should raise the suspicion of pelvic adhesions. The presence of pelvic adhesions at laparoscopy may be reliably predicted by preoperative history and physical examination.[29] Findings on physical examination associated with the presence of adhesions may include uterine immobility, adnexal masses, and tenderness. Other historical predictors associated with pelvic adhesions include a history of PID, endometriosis, previous pelvic adhesions, and tubal occlusions.

HSG is an adjunctive study in making the diagnosis of pelvic adhesions. Significant findings on HSG suggestive (but not strictly diagnostic) of pelvic adhesions include loculation of the contrast medium in a region surrounding the tube but no clear-cut demonstration of intraperitoneal spill and the presence of the tube high in the pelvis without movement on oblique films. Seventy-five percent of patients with these findings on HSG will have pelvic adhesions.[48] HSG may also be useful in the detection of peritubal adhesions without tubal occlusion.[49] Findings suggestive of peritubal adhesions on HSG include convoluted fallopian tube, loculation of spillage of contrast medium into the peritoneal cavity, ampullary dilatation, and peritubular halo effect (i.e., a double contour appearance of the tubal wall). There is a 25% false-positive rate for peritubal adhesions using HSG.[50] These data suggest that HSG may be a useful diagnostic procedure in the initial investigation of infertility to suggest adnexal pathology and both pelvic and peritubal adhesions.

Transvaginal ultrasound provides limited insight into the presence of adhesions.[51] Magnetic resonance imaging (MRI) has not been useful in the diagnosis of adhesions. Laparoscopy, laparotomy, or both are currently the only definitive procedures for identifying pelvic adhesions. Procedures to diagnose adhesions should also assess the exact extent of the pelvic adhesions, a predictor of the influence of this process on future fertility, and the likelihood of ectopic pregnancy. Outpatient clinical laparoscopy with a 2-mm laparoscope is a practical alternative for diagnosis of pelvic pathology, with excellent interobserver agreement.[52] The most sensitive and specific study for diagnosing pelvic adhesions continues to be laparoscopy.

Management

The decision to proceed with diagnostic laparoscopy and surgical management for pelvic adhesive disease depends on symptoms and fertility interests. Therapy should be individualized. The surgical goal of any procedure for pelvic adhesive disease is to restore pelvic anatomy to as nearly normal as possible and to minimize recurrence risk. The clinical goal is either to relieve pelvic pain or to restore fertility and minimize the likelihood of an ectopic pregnancy. The decision whether an operation is appropriate turns on an objective assessment of the degree of adhesions and condition of the tube. The decision to proceed with surgery for fertility enhancement is more objective and quantitative than for pain management. Objective scoring and classification guide decisions regarding the appropriateness of lysis of adhesions or referral for IVF for fertility enhancement. No definitive correlation has been described for guidance in pain management and procedures are frequently performed with a postoperative wait-and-see approach.

At diagnostic laparoscopy, tubal anatomy and extent of adhesive disease must be accurately and independently assessed. This assessment will influence the decision whether to proceed with adhesiolysis or abandon the procedure. Intraoperative assessment should evaluate the distal fallopian tube, including its diameter and patency, and the degree, character, and pelvic involvement of the adhesive process. If the tube is sufficiently damaged and mild pelvic adhesive disease is also present or if adhesions are severe regardless of tubal status, the surgical procedure should be abandoned and the patient referred for IVF. If the tubes are severely damaged or the adhesion so severe that any surgical procedure would not significantly enhance fertility, the procedure is best abandoned.

In circumstances in which surgical intervention is likely to yield reasonable outcomes for pregnancy and produce minimal risk of ectopic pregnancy, treatment decisions should focus on laparoscopic adhesiolysis, and in select cases laparotomy, and microsurgery.[55-58] A basic tenet guiding fertility surgery for pelvic adhesions is to refer for IVF if the adhesions are severe and require laparotomy. Management of pelvic pain uses a different paradigm in which laparotomy may be appropriate depending on history. Principles of management regardless of approach include precise visualization of tissue planes between the adhesions, the peritoneal tissue, and pelvic organs to enable a division of adhesive bands. Manipulation of tissue with fine atraumatic instruments reduces serosal abrasion and enables precise application of unipolar or bipolar forceps for precise hemostasis. The use of fine suture material precisely placed also decreases the likelihood of tissue damage.

The extent of adhesions dictates approach. At times, adhesions are so dense and vascular that they preclude a laparoscopic approach. Depending on a surgeon's experience and preference, a selection bias to laparoscopic adhesiolysis for simpler cases may exist. Cases that are easier to manage may be approached laparoscopically; more extensive adhesive processes may require laparotomy if pain is the indication. Referral for IVF is indicated for moderate and severe adhesions not surgically treated through laparoscopy. Comparison of adhesiolysis by laparoscopy and laparotomy suggests considerably different outcomes. Results vary because of different populations studied, the etiology of the adhesions, different staging of the adhesions, and surgical approaches. In fact, in dense adhesions where the adhesiolysis cannot be performed endoscopically, the patient is best referred for IVF, depending on the indications for the procedure (i.e., management pain or fertility enhancement). The rule of thumb is that *the safest, least invasive, but most effective approach should govern the decision.*

Prevention is a key to management. Adjuvant therapy for adhesion prevention with the use of systemically administered agents (locally instilled or applied) and barrier techniques are the main therapies (Table 17-2).[59-61] Each approach attempts to prevent adhesion formation through a different mechanism. These methods have all been variably effective. Adhesion-preventing agents are divided into two categories: intraperitoneal instillates and adhesion barriers. Intraperitoneal instillates include Ringer's lactate, dextran 70 (Hyskon®), and Intergel®. Adhesion barriers include Interceed® (TC7), absorbable adhesion barrier, Prelude®, Seprafilm®, and Sepragel®. Experimental adhesion barriers include Surgisis® (porcine submucosal ware), pericardial dome patch,

Table 17-2.
Historic Perspective of Treatment to Prevent Postoperative Adhesions

Category of Treatment	Specific Agent
Fibrinolytics	Streptokinases, urokinase, hyaluronidase, chymotrypsin, trypsin, pepsin
Anticoagulants	Heparin, citrates, oxalates
Anti-inflammatories	Corticosteroids, nonsteroidal anti-inflammatory agents, antihistamines
Antibiotics	Tetracyclines, cephalosporins
Intraperitoneal instillates	32% dextran-70, normal saline, Ringer's lactate solution
Intraperitoneal barriers	Endogenous grafts, omentum, peritoneum, amnion

siliconized nylon sheet, hyaluronate-based bioresorbable membrane, polypropylene mesh, and collagen membrane composite films.

Barriers

The most effective therapy for adhesion prevention is with barrier membranes (Table 17-3).[62] Three devices that are FDA approved for laparotomy use are Interceed® and Seprafilm®, which are site-specific, and Intergel®, which is broadly applied to an anatomic area. A variety of barrier membranes that demonstrated reduction in adhesion formation are available. One advantage of contemporary barriers is that they are site-specific and absorbable. They can be applied only at the operative site and do not require systemic administration or general intraperitoneal instillation. Applying the barrier only at the operative

Table 17-3.
Barrier Methods for Adhesion Prevention

Site Specific	Effectiveness	Comment
Oxidized-regenerated cellulose (Interceed)	• Significant reduction in extent and severity of reformed adhesions • May be applied laparoscopically	• Blood compromises effectiveness • Residual fluid in pelvis may dislodge barrier
Modified hyaluronic acid and carboxymethylcellulose (Seprafilm)	• Significant reduction in incidence, extent, and severity of postoperative adhesions • Cannot be applied laparoscopically	• Difficulty in application due to texture of barrier
Ferric hyaluronic gel (Intergel)	• Reduction in de novo and reformed adhesions	• Longer duration at operative site related to effectiveness

site provides the potential for specific control of adhesion formation in one location while avoiding the potential for systemic side effects of generalized therapy. These membranes also result in minimal inflammatory response. Barriers prevent the bonding of injured and exposed adjacent surfaces by producing either a slow-release lubricant or a non-stick surface.

Early studies using oxidized regenerated cellulose evaluated a hemostatic agent called Surgicel (Johnson & Johnson, Arlington, TX). These studies demonstrated no clear-cut efficacy in preventing adhesions, but the data were promising and suggested that some form of the agent might prove effective. A second-generation material also made of oxidized regenerated cellulose (Interceed, Johnson & Johnson) was designed. This is an effective barrier technique that is relatively easy to use, particularly through the laparoscope. However, it does have the disadvantage of being extremely sensitive to blood. Because of this, careful hemostasis is required prior to application of the barrier. It has a longer resorption time than Surgicel® and an ability to maintain its position without sutures. A significant reduction in adhesion formation was observed with this barrier for uterine and peritoneal side wall trauma.[62,63] In clinical trials, regenerated cellulose reduced adhesions after pelvic surgery. In a variety of clinical settings in which the barrier was used on one side and the opposite side served as control, Interceed® was associated with a reduction in the percentage of surface involved in adhesions.[64,65]

The most important steps for maximizing efficacy with regenerated cellulose barriers focus on its application, which may be limited by practical considerations. Essential to effective application is the removal of all intraperitoneal irrigants; a large enough piece of this barrier to completely cover the area at risk of adhesion formation must be used, and the fabric must be moistened with a small volume of irrigant. Adequate hemostasis is crucial. If hemostasis has not been achieved, this barrier turns black or brownish black. In these situations, the material must be removed, hemostasis again achieved, and a new piece applied.

Another barrier method for adhesion prevention that has been described is expanded polytetrafluoroethylene (Gore-Tex surgical membrane, Gore-Tex, W.L. Gore & Asso., Flagstaff, AZ). The nonabsorbable surgical membrane is a 0.1-mm sheet that has been used in cardiothoracic surgery as a substitute for the pericardium with a small pore size that inhibits cellular penetration. The membrane is nonabsorbable and inert and causes little foreign body reaction. It has been used for a variety of clinical products including sutures, vascular grafts, ligaments, and for reconstruction of the pericardium.[66–69] In clinical use, a multicenter, noncontrolled study evaluated ePTFE in patients treated for moderate to severe pelvic adhesive disease, significant deperitonealization after adhesiolysis, and myomas.[66,67] Adhesion reduction was noted.

Seprafilm® is a bioresorbable membrane (Genzyme Corporation, Cambridge, MA) composed of sodium hyaluronate and carboxymethylcellulose that acts as a site-specific device. It has been shown to be effective, but has the technical disadvantage of stickiness and the requirement that the film be held in place using special packaging. The barrier is resorbed from the peritoneal cavity within 7 days of placement and early studies showed this membrane to be an effective barrier in preventing pericardial and abdominal adhesions.[70–75,77] In a multicenter study to prevent adhesion formations after myomectomy, HAL-F significantly reduced the incidence, severity, extent, and area of postoperative adhesion formation without any associated morbidity.[76] Intergel® is made of hyaluronic acid, iron, and water (the purpose of the iron in the Intergel is to slow peritoneal absorption). Intergel provides a viscous coating of the peritoneal surfaces and may be applied throughout the pelvis at the time of any pelvic surgery. Intraperitoneal circulation appears to redistribute the solution throughout the pelvis reducing the need to have precise placement, which is a requirement of any barrier methods.[77]

Agents of Questionable Effectiveness

Intraperitoneal solutions are dextran and crystalloids. Dextran is a water-soluble, glucose polymer originally used as a plasma expander in a variety of molecular weights. Most research in adhesion prevention has used a 32% solution of dextran 70 (called dextran 70 because of its average molecular weight of 70,000). Dextran 70 is slowly absorbed from the peritoneal cavity during a period of 5 to 7 days in the critical healing phase. Dextran has been associated with significant clinical side effects that limits its use. The most common complication after intraperitoneal installation of dextran 70 is vulvar edema, which may occur in 2% of patients.[78] Edema of the leg, pleural effusions, and coagulopathy occur less frequently but are well described.[79] Disseminated intravascular coagulation, hypotension, anaphylactic shock, allergic symptoms, and adult respiratory distress syndrome have also been described in isolated case reports. Difficulty in using dextran solutions intraoperatively, secondary to their viscosity and stickiness, make them unacceptable to most physicians.

Crystalloid solutions, including Ringer's lactated solution, phosphate-buffered saline, and normal saline for hydroflotation, are the most commonly used adjuvant to reduce adhesion formation. They are administered as an instillate at the end of a surgical procedure. Volumes range from 100 to 400 ml, with 200 ml the most commonly used. This approach has the advantage of ease of use, low cost, and effectiveness. Several studies suggest that crystalloids reduce adhesion formation. However, in randomized studies this technique has not been shown to be effective. Aspects of peritoneal fluid dynamics and a rapid rate of absorption limit their use.[80]

Isotonic saline solutions are rapidly absorbed; other solutes are absorbed more slowly after equilibration with blood and peritoneal fluid. The rate of absorption during equilibration depends primarily on crystalloid osmotic pressure gradients across the peritoneal membrane and is most rapid when serum osmolality exceeds that of peritoneal fluid. Crystalloid solution is absorbed from the peritoneal cavity at approximately 35 ml/hour. Thus, 200 mL of solution is absorbed in 6 hours, and 500 ml of solution in 15 hours. Theoretical considerations of peritoneal fluid dynamics predict that crystalloid used as a peritoneal instillate at the end of surgery will not prevent adhesion formation. This prediction is consistent with clinical observations that fail to demonstrate a reduction in adhesions with crystalloids.[81]

Experimental Techniques of Unproven Effectiveness

Early studies focused on a reduction in the inflammatory response. Data from extensive animal studies to identify adjuvants that prevent the formation of adhesions suggested that anti-inflammatory drugs may be useful.[82] Anti-inflammatory drugs may limit the release of fibrinous exudate in response to inflammation at the surgical site and, thus, reduce the presence of fibrin clots.

Two classes of anti-inflammatory drugs have been evaluated: corticosteroids and nonsteroidal anti-inflammatory drugs (NSAIDs). Despite data suggesting that inhibitors of arachidonic acid metabolism, such as NSAIDs, reduce adhesion formation, their clinical efficacy is open to question. The pharmacologic prevention of adhesion formation may require better methods of delivery of the agent to the operative site. Delivery of these drugs when administered systemically is limited by surgical ischemia and devascularization. Investigations in the hamster to improve microvascular perfusion with nifedipine, verapamil, and diltiazem demonstrated a marked reduction in adhesion formation and positive influence on peritoneal repair.[83] Pentoxifylline, a methylxanthine derivative (used initially in peripheral vascular disease to improve perfusion in diabetics)[84] provided significant prevention of posttraumatic adhesions in an animal model. As yet, these approaches are experimental.

Tissue plasminogen activator, urokinase plasminogen activator, and streptokinase have also been evaluated in animal models.[74] Tissue plasminogen activator and urokinase plasminogen activator have been shown to be effective, while streptokinase and cyclosporine are not.[85,86] Octreotide, medroxyprogesterone acetate, and GnRH agonists have been shown to be effective methods of preventing adhesion formation in animal models.[87–90] Tolmetin, meclofenamate, and ibuprofen have been investigated in an attempt to prevent adhesion formation. None have been shown to be clearly efficacious.[91,92]

Operative Technique

Surgical treatment of adhesions, whether by operative laparoscopy or laparotomy, involves three critical aspects: (1) the technique used for adhesiolysis (i.e., laser, cautery, or sharp dissection), (2) placement of barriers at the surgical site at the time of the procedure, or (3) repeat (second-look) laparoscopy at various intervals to lyse any newly formed adhesions. Attention to detail and gentle tissue handling is essential. Extreme care should be taken in entering the abdomen in any patient considered at risk for abdominal and pelvic adhesions, especially patients with a midline incision. In laparoscopy, an open insertion with a Hasson cannula may be required. This procedure avoids the possibility of complications secondary to bowel or vessel damage if an occult loop of bowel or sheet of omentum adheres to the anterior peritoneum at the site of scope entry. Alternatively, in high-risk circumstances, especially if obesity may make abdominal entry through a limited incision difficult, a 3-mm scope may be inserted in a region well away from the infraumbilical area. Through this scope, assessment may be made of the proposed site of laparoscope insertion. In addition, if adhesions are present in this region, a secondary puncture may be placed and scissors, grasping forceps, or both may be inserted to free the proposed area from the adhesions.

After entry by laparotomy or insertion of the laparoscope, omental adhesions or loops of bowel may be adherent to the anterior abdominal wall or pelvic peritoneum and preclude adequate evaluation of the pelvic organs. These structures should be detached with sharp or blunt dissection to achieve a full panoramic view of the pelvic anatomy. The uterus should then be elevated from the pelvis by using an intrauterine manipulator. The adnexa should be placed on stretch to determine the character (i.e., filmy or dense) of the pelvic adhesions, the degree of mobility of the adnexal structures, and possible cleavage planes between the structures and the adhesions. An assessment of the degree of the adhesive process, the status of the fallopian tubes (especially the distal segment), and the relationship of the tubes to the ovaries should be made.

Chromotubation should be undertaken to rule out a proximal tubal obstruction. If this circumstance is evident in conjunction with distal tubal damage, the procedure should be abandoned because outcomes from bipolar obstruction are extremely poor. The patient is best referred for IVF. If proximal patency is established and the tube fills to its distal point, an assessment should be made of the diameter of the tube and any degree of dilatation. This information should be factored with the indications for the procedure (i.e., pain management or fertility enhancement). A decision should then be made regarding whether to proceed with operative laparoscopy, convert the procedure to a laparotomy and microsurgical procedure, or abandon the procedure.

With careful identification of serosal cleavage planes, adnexal adherences to the uterus are then separated, the tube is detached from the ovary with laterally directed movements, and the ovary is detached from the underlying peritoneum of the ovarian fossa or uterosacral ligament. Adhesions are identified and stretched with a probe or 3-mm grasping forceps are introduced through a second or third puncture (if necessary). Traction and countertraction may be used to place the adhesion on tension to better define tissue planes. Adhesions are divided individually, one layer at a time, with scissors, laser, or needle-tip cautery. Unipolar coagulation may be used for vascular adhesions. Adhesions should be excised when possible.

Adhesions are either removed or lysed until the pelvic anatomy is restored to as nearly normal as possible. Care must be taken to ensure complete hemostasis by use of needle-tip cautery or laser. The adnexal structures should be freely movable, the relationship of the tubes and ovaries restored, and free-flow of dye established by chromotubation. On completion of adhesiolysis, adjuvant therapy to prevent the formation of postoperative adhesions should be used.

Second-Look Laparoscopy

Laparoscopy between the time of serosal healing (i.e., 8 days) and established adhesion fibrosis (i.e., 21 days), may provide an effective way of reducing pelvic adhesions and ectopic pregnancy.[93,94] Use of adhesiolysis in this setting to improve pregnancy rates or long-term outcomes in patients with chronic pelvic pain is as yet unproven.

Evaluation Prior To ART

Management of pelvic adhesive disease prior to in vitro fertilization is relatively straightforward. Careful interpretation of hysterosalpingography is essential. In some circumstances, severe hydrosalpinges may give the appearance of spill of contrast media into areas of loculation. There is no imaging technique to clearly differentiate the two. In general, hysterosalpingography is a reliable method of distinguishing severe hydrosalpinges from accumulation of contrast into areas of loculation. However, depending on clinical circumstances and interpretation of the imaging, laparoscopy may be indicated to verify the condition of the tubes and for consideration of tubal ligation should severe hydrosalpinges be present. Should laparoscopy be undertaken in this setting, contingency plans should include the possible role of laparotomy should severe pelvic adhesive disease preclude adequate evaluation of the adnexae or, if severe hydrosalpinges are noted, preclude either salpingectomy or tubal ligation. Counseling regarding these two options is essential prior to embarking on any diagnostic laparoscopy. The role of hysteroscopic placement of cornual occlusive devices in this setting has not been adequately evaluated. There is no evidence that pelvic adhesive disease is associated with any diminution in responsiveness and ovarian reserve.

Outcomes Analysis

A lack of uniformity in patient populations and methodology has made the interpretation of clinical studies in the prevention of adhesions difficult. Barriers offer the best opportunity for adhesion prevention (Figure 17-1). Reduction in adhesion scores has been shown in a variety of circumstances.[94–97] Each of the three FDA approved devices have demonstrated a significant decrease in the extent of adhesions, as determined by surface area measurement, and a reduction in the recurrence of severe pelvic adhesions to adhesiolysis.[98] The two circumstances in which data describing success with barriers have been mixed are reduction in the frequency of adhesions at second-look laparoscopy and in reduction after the lysis of filmy adhesions. Regenerated cellulose has been shown to be most effective in reducing the amount of surface area involved in adhesion formation but may be of benefit only for patients with advanced severe pelvic adhesions.[99] Clear benefit could be attributed to the use of barriers in approximately one-third of cases. These findings thus question the role of barriers to enhance infertility.[94] In circumstances in which severe pelvic adhesions are present, the patient is best served by foregoing lysis of adhesions and referring instead for IVF. Barriers in reproductive surgery may be beneficial only for cases of severe adhesive disease after adhesiolysis. In cases of infertility, patients with significant adhesions clearly have improved outcomes from IVF rather than from surgery. From the standpoint of enhanced fertility, the exact role adhesiolysis has for severe adhesive disease is open to question.

Data are not yet forthcoming regarding the role that adhesion barriers play in the long-term reduction of pelvic pain symptomatology when adhesiolysis has been performed to manage chronic pelvic pain. It is essential that clinical

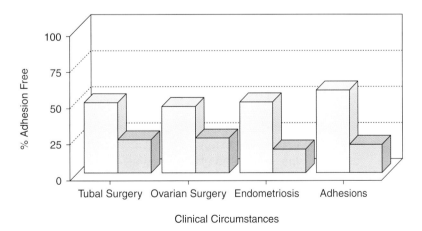

Figure 17-1   The effect of oxidized regenerated cellulose (red bars) compared with untreated controls in four clinical settings. Barrier methods have consistently demonstrated a reduction in adhesion formation.

performance and improvement in pregnancy rates for infertility patients and in the symptomatology of chronic pelvic pain in pain patients be used as the next step in the evaluation.

In spite of the proven effectiveness of various barriers in preventing adhesion formation, barrier use does not eliminate adhesions in all patients, limiting its effectiveness in extensive, lengthy procedures. In spite of the proven effectiveness of these barrier techniques in most studies, these studies have not assessed the clinical benefits of adhesion prevention in terms of limiting hospitalizations, recurrent pain, or enhancing fertility. Studies examining more definitive endpoints of cumulative pregnancy rates or pain improvement are required before a conclusive statement regarding the efficacy of synthetic surgical barriers can be made.

Despite careful surgical technique and the use of adjuvants, adhesions reform 50 to 100% of the time.[94,100,101] Reformation of adhesions at the site of a previous adhesion is independent of the original type of adhesion. De novo adhesions were identified in 51% of the patients at the time of second-look laparoscopy involving sites that were adhesion-free at the time of the initial surgery.[102,103] The extent and severity of the adhesions increases with the time that elapses after surgery. Because pelvic adhesions tend to reform, second-look laparoscopy after adhesiolysis may be advisable in select cases. The procedure enables a second adhesiolysis. In one series, second-look laparoscopy to clear fresh adhesions was performed 8 days after surgery. A third laparoscopy was also offered during the second postoperative year to patients who did not achieve a pregnancy. This relatively aggressive approach did not increase the pregnancy rate but did reduce the occurrence of ectopic pregnancies.[94] In another study, second-look laparoscopy significantly diminished the occurrence of permanent pelvic adhesions. The incidence of ectopic pregnancy after salpingostomy was significantly lower when first-look laparoscopy was performed on the eighth day after the procedure.[102] As a general rule however, failure to achieve a pregnancy 6 to 12 months after an adhesiolysis is indication for IVF.

Summary and Recommendations

There is still no panacea for pelvic adhesion prevention. No therapy has proven uniformly effective. Progress has been made in the reduction but not the prevention of pelvic adhesive disease. Despite the combined use of multiple adjuvants, there remains a disappointingly high rate of adhesion formation and reformation after surgery. Literature describing outcomes for barriers in the prevention of adhesion formation after surgery and reformation after lysis of adhesions presents an optimistic picture with gradual improvements in both study design and agents studied. Despite enthusiastic data suggesting that barrier techniques reduce adhesions, a clear-cut increase in pregnancy rates or reduction in pelvic pain has not been conclusively proven. Nonetheless, on the basis of previous observational data and current prospective, randomized, and controlled studies evaluating barriers, the following recommendations may be made.

- Extreme care must be made in recommending any surgical procedure to a patient whose fertility potential has not been completely realized.
- Meticulous surgical technique is essential, whether microsurgical or endoscopic.
- Intra-abdominal instillate has not been shown to reduce adhesion formation. Serious side effects, however, have limited use of dextran, and in some clinical settings, its use has fallen into disfavor.
- Barriers for the prevention of adhesions has provided the most effective method of reducing adhesion formation and reformation. Further prospective data are pending to define their use in broader clinical circumstances, and their exact impact on enhancing fertility and long-term reduction in pelvic pain.
- Adhesion prevention with barriers may be most effective in severe cases. For fertility therapy, such cases may best be managed by foregoing surgery and immediate referral for IVF.
- Three barriers have shown effectiveness: regenerated cellulose (Interceed), modified hyaluronic acid/carboxymethylcellulose (Seprafilm) and ferric hyaluronate gel (Intergel).

References

1. Boys F. The prophylaxis of peritoneal adhesions: a review of the literature. Surgery 1921;11:118–168.

2. Kuboto T. The prevention of peritoneal adhesions. Japan Med World 1922;11:226–234.

3. Johnson HL. Insulating patches and absorbable sutures made from fetal membranes. N Engl J Med 1937;216:878–882.

4. Gepfert JR, Stone ML. Further studies on the intraperitoneal use of bovine amnionic fluid in abdominal surgery. Am J Surg 1939;53:79–83.

5. Trelford JD, Trelford-Sauder M. The amnion in surgery, past and present. Am J Obstet Gynecol 1979;134:833–845.

6. Gepfert JR. Intraperitoneal use of amniotic fluid to promote smoother postoperative convalescence. Am J Surg 1936;32:40–44.

7. diZerega GS. The peritoneum and its response to surgical injury. In: diZerega GS, Malinak LR, Diamond MP, Linsky CB, eds. Treatment of post-surgical adhesions. Process in clinical and biological research, vol 358. New York: Wiley-Liss, 1989:1–11.

8. Liakakos T, Thomakos N, Fine PM, Dervenis C, Young RL. Peritoneal adhesions: etiology, pathophysiology, and clinical significance. Recent advances in prevention and management. Dig Surg 2001;18:260–273.

9.   Levrant SG, Bieber EJ, Barnes RB. Anterior wall adhesions after laparotomy or laparoscopy. J Am Assoc Gynecol Laparosc 1997;4:353–356.

10.   Ellis H, Harrison W, Hugh TV. The healing of peritoneum under normal and pathologic conditions. Br J Surg 1965;52:471–476.

11.   diZerega GS. Contemporary adhesion formation. Fertil Steril 1994;61:219–235.

12.   Whawell SA, Thompson JN. Cytokine-induced release of plasminogen activator inhibitor-1 by human mesothelial cells. Eur J Surg 1995;161:315–318.

13.   Hershlag A, Otterness IG, Bliven ML, et al. The effect of interleukin-1 on adhesion formation in the rat. Am J Obstet Gynecol 1991;165:771–774.

14.   Saltzman AK, Olson TA, Mohanraj D, et al. Prevention of postoperative adhesions by an antibody to vascular permeability factor/vascular endothelial growth factor in a murine model. Am J Obstet Gynecol 1996;174:1502–1506.

15.   Drollette CM, Badawy SZ. Pathophysiology of pelvic adhesions. Modern trends in preventing infertility. J Reprod Med 1992;37:107–121.

16.   Haney AF, Doty E. The formation of coalescing peritoneal adhesions requires injury to both contacting peritoneal surfaces. Fertil Steril 1994;61:767–775.

17.   Montz FJ, Shimanuki T, diZerega GS. Post-surgical mesothelial reepithelialization. In: DcCherney AH, Polan ML, eds. Reproductive surgery. Chicago: Year Book, 1987:31–48.

18.   Diamond MP, Daniell JF, Feste J, et al. Adhesion reformation and de novo adhesion formation after reproductive pelvic surgery. Fertil Steril 1987;47:864–866.

19.   Diamond MP, DeCherney AH. Pathogenesis of adhesion formation/reformation: application to reproductive pelvic surgery. Microsurgery 1987;8:103–107.

20.   McCormack WM. Pelvic inflammatory disease. N Engl J Med 1994;330:115–119.

21.   Cheong YC, Laird SM, Li TC, et al. Peritoneal healing and adhesion formation/reformation. Hum Reprod Update 2001;7:556–566.

22.   Westrom L. Incidence, prevalence, and trends of acute pelvic inflammatory disease and its consequences in industrialized countries. Am J Obstet Gynecol 1980;138:880–892.

23.   Westrom L, Joesoef R, Reynolds G, et al. Pelvic inflammatory disease and fertility. A cohort study of 1,844 women with laparoscopically verified disease and 657 control women with normal laparoscopic results. Sex Transm Dis 1992;19:185–192.

24.   Rapkin AJ. Adhesions and pelvic pain: a retrospective study. Obstet Gynecol 1986;68:13–15.

25.   Johnson AM, Grun L, Haines A. Controlling genital chlamydial infection. Br Med J 1996;313:1160.

26.   Bevan CD, Johal BJ, Mumtaz G, et al. Clinical, laparoscopic and microbiological findings in acute salpingitis: report on a United Kingdom cohort. Br J Obstet Gynaecol 1995;102:407–414.

27.   Centers for Disease Control and Prevention. Recommendations for the prevention and management of *Chlamydia trachomatis* infections, 1993. MMWR Recomm Rep 1993;42:1–39.

28. Stovall TG, Elder RF, Ling FW. Predictors of pelvic adhesions. J Reprod Med 1989;34:345–348.

29. Coste J, Laumon B, Bremond A, et al. Sexually transmitted diseases as major causes of ectopic pregnancy: results from a large case-control study in France. Fertil Steril 1994;62:289–295.

30. Wolner-Hanssen P. Silent pelvic inflammatory disease: is it overstated? Obstet Gynecol 1995;86:321–325.

31. Duffy DM, diZerega GS. Adhesion controversies: pelvic pain as a cause of adhesions, crystalloids in preventing them. J Reprod Med 1996;41:19–26.

32. Dodson NG. Antibiotic regimens for treating acute pelvic inflammatory disease. An evaluation. J Reprod Med 1994;39:285–296.

33. Ellis H, Moran BJ, Thompson JN, et al. Adhesion-related hospital readmissions after abdominal and pelvic surgery: a retrospective cohort study. Lancet 1999;353:1476–1480.

34. Washington AE, Katz P. Cost of and payment source for pelvic inflammatory disease. Trends and projections, 1983 through 2000. JAMA 1991;266:2565–2569.

35. Ray NF, Denton WG, Thamer M, Henderson SC, Perry S. Abdominal adhesiolysis: inpatient care and expenditures in the United States in 1994. J Am Coll Surg 1998;186:1–9.

36. Diamond MP, Freeman ML. Clinical implications of postsurgical adhesions. Hum Reprod Update 2001;7:567–576.

37. Mage G, Pouly JL, de Joliniere JB, et al. A preoperative classification to predict the intrauterine and ectopic pregnancy rates after distal tubal microsurgery. Fertil Steril 1986;46:807–810.

38. Caspi E, Halperin Y, Bukovsky I. The importance of periadnexal adhesions in tubal reconstructive surgery for infertility. Fertil Steril 1979;31:296–300.

39. Chan CL, Wood C. Pelvic adhesiolysis–the assessment of symptom relief by 100 patients. Aust N Z J Obstet Gynaecol 1985;25:295–298.

40. Kresch AJ, Seifer DB, Sachs LB, Barrese I. Laparoscopy in 100 women with chronic pelvic pain. Obstet Gynecol 1984;64:672–674.

41. Renaer M. Chronic pelvic pain without obvious pathology in women. Personal observations and review of the problem. Eur J Obstet Gynecol Reprod Biol 1980 Jul;10:415–463.

42. Steege JF, Stout AL. Resolution of chronic pelvic pain after laparoscopic lysis of adhesions. Am J Obstet Gynecol 1991;65:278–281.

43. Thompson JN, Whawell SA. Pathogenesis and prevention of adhesion formation. Br J Surg 1995;82:3–5.

44. The American Fertility Society. The American Fertility Society classifications of adnexal adhesions, distal tubal occlusion, tubal occlusion secondary to tubal ligation, tubal pregnancies, Müllerian abnormalities, and intrauterine adhesions. Fertil Steril 1988;49:944–955.

45. Bowman MC, Li TC, Cooke ID. Inter-observer variability at laparoscopic assessment of pelvic adhesions. Hum Reprod 1995;10:155–160.

46. Corson SL, Batzer FR, Gocial B, et al. Intra-observer and inter-observer variability in scoring laparoscopic diagnosis of pelvic adhesions. Hum Reprod 1995;10:161–164.

47. Marana R, Rizzi M, Muzii L, et al. Correlation between the American Fertility Society classifications of adnexal adhesions and distal tubal occlusion, salpingoscopy, and reproductive outcome in tubal surgery. Fertil Steril 1995;64:924–929.

48. Vasquez G, Boeckx W, Brosens I. No correlation between peritubal and mucosal adhesions in hydrosalpinges. Fertil Steril 1995;64:1032–1033.

49. Siegler AM. Hysterosalpingography. Fertil Steril 1983;40:139–158.

50. Fayez JA, Mutie G, Schneider PJ. The diagnostic value of hysterosalpingography and hysteroscopy in infertility investigation. Am J Obstet Gynecol 1987;156:558–560.

51. Guerriero S, Ajossa S, Lai MP, et al. Transvaginal ultrasonography in the diagnosis of pelvic adhesions. Hum Reprod 1997;12:2649–2653.

52. Seow KM, Lin YH, Hsieh BC, et al. Transvaginal three-dimensional ultrasonography combined with serum CA-125 level for the diagnosis of pelvic adhesions before laparoscopic surgery. J Am Assoc Gynecol Laparosc 2003;10:320–326.

53. Bevan CD, Johal BJ, Mumtaz G, et al. Clinical, laparoscopic and microbiological findings in acute salpingitis: report on a United Kingdom cohort. Br J Obstet Gynaecol 1995;102:407–414.

54. Faber BM, Coddington CC 3rd. Microlaparoscopy: a comparative study of diagnostic accuracy. Fertil Steril 1997;67:952–954.

55. Luciano AA, Maier DB, Koch EI, et al. A comparative study of postoperative adhesions following laser surgery by laparoscopy versus laparotomy in the rabbit model. Obstet Gynecol 1989;74:220–224.

56. Filmar S, Gomel V, McComb PF. Operative laparoscopy versus open abdominal surgery: a comparative study on postoperative adhesion formation in the rat model. Fertil Steril 1987;48:486–489.

57. Mettler L. Pelvic adhesions: Laparoscopic approach. Ann NY Acad Sci 2003;997:255–268.

58. Luber K, Beeson CC, Kennedy JF, et al. Results of microsurgical treatment of tubal infertility and early second-look laparoscopy in the post-pelvic inflammatory disease patient: implications for in vitro fertilization. Am J Obstet Gynecol 1986;154:1264–1270.

59. Tulandi T, Collins JA, Burrows E, et al. Treatment-dependent and treatment-independent pregnancy among women with periadnexal adhesions. Am J Obstet Gynecol 1990;162:354–357.

60. Horne HW Jr, Clyman M, Debrovner C, et al. The prevention of postoperative pelvic adhesions following conservative operative treatment for human infertility. A final 3-year follow-up report. Int J Fertil 1973;18:109–115.

61. Holtz G. Prevention and management of peritoneal adhesions. Fertil Steril 1984;41:497–507.

62. DeCherney AH. Preventing postoperative pelvic adhesions with intraperitoneal treatment. J Reprod Med 1984;29:157–161.

63. Interceed Adhesion Barrier Study Group. Prevention of postsurgical adhesions by INTERCEED(TC7), an absorbable adhesion barrier: a prospective randomized multicenter clinical study. INTERCEED(TC7) Adhesion Barrier Study Group. Fertil Steril 1989;51:933–938.

64. Sekiba K. Use of Interceed(TC7) absorbable adhesion barrier to reduce postoperative adhesion reformation in infertility and endometriosis surgery. Obstet Gynecol 1992;79:518–522.

65. Wiseman DM, Trout JR, Franklin RR, Diamond MP. Metaanalysis of the safety and efficacy of an adhesion barrier (Interceed TC7) in laparotomy. J Reprod Med 1999;44:325–331.

66. Li TC, Cooke ID. The value of an absorbable adhesion barrier, Interceed, in the prevention of adhesion reformation following microsurgical adhesiolysis. Br J Obstet Gynaecol 1994;101:335–359.

67. Haney AF, Doty E. The peritoneal response to expanded polytetrafluoroethylene and oxidized regenerated cellulose surgical adhesion barriers. Art Cells Blood Subst Immobil Biotechnol 1996;24:121–141.

68. Haney AF, Hesla J, Hurst BS, et al. Expanded polytetrafluoroethylene (Gore-Tex Surgical Membrane) is superior to oxidized regenerated cellulose (Interceed TC7+) in preventing adhesions. Fertil Steril 1995;63:1021–1026.

69. The Myomectomy Adhesion Multicenter Study Group. An expanded polytetrafluoroethylene barrier (Gore-Tex Surgical Membrane) reduces post-myomectomy adhesion formation. Fertil Steril 1995;63:491–493.

70. Risberg R. Adhesions: preventive strategies. Eur J Surg 1997;577 (suppl):32–39.

71. Haney AF, Doty E. Expanded-polytetrafluoroethylene but not oxidized regenerated cellulose prevents adhesion formation and reformation in a mouse uterine horn model of surgical injury. Fertil Steril 1993;60:550–558.

72. Carta G, Cerroni L, Iovenitti P. Postoperative adhesion prevention in gynecologic surgery with hyaluronic acid. Clin Exp Obstet Gynecol 2004;31:39–41.

73. Diamond MP. Reduction of adhesions after uterine myomectomy by Seprafilm membrane (HAL-F): a blinded, prospective, randomized, multicenter clinical study. Seprafilm Adhesion Study Group. Fertil Steril 1996;66:904–910.

74. Tsapanos VS, Stathopoulou LP, Papathanassopoulou VS, Tzingounis VA. The role of Seprafilm bioresorbable membrane in the prevention and therapy of endometrial synechiae. J Biomed Mat Res 2002;63:10–14.

75. Heidrick GW, Pippitt CH Jr, Morgan MA, Thurnau GR. Efficacy of intraperitoneal sodium carboxymethylcellulose in preventing postoperative adhesion formation. J Reprod Med 1994;39:575–578.

76. Becker JM, Dayton MT, Faxio VW, et al. Prevention of postoperative abdominal adhesions by a sodium hyaluronate-based bioresorbable membrane: a prospective, randomized, double-blind multicenter study. J Am Coll Surg 1996;183:297–306.

77. Johns DB, Keyport GM, Hoehler F, diZerega GS; Intergel Adhesion Prevention Study Group. Reduction of postsurgical adhesions with Intergel adhesion prevention solution: a multicenter study of safety and efficacy after conservative gynecologic surgery. Fertil Steril 2001;76:595–604.

78. Steinleitner A, Lambert H, Kazensky C, et al. Reduction of primary postoperative adhesion formation under calcium channel blockade in the rabbit. J Surg Res 1990;48:42–45.

79. Steinleitner A, Lambert H, Kazensky C, et al. Use of pentoxifylline as an adjuvant to prevent postsurgical adhesion formation: preliminary investigations in a rodent model. J Gynecol Surg 1989;5:367–373.

80. Rosenberg SM, Board JA. High-molecular weight dextran in human infertility surgery. Am J Obstet Gynecol 1984;148:380–385.

81. McLucas B. Hyskon complications in hysteroscopic surgery. Obstet Gynecol Surv 1991;46:196–200.

82. Saravelos HG, Li TC. Physical barriers in adhesion prevention. J Reprod Med 1996;41:42–51.

83. Pagidas K, Tulandi T. Effects of Ringer's lactate, Interceed(TC7) and Gore-Tex Surgical Membrane on postsurgical adhesion formation. Fertil Steril 1992;57:109–201.

84. Rodgers KE. Non-steroidal anti-inflammatory drugs (NSAIDs) in the treatment of post-surgical adhesion. In: diZerega GS, Malinak LR, Diamond MP, Linsky CB, eds. Treatment of post-surgical adhesions. New York: Wiley-Liss, 1990.

85. Shushan A, Mor-Yosef S, Avgar A, Laufer N. Hyaluronic acid for preventing experimental postoperative intraperitoneal adhesions. J Reprod Med 1994;39:398–402.

86. Hill-West JL, Dunn RC, Hubbell JA. Local release of fibrinolytic agents for adhesion prevention. J Surg Res 1995;59:759–763.

87. Leondires MP, Stubblefield PG, Tarraza HM, Jones MA. A pilot study of cyclosporine for the prevention of postsurgical adhesion formation in rats. Am J Obstet Gynecol 1995;172:1537–1539.

88. Montanino-Oliva M, Metzger DA, Luciano AA. Use of medroxyprogesterone acetate in the prevention of postoperative adhesions. Fertil Steril 1996;65:650–654.

89. Lai HS, Chen Y. Effect of octreotide on postoperative intraperitoneal adhesions in rats. Scand J Gastroenterol 1996;31:678–681.

90. Grow DR, Coddington CC, Hsiu JG, Mikich Y, Hodgen GD. Role of hypoestrogenism or sex steroid antagonism in adhesion formation after myometrial surgery in primates. Fertil Steril 1996;66:140–147.

91. Wright JA, Sharpe-Timms KL. Gonadotropin-releasing hormone agonist therapy reduces postoperative adhesion formation and reformation after adhesiolysis in rat models for adhesion formation and endometriosis. Fertil Steril 1995;63:1094–1100.

92. LeGrand EK, Rodgers KE, Girgis W, et al. Efficacy of tolmetin sodium for adhesion prevention in rabbit and rat models. J Surg Res 1994;56:67–71.

93. Cofer KF, Himebaugh KS, Gauvin JM, Hurd WW. Inhibition of adhesion reformation in the rabbit model by meclofenamate: an inhibitor of both prostaglandin and leukotriene production. Fertil Steril 1994;62:1262–1265.

94. Operative Laparoscopy Study Group. Postoperative adhesion development after operative laparoscopy: evaluation at early second-look procedures. Fertil Steril 1991;55:700–704.

95. Bowman MC, Cooke I. The efficacy of synthetic adhesion barriers in infertility surgery. Br J Obstet Gynecol 1994;101:3–6.

96. Pagidas K, Tulandi T. Effects of Ringer's lactate, Interceed (TC) and Gore-Tex Surgical Membrane on postsurgical adhesion formation. Fertil Steril 1992;57:199–201.

97. Nordic Adhesion Prevention Study Group. The efficacy of Interceed (TC 7) for prevention of reforma-

tion of postoperative adhesions on ovaries, fallopian tubes, and fimbriae in microsurgical operations for fertility: a multicenter study. Fertil Steril 1995;63:709–714.

98. Gomel V, Urman B, Gurgan T. Pathophysiology of adhesion formation and strategies for prevention. J Reprod Med 1996;41:35–41.

99. Azziz R. Microsurgery alone or with Interceed Absorbable Adhesion Barrier for pelvic sidewall adhesion re-formation. The Interceed (TC 7) Adhesion Barrier Study Group II. Surg Gynecol Obstet 1993;177:135–139.

100. Daniell JF, Pittaway DE. Short-interval second-look laparoscopy after infertility surgery: a preliminary report. J Reprod Med 1983;28:281–283.

101. Larsson B. Efficacy of Interceed in adhesion prevention in gynecologic surgery: a review of 13 clinical studies. J Reprod Med 1996;41:27–34.

102. Surrey MW, Friedman S. Second-look laparoscopy after reconstructive pelvic surgery for infertility. J Reprod Med 1982;27:658–660.

103. Jansen RPS. Early laparoscopy after pelvic operations to prevent adhesions: safety and efficacy. Fertil Steril 1988;49:26–31.

Index

Note: Page references in *italics* indicate figures and tables